W9-BXU-068

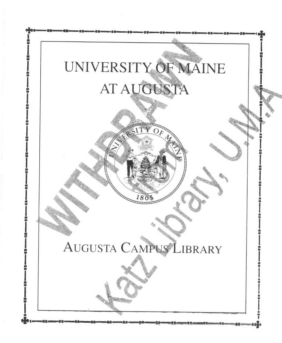

UNIVERSITY OF MAINE
AT AUGUSTA

AUGUSTA CAMPUS LIBRARY

WITHDRAWN

Katz Library, U.M.A.

UNDERSTANDING AIDS

UNDERSTANDING AIDS

SECOND EDITION
Advances in Research and Treatment

SETH C. KALICHMAN

American Psychological Association
Washington, DC

Copyright © 1998 by the American Psychological Association. All rights reserved. Except as permitted under the United States Copyright Act of 1976, no part of this publication may be reproduced or distributed in any form or by any means, or stored in a database or retrieval system, without the prior written permission of the publisher.

Published by
American Psychological Association
750 First Street, NE
Washington, DC 20002

Copies may be ordered from
APA Order Department
P.O. Box 92984
Washington, DC 20090-2984

In the U.K., Europe, Africa, and the Middle East, copies may be ordered from
American Psychological Association
3 Henrietta Street
Covent Garden, London
WC2E 8LU England

Typeset in Minion by EPS Group Inc., Easton, MD

Printer: Braun-Brumfield, Ann Arbor, MI
Cover Designer: Supon Design Group, Washington, DC
Technical/Production Editor: Catherine R. W. Hudson
Cover Illustration: Elizabeth Wolf, Washington, DC

Library of Congress Cataloging-in-Publication Data
Kalichman, Seth C.
    Understanding AIDS : advances in research and treatment / Seth C.
    Kalichman. — 2nd ed.
        p.   cm.
    Includes bibliographical references and index.
    ISBN 1-55798-529-4. — ISBN 1-55798-530-8 (pbk.; acid-free paper)
    1. AIDS (Disease)   2. AIDS (Disease)—Psychological aspects.
3. AIDS (Disease)—Social aspects.   4. AIDS (Disease)—Patients—
Counseling of.   5. Mental health personnel.   I. Title.
RC607.A26K356   1998
616.97'92'0019—dc21   98-7455
                                                                                        CIP

British Library Cataloguing-in-Publication Data
A CIP record is available from the British Library.

Printed in the United States of America
First Edition

This book is dedicated to
Hannah Fay,
in the hope that she will
know of AIDS
only as we now know
of polio.

Contents

Foreword to the Second Edition

In most fields, a book written 4 years ago continues to be timely. However, since the first version of this book was published in 1995, the story of AIDS has changed dramatically in multiple and fundamental aspects. Consequently, a second edition is truly necessary and useful for today's world of HIV–AIDS.

Since 1995, it has become increasingly common for clinicians to prescribe combination antiviral therapy to HIV-positive patients, rather than a single medication at a time. This alteration in itself has positive effects on health and survival. In addition, the appearance of two major treatment developments has created even more profound changes in therapeutic options and outlook, with corresponding changes in morbidity and mortality rates. The first development is an assay of serum levels of HIV copies (viral load), providing a critical tool for clinical decision making. The second is the marketing, since December 1995, of HIV protease inhibitors, a class of drugs that achieves a new level of efficacy when combined with previously available antiviral medication.

Changes in mortality and morbidity figures have made headline news since the beginning of 1996. Large-scale national and international studies, published in 1998, have documented declines in mortality of up to 75% even in patients with advanced immunosuppression, and declines in the incidence of opportunistic infections of 73%. This is true across gender, risk, and age groups.

With the advent of such changes come multiple challenges. For those who expected to die and who are now offered the prospect of extended survival, readjustment of plans, goals, and expectations is complex. For the nontrivial minority who do not benefit at all, or who do not maintain an initial benefit from the new drugs, there are other kinds of complicated psychological issues to confront. New complex issues concern the effect of these new treatments and improving health on risk behaviors, on neuropsychological function, and on maintenance of demanding and unforgiving medication regimens for the indefinite future. Because there are now effective treatments starting with the on-set of HIV infection, new uncertainties arise in the context of protection of individual confidentiality versus partner notification and contact tracing, as well as the possibility of postexposure prophylaxis. These are some but by no means all of the issues that arose in the past 3 years, which require extensive rethinking of assumptions, of educational mes-sages, of clinical management, that this new edition undertakes to ad-dress.

In the past 3 years, when graduate and postdoctoral fellows have sought an introduction to the field of HIV–AIDS, Dr. Kalichman's book was the book I gave everyone. I chose this book because of its concep-tual clarity, even handling of complex issues, breadth, and exhaustive citation. By covering biomedical as well as psychiatric and psychosocial arenas in the field of HIV–AIDS, this book provides a wonderful over-view and frame of reference for readers in many disciplines.

I look forward to the opportunity to distribute this new edition to the next generation of students seeking to inform themselves about the biomedical, clinical, social, and research issues in the field of HIV–AIDS.

JUDITH G. RABKIN, PhD, MPH

Foreword to the First Edition

HIV is here to stay. Great strides have been made in preventing new infections, and the day will come when an effective vaccine will be added to the arsenal of preventive strategies. But the recent disheartening news about the pace of vaccine development and ongoing difficulties in securing sufficient resources for HIV prevention mean that people with HIV will need care from professionals qualified to meet their numerous and complicated needs.

The easiest work in HIV is behind us, and the really difficult work lies ahead. A headline appeared recently in the *San Francisco Examiner* that read, "AIDS Loses Urgency in Nation's List of Worries." Two days later, another headline ran: "AIDS Is Leading Cause of Death for Ages 25–44." Together, these headlines sum up the enormous challenges in front of us. The AIDS epidemic marches on. It continues to devastate the vulnerable populations of the United States and of the world.

The HIV epidemic has taken many people from us. But the HIV epidemic is also an inspiring story of care and commitment. Dr. Kalichman's volume, *Understanding AIDS: A Guide for Mental Health Professionals*, speaks to this care and commitment. It outlines many of the problems so evident in AIDS, but it also presents hope, in that it demonstrates what can be done. It points to the fact that people with HIV experience devastation in most of their organ systems, as well as in their psychological and social welfare. It demonstrates that treatments and interventions are available to maintain health as long as possible. It demonstrates that quality of life can be maintained, even when health declines. It demonstrates that individuals with HIV and AIDS can be helped in very specific ways and that they can have good lives even in the presence of their disabilities.

This book is remarkable in its comprehensiveness. No one can work with people with HIV and AIDS without having an understanding of the biological, psychological, and social factors at work. This book reminds mental health professionals that they need to understand the basic pathophysiology of the disease. It reminds them that they need to be well conversant with developments in treatments so that they can help their patients make wise health care choices. It reminds them that they need to understand the myriad causes of cognitive, emotional, and behavioral difficulties people with HIV may experience, so that they can provide the best care possible for individuals with this complicated disease.

This book is important in bridging the often artificial gap between primary prevention and care. It reminds the provider that good care and good prevention go hand in hand, and that attention to issues of prevention is necessary in any comprehensive care plan. It also reminds the provider that a wide variety of strategies are available and can be used, depending on the needs of the patient.

The HIV epidemic has changed our world. It has devastated many of us and many of our communities. But there have been positive benefits as well. There now exists a vast network of community-based organizations devoted to HIV prevention in various vulnerable communities. We are now talking about things that were not talked about so openly before the epidemic: topics like homosexuality, oral and anal sex, adolescent and teen sexuality, the relative merits of teenage sex education, the importance and stability of same-sex partnerships, the wonderful caregiving so evident in traumatized communities, and the lives of injection drug users. No one can pretend any more that these topics are not important.

Committed and caring mental health professionals are essential in the fight to prevent the further spread of HIV and in the struggle to help individuals with the disease maintain quality of life. As Prior Walter, the main character with AIDS in Tony Kushner's *Angels in America* says, "This disease will be the end of us, but not nearly all, and the dead will be commemorated and will struggle on with the living. We are not going away. We won't die secret deaths any longer. The world only spins forward. We will be citizens. The time has come." This text, and the mental health professionals who use it, are key to helping the world spin forward, to helping the time come when all citizens experience the best that can be offered.

THOMAS J. COATES, PhD
Director, Center for AIDS Prevention Studies
University of California, San Francisco

Acknowledgments

Understanding AIDS would not have been possible without the help of many people to whom I am deeply indebted. I received helpful comments and encouragement early in the development of the first edition of *Understanding AIDS* from Tom Coates, PhD, at the Center for AIDS Prevention Studies at the University of California, San Francisco. Joe Ricker, PhD, a neuropsychologist, and Laura Radke, MD, an infectious disease physician, reviewed chapters for technical accuracy in the first edition. Ann O'Leary, PhD, John C. Markowitz, MD, and Margaret Nettles, PhD, provided detailed and extensive reviews. Susan Chuck provided invaluable feedback on the HIV treatments chapter. The insightful comments of these highly valued researchers made substantial contributions to the refinement and completeness of the text. I am fortunate to have written the first edition at the Center for AIDS Intervention Research (CAIR), supported by National Institute of Mental Health (NIMH) Center grant P30 MH 52776 and grant R01 MH 57624. My colleagues Kathy Sikkema, PhD, and Tony Somlai, EdD, provided countless suggestions and resources; Allan Hauth assured that I had available to me all of the current research; Tami Payne assisted in preparing the original manuscript; and Jeff Kelly, PhD, David Ostrow, MD, David Rompa, and Michael Morgan provided helpful suggestions and pointed me to many valuable resources. Thanks to Judith Rabkin, PhD, for her many thoughtful comments. The second edition has benefited from resources provided by Dan Dunable, Leslie Brogen, Jeff Graham, and the Peer Counseling Program of the AIDS Survival Project, Atlanta, GA. Bineetha Ramachandran assisted me in researching the literature on HIV treatment adherence for chapter 3, and Moira Kalichman prepared the manuscript for the second edition. I am grateful to Moira, my parents, and the rest of my family for their endless patience and support. I also thank the men and women who participated in the "Health Needs Assessment" interviews and the "Health Surveys of Atlanta," which helped clarify issues and assure external validity of the presentation of research findings. I also which to thank Catherine R. W. Hudson of APA Books for her excellent work as production editor. Finally, I am indebted to Ted Baroody and Julia Frank-McNeil of APA Books who are once again thanked for their continued support, collaboration, encouragement, and friendship.

UNDERSTANDING AIDS

Introduction

The uncertainties of human immunodeficiency virus (HIV) infection and its relentless progression to AIDS are the source of enormous psychological and social burdens. Like all previous epidemics, AIDS devastates individuals, families, communities, and societies. AIDS cannot be thought of as a single stressful life event, but rather as an unremitting force with an uncertain course. Nearing the end of its second decade, AIDS has established a permanent place for itself in the scope of world health. When a preventive vaccine becomes available it will not be one hundred percent effective and when there is a cure it will not be universally accessible. Unlike the early years of AIDS, when immediate but temporary solutions were sought, AIDS must now be dealt with in the long haul.

Human service professionals caring for people with HIV–AIDS confront many challenges directly resulting from HIV disease, medical treatments, and the social problems within which HIV–AIDS is embedded. Although not expected to be expert in the medical aspects of AIDS, counselors, therapists, social workers, case managers, and others who provide services to people affected by AIDS should have a basic understanding of HIV–AIDS and its manifestations. Because the biological aspects of HIV–AIDS directly affect the psychological experience of HIV infection, psychosocial interventions must be sensitive to the biomedical underpinnings of HIV disease. For these reasons, the biological and medical aspects of AIDS are the focus of Part One of this book. HIV and its actions against the immune system are discussed first, emphasizing the aspects of viral transmission dynamics and epidemiology that are most relevant to the psychological aspects of AIDS. In chapter 2, illness-related aspects of HIV–AIDS are discussed, highlighting the psychosocial implications of HIV antibody testing and the

3

natural history of HIV infection. Chapter 3 discusses medical treatments for HIV infection and AIDS-associated opportunistic illnesses, emphasizing the recent advances in anti-HIV treatments.

Part Two reviews the psychological, neuropsychological, and social sequelae of HIV–AIDS. Although AIDS shares many things in common with other chronic and life threatening illnesses, several events are unique to the experience of having HIV–AIDS. Unlike most other life-threatening illnesses, HIV infection primarily strikes young and middle-aged adults. AIDS involves social discrimination, prejudice, isolation, and disruptions to social and sexual relationships. Chapter 4 reviews the psychological sequelae of HIV infection across phases of the disease, focusing on emotional distress, maladaptive behaviors, and the health implications of stress. Chapter 5 discusses the central and peripheral nervous system involvement of HIV infection and its implications for cognitive functioning, neuropsychological impairment, and everyday living. Chapter 6 discusses the adverse social consequences of HIV infection, focusing on social stigmatization and isolation.

Part Three reviews the adjustment and coping processes of people with HIV–AIDS and the means by which professional services may facilitate adaptation. Specifically, these three chapters focus on HIV-related adjustment, coping, social support, and mental health services. Chapter 7 discusses the complex issues of sexual adjustment to HIV–AIDS, including sexual behavior, serostatus disclosure to sex partners, and sexual functioning. Chapter 8 reviews the coping processes identified in people with HIV–AIDS, including the roles of meaning, control, self-esteem, coping strategies, optimism, and spirituality. Chapter 8 also discusses the structural and functional aspects of support over the course of HIV infection. Finally, chapter 9 focuses on HIV-related counseling, psychotherapy, and social support interventions. Clinical assessment, themes in psychotherapy, pharmacological treatments, and ethical issues that arise with HIV-seropositive people are also discussed in chapter 9.

Understanding AIDS was written to provide a broad overview of the research literature on the psychological and social aspects of HIV–AIDS. The book is not solely intended for practitioners who specialize in caring for people affected by AIDS. Rather, my hope is that all human service professionals will have adequate knowledge of and sensitivity to the issues of HIV–AIDS. The purpose of *Understanding AIDS* is to help achieve these goals.

NOTE ON THE SECOND EDITION

This second edition of *Understanding AIDS* differs in several ways from the first edition. Aside from completely updating all of the sections of the book to include advances in research and emerging issues in AIDS, several major changes appear in this edition. First, chapter 3 is now dedicated entirely to issues in the medical treatment of HIV–AIDS. Revolutionary and rapid advances in treatments prompted inclusion of this chapter. The material on stress and its health effects that were previously in this chapter now appear in chapter 4, along with other psychological sequelae of HIV–AIDS. In addition, chapter 7 now concerns sexual adjustment to AIDS. It has been common to neglect the sexual aspects of AIDS, and the first edition of *Understanding AIDS* was guilty of these omissions. However, this edition overviews these important issues. Information on social support previously covered in its own chapter is now included in chapter 8 with other aspects of coping and adjustment, and social support interventions are included in chapter 9 along with counseling and psychotherapy. Chapter 9 has been further revised to discuss several schools of psychotherapy that were not included in the first edition, such as interpersonal therapy, psychodynamic therapy, and supportive psychotherapy. These changes to the second edition were meant to improve and update the text, while retaining the original structure and content of the first edition. The second edition of *Understanding AIDS* includes over one hundred citations to works from 1995 to 1998, and the appendixes include an updated glossary and resource guide, including internet HIV–AIDS information web sites. Finally, the subtitle has changed from *A Guide for Mental Health Professionals* to *Advances in Research and Treatment* to reflect the broader content of this book.

PART ONE

Virology, Epidemiology, and Clinical Manifestations

Thus, the disease, which apparently had forced on us the solidarity of a beleaguered town, disrupted at the same time long-established communities and sent men out to live, as individuals, in relative isolation. This, too, added to the general feeling of unrest

(Camus, *The Plague*, 1948, p. 160).

Yet the virus would continually find vulnerable Homo sapiens all over the world, for the human factors responsible for spread of the virus would resist change. Governments of countries without AIDS would smugly deny the correlation of such behaviors with the inevitable arrival of the virus. And in nation after nation, when AIDS arrived it would find conditions ideal for rapid spread, and politicians would be unwilling to take unpopular steps to acknowledge the threat, thereby possibly altering the epidemic's course

(Garrett, *The Coming Plague*, 1994, p. 389).

1

The HIV–AIDS Pandemic

The devastation caused by epidemic infectious diseases, including syphilis, smallpox, leprosy, influenza, tuberculosis, and polio are well recorded throughout history. For example, the epidemic that became known as the Black Death, a combination of bubonic, spectemic, and pneumonic plague, swept across 14th-century Europe between 1347 and 1352, killing an estimated one third of Europe's population (Kishlansky, Geary, & O'Brien, 1991; Ziegler, 1969). Today the word *plague* is reserved for a specific class of infectious disease, but plagues historically refer to widespread contagious diseases associated with significant death. *Plague* can therefore be used to describe widespread loss of life because of any infectious disease. Beyond the scope of previous global epidemics, HIV infection, the cause of AIDS, has reached the proportions of a pandemic, having infected millions and promising to infect millions more.

Understanding how HIV rapidly grew to its current status of a global health crisis is just beginning. There is substantial evidence that HIV infection has occurred in central Africa since the mid-1950s, where antibodies specific to HIV were identified in stored blood specimens (Gallo, 1987, 1988). However, HIV infection was overshadowed at the time by numerous other fatal illnesses that afflict developing countries. AIDS also remained hidden because its clinical manifestations are expressed as other, more readily recognizable infections.

The exact origin of HIV and its introduction to humans is unknown, but there is much speculation and theorizing about where and how HIV first evolved. One line of thought is that HIV was well established in all areas of the world but has only recently been recognized. However, this theory has not been well substantiated. A second proposition holds that HIV evolved through the mutation of an older and nonpathogenic virus. Virologists, however, have dismissed this explanation for HIV on the basis of specific characteristics of the virus and its relationship to other viruses. A third and widely discussed possible origin of HIV is zoonosis, the recent entry of a nonhuman virus into human populations. Zoonosis is a probable explanation for HIV for several reasons, especially because similar viruses exist in old-world apes living in areas that surround regions of Africa where HIV is endemic (Goudsmit, 1997). Still, zoonosis has not been universally accepted as the source of HIV. The most widely held view of HIV is that it represents a virus that developed in humans in Central Africa and only recently spread to other regions of the world, primarily through global travel and transcontinental commerce. Epidemiological data provide the strongest support for this last theory (Gallo, 1988; Mann & Tarantola, 1996).

The first identified cases of AIDS in the United States occurred in the spring of 1981, when the Centers for Disease Control and Prevention (CDC) reported that five young, previously healthy, homosexually active men in Los Angeles exhibited a rare upper respiratory infection, *Pneumocystis carinii* pneumonia (Fauci et al., 1984; Gallo, 1987). One month later, the CDC reported another 10 cases of this illness and 26 cases of Kaposi's sarcoma, a rare cancer of connective and vascular tissues. All of these cases occurred in New York City, San Francisco, and Los Angeles among previously healthy young homosexual men. The earliest cases of AIDS were traced to a man who became known as *Patient Zero*, who had links to numerous documented sexual contacts, some of whom are depicted in Figure 1.1. By the end of 1981, the

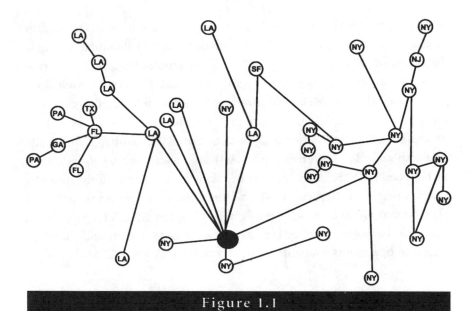

Figure 1.1

Approximate representation of Patient Zero's sexual network and his association to the first cases of AIDS. Circles with LA represent cases in Los Angeles; GA, Georgia; PA, Pennsylvania; FL, Florida; TX, Texas; NY, New York; SF, San Francisco; NJ, New Jersey.

number of AIDS cases grew to 257, and to over 2,000 by the end of 1983, setting into motion the rapid accumulation of over 100,000 AIDS cases in the first decade of the epidemic, reaching 360,000 cases by the end of 1993, and over 600,000 cases by the start of 1998. A new case of AIDS is reported in the United States every 15 minutes, more than 5,000 people in the world become infected with HIV each day, approximately 1,000 babies are born with HIV each day worldwide, and a person in the world dies of AIDS complications every 30 minutes.

Evidence that AIDS is caused by a new human virus emerged between late 1983 and early 1984. Considered the most rapid progression of scientific advances in response to a new disease in the history of biology and medicine, the accelerated pace of understanding AIDS is embodied in a rich literature. The 24 published papers on HIV—AIDS in 1982 contrasts with the 8,300 articles published in 1990 (Elford, Bor,

& Summers, 1991). The proliferation of HIV–AIDS research is also evident by the emergence of several scientific and professional journals dedicated solely to publishing AIDS-related articles (e.g., *AIDS, Journal of Acquired Immune Deficiency Syndromes and Human Retrovirology, AIDS and Behavior, AIDS Education and Prevention, International Journal of STD and AIDS, AIDS Patient Care*, and *AIDS Care*), as well as by the biannual International Conference on AIDS, which includes literally thousands of presentations. Articles concerning various aspects of HIV and AIDS regularly appear in scientific and professional journals across disciplines. Between 1981 and 1990 there were more than 32,700 HIV-related scientific articles published (Elford et al., 1991). As a result, many of the mysteries of AIDS have now become known and there are multiple treatments available to fight against HIV–AIDS.

DISCOVERY OF THE HUMAN IMMUNODEFICIENCY VIRUS

Human immunodeficiency virus is a retrovirus belonging to a group of *cytopathic lentiviruses.* Lentiviruses integrate their genetic material with a cell's genetic material through the complicated process of reverse transcription (Z. F. Rosenberg & Fauci, 1991). There are several known retroviruses in the animal kingdom, including the visna virus that infects sheep, feline immunodeficiency virus in cats, and avian sarcoma virus in chickens (Fauci, 1988; Gallo, 1988). Retroviruses are often communicable, as is the case with feline leukemia virus, which causes immune deficiency and malignancies (Gallo, 1986, 1991). Whereas animal retroviruses have been studied since the early part of the century and pose no threat to humans, human retroviruses have only recently been identified.

The first human retrovirus was discovered by Robert Gallo and his associates at the National Cancer Institute (NCI). Uncertain that retroviruses existed in humans, NCI researchers identified the first human retrovirus, the human T-cell lymphotropic virus type I (HTLV-I) in the late 1970s. The clinical importance of HTLV-I is that it causes a type of leukemia involving T-helper lymphocyte cells, which play an integral role in the human immune system. HTLV-I also causes progressive mye-lopathy, a disease of the spinal cord, as well as certain lymphatic cancers. Subsequently, NCI labs discovered a second human leukemia-causing retrovirus, HTLV-II, establishing the likelihood that other undiscovered human retroviruses exist. The discovery of two leukemia-causing hu-man retroviruses held answers to many questions raised nearly a decade later by AIDS.

On the basis of epidemiologic evidence and disease symptoms, it was believed that AIDS resulted from a viral infection (Levy, Kaminsky, et al., 1985). AIDS appeared to be caused by a human retrovirus because it shares several characteristics with HTLV-I and HTLV-II, including the fact that it results in a loss of T-helper lymphocyte cells and it is spread through blood, perinatal events, and sexual contact. Between 1983 and 1984, the virus that causes AIDS was discovered by three laboratories and given three different names: *lymphadenopathy associated virus (LAV)*, discovered by Luc Montagnier of the Pasteur Institute of France; *human T-cell lymphotropic virus type-III (HTLV-III)*, identified by Rob-ert Gallo at the National Cancer Institute; and *AIDS-associated retro-virus (ARV)*, discovered by Jay Levy of the Cancer Research Institute of the University of California at San Francisco. All three virus isolates were essentially the same in terms of structure, apparent mechanisms of transmission, and disease manifestations. Because they were actually variants of the same virus, they were renamed in 1986, the *human immunodeficiency virus type-1* (HIV-1; Fauci, 1986; Gallo, 1987; Levy, 1992).

Subsequently, a second AIDS-causing virus, HIV-2, was discovered in 1986 in West Africa. The differences between HIV-1 and HIV-2 are mostly molecular, with few differences in clinical symptomatology. It is thought that HIV-2 is evolutionarily related to HIV-1, because the two viruses share several molecular and pathogenic characteristics (Gallo & Montagnier, 1988). However, HIV-2 has not spread across populations to cause disease at nearly the magnitude of HIV-1 and remains relatively contained to West Africa. Concerns about potential increases in North American HIV-2, however, have led to screening for HIV-2 antibodies in addition to HIV-1 antibodies in the national blood supply (S. A.

Myers, Prose, & Bartlett, 1993). Although HIV-2 may become a greater health threat in the future, HIV-1 accounts for the majority of AIDS cases in the world (Glasner & Kaslow, 1990).

There is great diversity found among laboratory isolates of HIV-1, both when samples are taken from different infected persons as well as when isolates come from a single source patient. HIV has been classified into 10 genetic subtypes, designated by the letters A through J, as well as isolated highly divergent strains, or *outliers* (Expert Group of the Joint United Nations Programme on HIV/AIDS, 1997). The various subtypes of HIV have different geographic distributions and many differ in their transmission properties. Variations within infected individuals make HIV particularly difficult for the immune system to manage because alterations in its biochemistry evade targeted immune responses. Similar but distinct HIV-1 substrains cause deterioration of the immune system because each variant of the virus kills T-helper cells. The profusion of biochemically different strains of HIV-1 poses great obstacles to developing effective treatments, especially preventive vaccines.

In summary, there are two known groups of human retroviruses, the leukemia-causing retroviruses, HTLV-I and HTLV-II, and the viruses that cause AIDS, HIV-1 and HIV-2. Both groups are transmitted through close intimate contacts where blood, semen, or vaginal fluids are exchanged; both groups share T-helper cells as a common pathogenic target; both become dormant and integrated into the genetic material of infected cells; and both are related to viruses found in old-world primates. These commonalities suggest that HTLVs and HIVs have a common origin (Gallo, 1988). However, the clinical manifestations of HTLV and HIV are distinct, with the HTLVs causing leukemia, which is characterized by unrestrained growth and proliferation of white blood cells and the HIVs causing profound deterioration of the immune system because of loss and dysfunction of T-helper lymphocytes. The global AIDS epidemic is the result of HIV-1 infection. How HIV-1 destroys the immune system is the key to understanding AIDS.[1]

---

[1]From here forward HIV will refer to HIV-1 unless otherwise noted.

VIRAL CYCLE OF HIV

A virus consists of core genetic material, most often deoxyribonucleic acid (DNA), and a surrounding protein coat. Retroviruses, however, have at their genetic core a strand of ribonucleic acid (RNA). Following retroviral infection of a target cell, RNA is converted into DNA through reverse transcription, a process that relies on the enzyme *reverse transcriptase*. The new viral DNA then either proliferates in the infected cell or integrates itself directly with the cell's genetic material. The ability of retroviral RNA to transcribe itself into a DNA copy and integrate with host cell DNA is the hallmark of a retrovirus. The virus can then lay dormant for long periods of time, safely hidden within host cells. To complete its cycle, a virus must also assemble, package, and replicate itself as a free virus, using the host cell's resources.

The viral cycle of HIV has eight principal steps, shown in Figure 1.2: (a) Upon entry into the bloodstream of an infected person, HIV becomes attached to the membrane of a target cell. HIV is highly selective in its binding properties, only targeting cells that express a surface molecule designated *cluster determinant-4* (CD4), that usually acts as a receptor for infectious agents (antigens). T-helper lymphocytes are one type of cell that expresses the surface molecule CD4, which has an extremely high affinity for the HIV envelope surface protein *gp*120. In fact, the binding between HIV *gp*120 and CD4 is stronger than between CD4 and most non-HIV infectious agents (Hamburg, Koenig, & Fauci, 1990; Z. F. Rosenberg & Fauci, 1991). HIV–CD4 binding is also mediated by other molecules. Chemokine receptors, such as CCR5 or CXCR4 depending on the strain of the virus, mediate the fusion of HIV envelope proteins to cell membranes (Berger, 1997). HIV may bind with CCR5, for example, and activate the targeted cell, increasing its vulnerability to HIV infection and stimulating the production of HIV in an already infected cell (Weissman, 1997). In addition, HIV can bind with surface molecules found on immune cells other than CD4 using similar processes (Levy, 1996). (b) After binding with the cell membrane, the virus enters the host cell by means of the same CD4 surface molecule involved in viral attachment. (c) Once in the cell, the viral genetic material, RNA, is reverse transcribed into a DNA copy. Reverse transcrip-

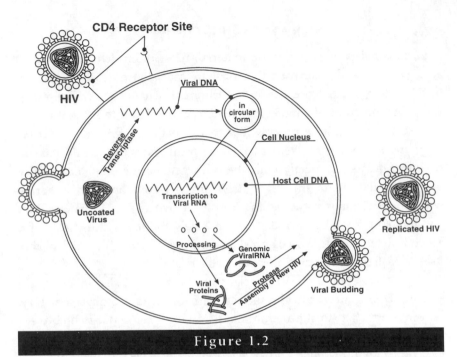

Figure 1.2

The HIV replication cycle. HIV binds with CD4 receptors and enters the cell where its RNA is transcribed to DNA using the cell's resources to produce new HIV particles.

tion of RNA to DNA requires the enzyme reverse transcriptase, a process that is distinctive to retroviruses, not found in DNA viruses. (d) Using the enzyme integrase, the retroviral DNA becomes integrated with the genetic material of the host cell. (e) The integrated viral DNA, or proviral DNA, works in the cell to transcribe viral messenger-RNA, which serves to produce more retrovirus. (f) Viral messenger-RNA produces structural proteins for the production of HIV RNA and envelope proteins. (g) The new viral RNA is encapsulated as the core of newly produced proteins in the assembly of new HIV. The enzyme protease plays a critical role in splicing proteins for the assembly of new virus particles. (h) Replicated virus particles eventually bud and release from the host cell, infecting a multitude of new host cells. Thus, the natural flow of genetic information, from DNA to RNA, is reversed in the case of retroviruses, going from RNA to DNA, making retroviruses extremely complicated to understand and treat.

Shortly after infection with HIV, there is a brief period of intensive viral replication, where HIV rapidly multiplies and disseminates. This period is characterized by high concentrations of virus, or *viremia*, and is followed by a decline in virus replication (Tindall, Imrie, Donovan, Penny, & Cooper, 1992). HIV replicates at a rate of a billion new virus *particles each day*, therefore doubling the viral population every two days in untreated people (Ho, 1996). Thus, the viral burden in people with AIDS can be 100 times greater than the viral burden in asymptomatic HIV seropositive persons (Henrad et al., 1995). When not replicating, HIV hides within cells in a latent phase. HIV can exist in latent form in T-helper lymphocytes, as well as in other infected cells, for long periods of time. Latent HIV infection occurs while the viral genetic material (provirus) is integrated within the host cell system (Bednarik & Folks, 1992; Fauci, 1986; Weber & Weiss, 1988). Viral latency should not, however, be confused with clinically asymptomatic periods. Although there may be an absence of clinical symptoms during viral latency, viral replication is occurring in host cells during asymptomatic periods (Maddox, 1993). Thus, HIV can be latent during periods of symptomatic illness and can actively replicate during asymptomatic periods.

Activation of dormant HIV in T-helper lymphocytes can occur under a number of conditions. The slow and persistent progression of immunologic destruction and clinical symptomatology characteristic of HIV infection results from its complex genetic regulation as well as the interaction between HIV, its host cell, and networks of modulating cofactors. Infectious agents likely to facilitate HIV activation include herpes simplex virus type-2, HTLV-I, HTLV-II, Epstein-Barr virus, and hepatitis B virus (Hamburg et al., 1990; Hirsch, Schooley, Ho, & Kaplan, 1984; Laurence, 1992; Pantaleo, Graziosi, & Fauci, 1993). Thus, stimulation of the immune system and activation of HIV are intricately connected. When activated, proviral DNA in host cells transcribe messenger-RNA, which in turn initiates protein synthesis and the assembling of new HIV.

The amount of HIV detected in blood and other body systems varies over the course of infection. Quantities of HIV (also referred to as *viral load, viral burden,* and *viremia*), rapidly escalate during the onset of HIV infection. A person newly infected with HIV can have millions of copies of HIV RNA per milliliter of blood. Viral load is reduced, however, as a result of immune responses to HIV infection. Viral replication occurs during all phases of infection, and viral load appears stable through untreated asymptomatic periods (Henrad et al., 1995). Tests for viral load that measure HIV RNA include polymerace chain reaction (PCR) and branched DNA (bDNA) analyses. Monitoring viral load is critical to assessing the health of people with HIV (Vlahov et al., 1998). At later phases of infection, however, viral load once again increases. Figure 1.3 illustrates the relationship between viral load, T-helper lymphocyte counts, stage of illness, and time of HIV infection.

HIV AND THE IMMUNE SYSTEM

T-helper lymphocytes are destroyed when HIV erupts, or buds, from host cells. However, there are a number of other mechanisms by which HIV destroys lymphocytes (see Table 1.1). When HIV erupts from an infected cell, the virus sheds fragments of envelope protein *gp*120, which can adhere to the CD4 surface molecules of neighboring T-helper cells. HIV *gp*120 binding with uninfected T-helper cells can cause several adverse effects. First, *gp*120 can adhere uninfected T-helper cells together, forming a giant multinucleated clump of incapacitated cells called *syncytia* (Gallo & Montagnier, 1988; Weber & Weiss, 1988). Syncytia are commonly found in the lymphatic systems and brains of HIV-infected patients (Hamburg et al., 1990). Another effect of binding *gp*120 to the surface of T-helper cells is the triggering of an immune response against the host cell itself. When *gp*120 is detected as a foreign particle by the immune system, it is destroyed along with uninfected lymphocytes. In addition to killing cells, HIV can interfere with fundamental functions of T-helper cells. Unintegrated DNA within infected cells, for example, can have significant effects on T-helper lymphocytes (Hamburg et al., 1990). Several other means by which HIV destroys T-helper cells have been well established (Pantaleo et al., 1993).

18

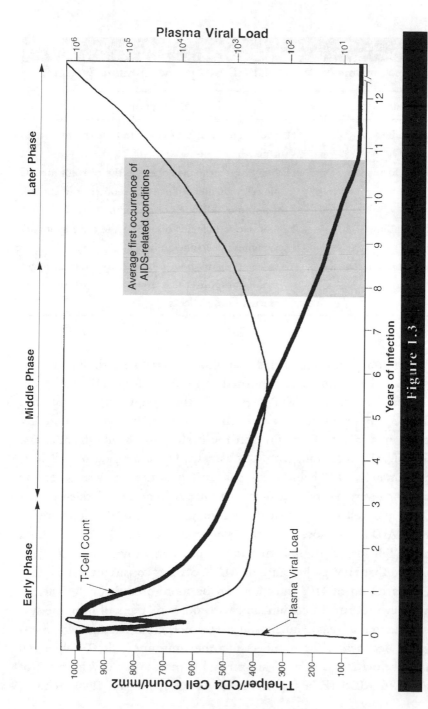

Figure 1.3

Relationship between viral load, T-helper lymphocyte counts, stage of illness, and time of HIV infection.

Table 1.1
Mechanisms by Which HIV Destroys the Immune System

Mechanism	Description
HIV budding	HIV reproduced in cells erupt and infect a multitude of new host cells
Syncytia formation	HIV envelope proteins adhere to the receptor area of one cell that then adheres to another until clusters of immune cells are bound together
gp120 binding	HIV envelope proteins bound to the cell membrane can impair cell functioning
Autoimmune responses	Virus components bound to cell membranes trigger immune responses that eventually attack the infected immune cells

Quantitative loss of T-helper lymphocytes was the earliest and most widely cited immunologic abnormality resulting from HIV infection, and it is the depletion of T-helper cells that results in the profound immune suppression that causes AIDS. T-helper lymphocytes rapidly decline by a factor of one third in the first 12 to 18 months after the onset of HIV infection, with a subsequently slower rate of cell loss, approximately 80 T-helper cells per unit measure per year, over the course of several years (McCutchan, 1990). A second accelerated period of T-helper cell decline usually occurs prior to the development of clinical AIDS. The close associations among duration of HIV infection, loss of T-helper cells, and immunosuppression provide the strongest evidence that HIV is the cause of AIDS. Studies consistently show that the progression of HIV infection can be monitored through T-helper lymphocyte counts in conjunction with other markers of immune system functioning (e.g., Hutchinson et al., 1991). For example, independent of declines in the numbers of other immune cells, T-helper cell counts below 200 cells/mm^3 are a reliable marker for development of full-blown AIDS (Fahey et al., 1984; Hamburg et al., 1990; Schoub,

1993) and have, therefore, been included as a diagnostic criterion in AIDS case definitions.

In addition to absolute numbers of T-helper cells, the ratio between T-helper and T-suppressor (CD4) cells is a key indicator of immune system functioning. Healthy people have more T-helper lymphocytes at any given time than T-suppressor cells, with 60% of peripheral lymphocytes being T-helper cells and 30% T-suppressor cells (Fauci et al., 1984). However, with HIV infection, the ratio is often inverted. Although other infections may result in increased numbers of T-suppressor cells relative to T-helper cells, HIV causes the inversion because of the loss of T-helper cells rather than because of an increase in T-suppressor cells. This immune system abnormality suppresses immunity and results in a substantial increase in susceptibility to infectious diseases.

Aside from direct damage to T-helper cells, immune dysfunction occurs as an indirect result of HIV infection. As a part of the cell-mediated branch of the immune system that deals with infection-causing microorganisms, T-helper lymphocytes coordinate immune responses to viruses. T-helper cells become impaired when HIV envelope proteins adhere to their cell membrane (Z. F. Rosenberg & Fauci, 1991), disrupting the normal cell signaling and feedback systems. Progressive T-helper cell dysfunction, therefore, accounts for immune disturbances caused by HIV infection, which ultimately interfere with multiple branches of immune functioning. The widespread and diffuse effects of HIV were at first surprising because it selectively infects a single type of immune cell, the T-helper lymphocyte. However, the effects of HIV infection are pronounced because losing T-helper cells and the accompanying cell disturbances result in dysfunction across several branches of the immune system.

Although the primary target of HIV is the T-helper lymphocyte, several other immune system cells are indirectly affected by HIV infection. For example, although there is not a significant loss of T-suppressor cells or natural killer cells, these cells are coordinated by T-helpers. Also of particular importance are the monocyte macrophages, which also express the CD4 surface molecule to which HIV selectively binds. Monocyte macrophage cells are phagocytes; they engulf and destroy infectious agents. Thus, HIV may enter macrophages after binding with the CD4 surface molecule, or HIV may be engulfed through phagocytosis. HIV-infected macrophages are unable to attack and destroy other microorganisms (Hamburg et al., 1990). HIV that is harbored inside of host macrophage cells is also protected from immunologic responses and may be disseminated throughout the body, particularly to the lungs and brain (Hamburg et al., 1990; Z. F. Rosenberg & Fauci, 1991).

HIV effectively evades the immune system by harboring inside immune cells and destroying the branches of the immune system that typically protect against viral infections. Another critical aspect of HIV's ability to destroy the immune system is its mutation into multiple genetic strains. Nowak and McMichael (1995) described how HIV's mutation rate gives rise to genetic variability that evades immune responses and, therefore, promotes its survival. This evolutionary perspective suggests that it is HIV's mutation rate that creates a survival advantage; the production of new genetic strains eventually overwhelms the immune system. Rates of HIV replication and mutation translate to several thousands of generations of virus particles over a 10-year period, representing as much genetic change as humans may experience over the course of 1 million years (Nowak & McMichael, 1995).

Whereas the scientific community has mostly accepted HIV as the cause of AIDS, there have been alternative etiological theories. For example, molecular biologist Peter Duesberg, of the University of California at Berkeley, has suggested that AIDS is the end result of a combination of health-related problems of which HIV infection plays only a minor role. Appearing mostly in the popular press (e.g., Guccione, 1993), Duesberg's views and those of others stimulated a wide-scale debate on the cause of AIDS. Alternative perspectives discount HIV as being a sufficient cause of disease and place greater weight on other infectious agents and life-style factors, particularly substance abuse and malnutrition, working together to impede the immune system (Root-Bernstein, 1990). Theories of AIDS that de-emphasize the role of HIV have, thus far, lacked scientific verification and have been considered a form of AIDS denial (Essex, 1997).

In summary, although many unanswered questions remain, much has been learned about HIV infection. The link between HIV on the one hand and immunologic impairment and AIDS on the other is well established. As the immune system deteriorates, the body becomes susceptible to infections and other disease processes that are normally controlled by immune responsiveness. HIV affects immunity through several pathways, including the direct loss of T-helper cell functions and impairment of other immune system cells whose functions are mediated by T-helper cells. Similar to other retroviruses, such as HTLV-I and HTLV-II, HIV is contracted through only a few very specific behavioral practices.

ROUTES OF HIV TRANSMISSION

Early epidemiological studies demonstrated that AIDS resulted from an infectious disease. Because the first U.S. AIDS cases almost exclusively involved men who had sex with men, the causal agent, not yet known, was thought to spread through sexual practices. At that time, any possible means of contracting the disease through intimate as well as casual contact were considered possible and there was much speculation about how a person might get AIDS. Hysteria was commonplace and understandable given the unknown cause of a new and devastating illness. Careful epidemiological study over the past decade, however, has provided conclusive findings on how HIV is and is not transmitted. To date, HIV and HIV-infected cells have been isolated in substantial quantities from human blood, vaginal secretions, semen, and breast milk, with significantly lower quantities in saliva and urine (Glasner & Kaslow, 1990; Levy, 1992). Thus, there are four principal modes of HIV transmission: person to person through fluid-exchanging sexual behaviors; person to person through use of HIV-contaminated injection equipment; mother to infant during pregnancy, labor and delivery, or breast feeding; and person to person through transfusion with infected blood or blood products.

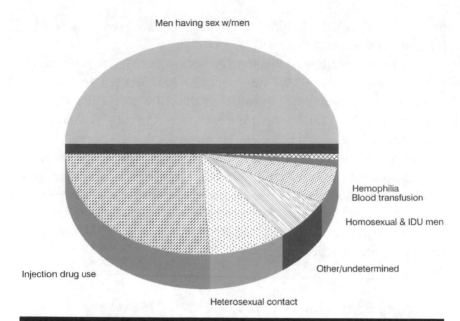

Men having sex w/men

Hemophilia
Blood transfusion

Homosexual & IDU men

Other/undetermined

Heterosexual contact

Injection drug use

Figure 1.4

Proportions of U.S. adult AIDS cases attributed to the most frequent HIV transmission categories: N = 604,176, through June 1997. IDU = Injection drug using.

Figure 1.4 presents the percentages of U.S. adult AIDS cases attributed to the most frequent HIV transmission categories. Figure 1.5 presents the percentages of worldwide adult AIDS cases attributed to various modes of HIV transmission. As shown, the U.S. epidemic has been driven by homosexual activity among men, whereas heterosexual contact accounts for the majority of AIDS cases worldwide. Table 1.2 summarizes the most common routes of HIV transmission, each of which is described below.

Anal Intercourse

Anal intercourse was the first identified route of HIV transmission in North America. Among men who have sex with men, anal intercourse is the primary reason for the large number of AIDS cases in this pop-

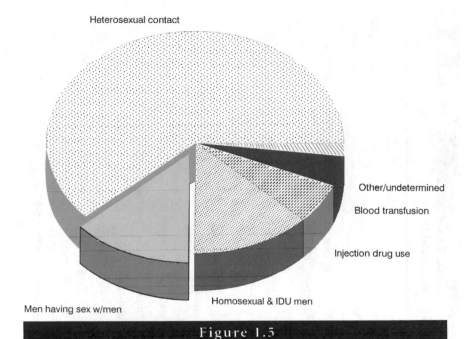

Heterosexual contact

Other/undetermined

Blood transfusion

Injection drug use

Homosexual & IDU men

Men having sex w/men

Figure 1.5

Proportions of worldwide adult AIDS cases attributed to modes of HIV transmission. IDU = Injection drug using.

ulation. Longitudinal cohort studies of gay men residing in U.S. HIV epidemic centers showed close associations between the practice of anal intercourse and HIV infection. For example, Kingsley et al. (1987) followed 2,507 men enrolled in the Multicenter AIDS Cohort Study and found that receptive anal intercourse was the primary sexual behavior related to HIV infection. Receptive anal intercourse is the only male homosexual practice that is definitively associated with contracting HIV. The risk of becoming infected with HIV accelerates in direct proportion to the number of receptive anal intercourse partners men report (Kingsley et al., 1987). Men who engaged in receptive anal intercourse with one partner were three times more likely to be HIV antibody positive than were men who did not practice receptive anal intercourse, and men with five or more such partners demonstrated an 18-fold increase in risk. Kingsley et al. further showed that men who reduced their

Table 1.2
Common Routes of HIV Transmission

Route	Transmission Mechanism	Per-Contact Probability of HIV Transmission[a]
Anal intercourse	Infected semen or blood enters the anal–rectal mucosa or penis through absorption or micro-openings. Varies with presence of blood, STIs, lacerations, and stage of HIV infection.	.0001–.3
Vaginal intercourse	Infected vaginal fluids, semen, or blood enters the vaginal or penile mucosa or through micro-openings. Varies with presence of blood, STIs, lacerations, and stage of HIV infection.	.0001–.056
Oral–genital contact	Infected semen or vaginal fluids enter blood stream through micro-openings in oral cavity or infected cells enter vagina or penis through micro-openings.	Unknown
Perinatal transmission	Transplacental transfer of virus during gestation, transfer of virus or maternal blood during labor and delivery, breast feeding.	.15–.30[b]
Injection drug use with sharing	Use of needles and other injection equipment previously used by an infected person exposes HIV directly to the blood stream.	.067
Needle-stick injury	Occupational injury in medical setting.	.0001–.003
Blood transfusion	Principal risk in United States occurred prior to 1984 blood screening programs, blood or blood parts from an infected person enter blood stream.	.95

NOTE: [a]Data from Centers for Disease Control and Prevention, 1997, unpublished summary statistics. [b]Reduced by 67% with antiretroviral treatment.

practice of receptive anal intercourse substantially reduced their risk for HIV infection.

Prospective studies of gay men also show increased risks for infection when there is rectal tissue damage during anal intercourse (O'Brien, Shaffer, & Jaffe, 1992). Chmiel et al. (1987) found that rectal trauma resulting from anal sex provides highly efficient access for HIV to enter the bloodstream. Of the men in the large Chmiel et al. sample who experienced rectal injuries or bleeding caused by anal sex acts, 90% were HIV infected. In another longitudinal study, Keet, van Lent, Sandfort, Coutinho, and van Griensven (1992) followed 102 men who contracted HIV infection and found that the majority attributed becoming infected to having engaged in anal intercourse. Thus, there is conclusive evidence that anal intercourse affords highly efficient transmission of HIV, and the risk is greatest for receptive partners who experience rectal trauma. It should be noted, however, that proceptive, or insertive, anal intercourse also carries substantial risk for HIV infection and should not be dismissed as a low-risk sexual activity.

Risk associated with anal intercourse results from the high degree of vascularization of anal-rectal tissue and its relatively thin mucosal lining. The practice of anal intercourse is not found exclusively among gay and bisexual men. Gayle and D'Angelo (1991) reported that 25% of female adolescents engage in anal intercourse and that anal intercourse is often practiced among adolescents as a method of avoiding pregnancy and "maintaining virginity." Padian et al. (1987) found that women infected with HIV frequently practiced anal intercourse, and this was most commonly when their partner was bisexual. Finally, in a national sample of men, of which only 2% reported homosexual experiences, Billy, Tanfer, Grady, and Klepinger (1993) found that 20% of respondents reported engaging in anal intercourse.

Vaginal Intercourse

Penile–vaginal intercourse accounts for the greatest number of HIV infections in the world. Heterosexual transmission of HIV, primarily through vaginal intercourse, has been widely documented in North America, and HIV transmission between men and women is bidirectional (J. B. Glaser, Strange, & Rosati, 1989; Nicolosi et al., 1994). Between 1989 and 1992, the number of U.S. AIDS cases attributable to heterosexual contact more than doubled for men and women (Haverkos & Quinn, 1995). During the course of one prospective study, approximately 10% to 20% of women married to HIV infected men contracted HIV infection (Padian, Shiboski, & Jewell, 1991). Although HIV transmission from women to men occurs during vaginal intercourse, the rates of transmission are not as high as those for men to women (Padian et al., 1991). One study that followed 730 couples with one HIV-seropositive partner found that the risk of male-to-female infection is more than double that of female-to-male transmission (Nicolosi et al., 1994). Exact rates of male-to-female and female-to-male HIV transmission are not known, but two possible reasons for higher male-to-female transmission efficiency are (a) the greater mucosal surface area of the female genital tract and (b) the large number of potentially infected cells in seminal fluids. Although there may be differential rates of infection for receptive and proceptive partners, as in anal intercourse, there are no exact probabilities available for calculating risk for HIV infection from vaginal intercourse. In fact, multiple cofactors and variations in infectivity prohibit reliable estimates of risk over multiple occurrences of vaginal intercourse (Downs & De Vincenzi, 1996).

It is well documented that HIV infection can occur after a single heterosexual exposure (May, 1988). In a classic example of how rapidly HIV can spread among heterosexuals, Clumeck et al. (1989) discussed one African man living in Belgium who infected 11 of 18 of his female sex partners. A portion of these women in turn reported subsequent sexual contact with other men who may have also become infected.

Oral–Genital Contact

Despite the fact that oral–genital HIV transmission is biologically plausible when HIV infected semen or vaginal fluids are exposed to oral mucosa (Baba et al., 1996), early epidemiological studies failed to find associations between oral sex and HIV infection. Laboratory research supported the low probability of HIV transmission during oral sex by identifying only small amounts of the virus in saliva, as well as by identifying enzymes in saliva that inactivate HIV (Bergey et al., 1994; Fox, Wolff, Yeh, Atkinson, & Baum, 1989; McNeely et al., 1995). Later studies of couples where one partner was HIV infected and the couple only engaged in oral sex without condoms further failed to substantiate risks for HIV transmission posed by oral sex (De Vincenzi, 1994). Additional cohort studies have reported similar findings (e.g., Ostrow, DiFranceisco, Chmeil, Wagstaff, & Wesch, 1995), suggesting that risks of HIV infection through oral sex must be considered minimal.

Oral–genital contact, particularly oral–penile intercourse, however remains controversial for HIV transmission risk. Exposure of semen to the oral cavity has been reported as the sole risk behavior in a relatively small but growing number of cases. Lifson et al. (1990) described two men who indicated semen in their mouth as their only possible risk for HIV infection over a 5-year observation period. Samuel et al. (1993) reported an additional four men from the same cohort as Lifson et al. who became HIV infected by practicing receptive oral intercourse and had no history of engaging in unprotected anal intercourse. Keet et al. (1992) identified four cases, and Edwards and White (1995) reported one case of orally contracted HIV infection. Another epidemiological study has reported four persons who seroconverted and only reported oral–genital contact as a risk factor while under observation in a longitudinal cohort (Schacker, Collier, Hughes, Shea, & Corey, 1996). These case reports have led to considerable debate over the potential risks for HIV transmission posed by oral sex.

HIV transmission during oral sex may be obscured by anal or vaginal intercourse. When oral sex occurs in the same sexual encounter as anal and vaginal intercourse, the higher-risk activities are considered the cause of infection. Social pressures to deny engaging in any anal intercourse also complicate efforts to estimate the risk of oral sex. Thus, a small number of people who admit oral sex practices and lie about anal or vaginal intercourse raise false concerns. Another problem with case reports is that they do not provide information necessary for determining proportions of people infected through oral–genital contact because the proper denominator is not known. Risks for oral transmission of HIV are clearly increased with oral or genital lacerations, abrasions, or bleeding.

Despite its biological plausibility, perceptions of low risks of oral sex appear to have resulted in increased rates of unprotected oral intercourse in New York City (Dean & Meyer, 1995) and San Francisco (Schwarcz et al., 1995). A study of gay and bisexual men surveyed at a large gay pride festival in Atlanta found that 32% of men felt anxious over the potential risks of oral sex and oral sex anxious men were significantly more likely to report using condoms during oral sex than were nonanxious men (Kalichman, Cherry, et al., 1997).

In terms of oral–vaginal contact, there is no epidemiological evidence that suggests HIV transmission occurs through this activity. Although also biologically plausible, women who exclusively engage in sexual acts with other women have not been found at risk for HIV infection (H. Cohen, Marmor, Wolfe, & Ribble, 1993; Kennedy, Scarletti, Duerr, & Chu, 1995). Most striking, a study of 960,000 female U.S. blood donors did not find a single case of HIV infection among women having exclusive sexual contact with other women (Petersen et al., 1992). These findings are supported by a study of over 1,000 women with HIV infection, which found that only one woman reported sexual contact with women as her sole risk factor (Chu, Conti, Schable, & Diaz, 1994). Oral–vaginal contact therefore appears to carry even lower risks than oral-penile contact, which itself is apparently low risk.

Cofactors for Sexual Transmission of HIV

Several factors are known to influence the relative risks of HIV transmission. Lesions caused by trauma to mucous membranes can increase access of HIV to infectable cells. Of particular importance are other sexually transmitted infections, especially those that degrade the integrity of mucous linings. Syphilis, chancroid, and herpes simplex virus cause ulcers associated with increased HIV transmission (Eng & Butler, 1997). Chlamydia, gonorrhea, and trichomoniasis do not necessarily cause ulcers, but they do degrade mucous membranes and result in increased exposure of HIV-susceptible cells in the genital tract (E. J. Beck et al., 1996; Weir, Feldblum, Roddy, & Zekeng, 1994). Lesions are not necessary for HIV transmission, however, because mucous membranes contain Langerhans cells that carry CD4 on their surface. Langerhans cells transfer infectious particles to immune cells; unfortunately, they also transport HIV (Ayehunie et al., 1995; Soto-Ramirez et al., 1996).

Other factors that influence sexually transmitted HIV include genetic characteristics of host cells, strains of the virus, and stage of HIV infection (Royce, Sena, Cates, & Cohen, 1997). In addition, male circumcision has been associated with HIV transmission risk. Uncircumcised men appear to have lower risk behavior histories, including rates of intercourse and numbers of sex partners, than do circumcised men (Laumann, Masi, & Zuckerman, 1997; Seed et al., 1995). However, despite their lower risk profile, uncircumcised men appear more susceptible to contracting HIV (Moses et al., 1994; Urassa, Todd, Boerma, Hayes, & Isingo, 1997). Uncircumcised men's risks may be attributed to infectable cells found in foreskin or differences in tissues of the glans-penis. Intercourse during menses and other blood-related sex practices will also increase transmission risks for HIV (Royce et al., 1997). Women who douche, particularly with noncommercial solutions, also appear at increased risk (Gresenguet, Kreiss, Chapko, Hillier, & Weiss, 1997). These and other cofactors likely increase and decrease relative risks of HIV transmission.

Condoms and Other Protection Against Sexual Transmission

Once HIV was determined to cause AIDS and it was established that HIV was transmitted through sexual contact, studies evaluated the effectiveness of condoms as barriers against HIV transmission. Laboratory tests conclusively showed that intact latex condoms are impermeable to HIV and other retroviruses (Conant, Hardy, Sernatinger, Spicer, & Levy, 1986). The effectiveness of latex condoms as a primary means of preventing HIV transmission has resulted in the widespread distribution of condoms and mass media promotion of condom use. To increase the use of barrier methods of protection further, and to offset power differentials in condom-use decision making in heterosexual relationships, the female condom, an insertive condom-like lubricated polyurethane sheath, is also available. There is also evidence that some spermicidal applications, in particular nonoxynol-9, may have virucidal effects and may add to the protective value of condoms. Laboratory studies have shown that some spermicides have virus-deactivating properties that disrupt the viral envelope (M. J. Rosenberg et al., 1993). Spermicides may also, however, thin mucous linings, and allergic reactions to spermicides can actually increase HIV transmission risks. Thus, until proven otherwise, spermicides should only be used in combination with condoms for protection against HIV transmission.

Population-based surveys consistently show that frequency of condom use tends to be quite low even among persons with identifiable high-risk behavior histories. In a nationally representative study, Tanfer, Grady, Klepinger, and Billy (1993) found that nearly two thirds of sexually active men did not use condoms at all in the previous month. Studies of women living in inner-cities find that women with high-risk behavior histories are no more likely to use condoms than women at lower behavioral risk (Kalichman, Hunter, & Kelly, 1992; Sikkema et al., 1995). Among men who have sex with men, Kelly, Murphy, Bahr, Koob, et al. (1993) reported that men who engaged in unprotected anal intercourse were not intending to use condoms in the future. Condom use is also infrequent among injection drug users, with 46% of men who inject drugs reporting never using condoms with their steady sex partners and 52% never using them with casual partners (Centers for Disease Control and Prevention [CDC], 1992a, 1992b). Individuals with multiple sex partners are more likely to use condoms than those who have one long-term partner, even among injection drug users whose partners may be at high-risk (Upchurch et al., 1992).

It should be noted that when latex condoms are used they reduce but do not eliminate risk for HIV transmission. Condom failures in people using them for protecting against HIV, as well as other sexually transmitted infections and pregnancy, are well known. Condom failure frequently occurs during vaginal intercourse (Grady, Klepinger, Billy, & Tanfer, 1993; Richters, Donovan, & Gerofi, 1993) and anal intercourse

(Golombok, Sketchley, & Rust, 1989). A national survey found that over a 6-month period, 13% of men using condoms experienced breaks or tears, and 14% had condoms slip off during intercourse (Grady et al., 1993). As many as 79% of heterosexual couples who consistently use condoms experience breaks (Hatcher et al., 1988). One study showed that even with consistent use of condoms, HIV infection occurred among 17% of heterosexual couples with an HIV-infected partner, compared with 82% for those who inconsistently used condoms (Hatcher et al., 1988). Condoms commonly fail among men who have sex with men, with 31% reporting condom breaks at least once during anal intercourse (Golombok et al., 1989). Similarly, a study of over 500 male commercial sex workers in San Francisco found that 58% experienced condom breaks and 47% had condoms slip off, usually during anal intercourse (Waldorf & Lauderback, 1993). With respect to the female condom, there is an overall estimated 26% failure rate for pregnancy, and the failure rate is 11% when used consistently and correctly (CDC, 1993b).

Microscopic tears in latex condoms permit HIV transmission because HIV is considerably smaller than other sexually transmitted viruses, including herpes simplex viruses and cytomegalovirus (Feldblum & Fortney, 1988). Thus, it is not only essential that condoms be used, but that they be used correctly, including using a new condom for each occurrence of sexual intercourse, keeping the condom on for the entire duration of the sex act, leaving an adequate reservoir at the tip to collect semen, ensuring that there is no air between the condom and penis, and using adequate and proper lubrication to reduce strain on the latex.

A common factor in condom failure is the use of oil-containing lubricants. Because oil-containing products, even if water-soluble, quickly deteriorate latex, only oil-free, water-based lubricants should be used to lubricate latex condoms. Unfortunately, the mistaken use of oil-containing lubricants is common, with 60% of gay and bisexual men reporting use of oil-containing products to lubricate latex condoms during anal intercourse (D. J. Martin, 1992). It is common for people to mistake water-soluble products, which may contain oils, with the necessary water-based lubricants. Thus, although condom-use promotion is essential to prevent the spread of HIV, condoms are not foolproof and require instruction for proper use.

Injection Drug Use

Transmission of HIV occurs when needles, syringes, and other injection equipment is used by an infected person and shared with other injectors. Residual blood contaminates the injection apparatus and can directly transmit HIV to a sharing partner. As many as 40% of injection drug users had shared needles and syringes during the first decade of AIDS (Magura et al., 1989). Rates of infection had declined since the threat of contracting HIV through contaminated needles was first publicized (Des Jarlais, Freidman, & Casriel, 1990). Legal exchange of needles clearly prevents HIV infections (National Institutes of Health, 1997). Unfortunately, the public health benefits of syringe exchange are often overshadowed by the politics of substance abuse.

Sharing injection equipment occurs within the sociocultural and economic contexts of injected drug addictions. Users share equipment when learning how to inject, showing others how to inject, and as a part of close and intimate relationships. Syringe sharing can also occur because addicts are reluctant to carry clean needles and syringes with them because of the potential for criminal charges if caught (Booth, 1988). Renting or selling used needles and syringes can also be a way to financially support addictions. Used injection drug equipment is also obtained through *shooting galleries*, where injectors rent or borrow injection equipment. Thus, HIV has been widely transmitted among injection drug users by way of injection equipment shared by a circle of friends as well as strangers. Once infected, injection drug users can transmit HIV to sexual partners, who may or may not also inject drugs.

Perinatal HIV Transmission

Pregnant women infected with HIV can transmit the virus to their unborn or newly born children. In developing countries, between 18% and 40% of infants born to HIV-1 infected women acquire HIV-1 infection, although the risk for HIV-2 transmission is much lower (Adjorolo-Johnson et al., 1994). The first cases of AIDS in children were reported in 1982, and AIDS is now among the leading causes of death in children older than 1 year. Infection from mother to offspring occurs by HIV crossing the placenta, usually during the second and third trimesters, and through contact with infected maternal blood and vaginal fluids during labor and delivery (Z. F. Rosenberg & Fauci, 1991; Ryder & Hassig, 1988). Studies have shown that newly infected women and women with advanced HIV infection are more likely to transmit HIV to their fetus than are women who are pregnant during times when viral load may be lower (O'Brien et al., 1992). In addition, HIV is present in breast milk, making it possible for transmission to occur during breast-feeding. Risk for perinatal HIV transmission is, however, reduced by maternal use of antiretroviral medications (Baba, Sampson, Fratazzi, Greene, & Ruprecht, 1993). The results of AIDS Clinical Trial Group Protocol 076 demonstrated that the antiretroviral drug zidovudine (AZT) administered to pregnant women and their infants resulted in a two-thirds reduction in risk for HIV transmission, demonstrating an effective means of preventing perinatal HIV transmission. However, the cost of antiretroviral drugs limits their impact on perinatal HIV infection worldwide.

An estimated 6,000 births to HIV-infected women occur each year in the United States (Gwinn et al., 1991; Rogers & Kilbourne, 1992). The majority of infants born to HIV-infected mothers test HIV antibody positive because maternal antibodies, although not necessarily the virus, cross the placenta during gestation. HIV infection actually occurs in 20% to 40% of infants born to untreated HIV infected mothers. Conclusive testing for HIV antibodies in newborns, therefore, can only occur after maternal antibodies dissipate from the infant's bloodstream and are replaced with the infant's own HIV antibodies, if the infant has indeed been infected. However, tests for the presence of HIV itself, such as with PCR, can be conducted earlier.

Blood Transfusions and Blood Products

Early in the U.S. AIDS epidemic donated blood could not be tested for HIV antibodies, and HIV was unknowingly transmitted to transfusion recipients. Receiving a single unit of HIV-infected blood carries a 95%

chance of HIV infection. Persons at greatest risk for HIV infection through U.S. blood transfusions are those who received blood or blood products between 1978, when the U.S. HIV epidemic began, and 1984, when the HIV-antibody test became available and blood screening programs were initiated. Prior to screening blood, hemophiliacs were vulnerable to HIV infection because of multiple blood transfusions and treatments with blood components combined from multiple donors. As a result of exposure to contaminated blood products in the early 1980s, 50% to 65% of U.S. hemophiliacs were HIV infected, and AIDS is the leading cause of death in this population (Dew, Ragni, & Nimorwicz, 1991). Furthermore, HIV-infected hemophiliacs unknowingly transmitted HIV to their sex partners, and women infected with HIV through blood transfusions often infected their newborns (Chorba, Holman, & Evatt, 1993). However, blood-donor screening programs were implemented in March 1985 in the United States, the result of which has been to dramatically reduce HIV infection through blood transfusions. A study of over 4 million blood donations from 19 regions in the United States during 1992 and 1993 found that 1 donation in every 360,000 was made during the brief window period between exposure to HIV and development of HIV antibodies. In addition, 1 in 2,600,000 HIV seropositive donations may go undetected because of laboratory error. Thus, it was estimated that the risk of HIV infection from blood transfusion is between 1 in 450,000 to 1 in 660,000, a much lower risk than once thought (Lackritz et al., 1995). Unfortunately, most developing countries have not established widespread donor screening programs, making HIV transmission through blood transfusion a continued global threat (Mann & Tarantola, 1996).

HIV Transmission to and From
Health-Care Professionals

Invasive medical and dental procedures may allow for bidirectional exposure to HIV. Health-care workers serving HIV-infected patients can become infected when professionals have open wounds exposed to patient blood or when patient blood splashes on mucous membranes. Occupational HIV infection has occurred in people in several health-care professions, including nurses, lab technicians, health aides, physicians, and surgeons. However, few health providers have been infected from patients. Among all occupationally infected health-care workers, 84% were exposed through percutaneous injury, such as a cut or needle-stick puncture, and 13% through mucous-membrane exposure, such as through the mouth or eyes (CDC, 1992i). Still, the risk for occupational HIV infection is very low.

Among phlebotomists, professionals who draw blood samples, needle-stick injuries are infrequent, with about one injury occurring for every 6,000 collected specimens. Among those who experience needle-stick injuries, few people become HIV infected. Several prospective studies of other health-care professions show similar low rates of occupationally acquired HIV infection. Among more than 4,000 health-care workers, of whom half experienced percutaneous exposure to HIV-infected materials, there were minimal risks for infection (Gerberding, 1992). In an early study, Hirsch et al. (1985) found no cases of occupational HIV transmission among hospital employees, including 33 with accidental needle-stick injuries and other open wounds exposed to patient blood. Henderson et al. (1986) reported that of 150 health-care workers with percutaneous or mucous-membrane exposure to HIV, none became HIV infected. Thus, although health-care occupational risk for HIV infection does exist, the overall rate of transmission is extremely low for both percutaneous and mucous-membrane exposures.

HIV transmission can also occur from health-care workers to patients. Provider-to-patient transmission can result from direct exposure to an infected provider's blood during an invasive procedure or through the use of contaminated medical instruments. For example, two people in the United States and one in Europe have been infected with HIV as a result of invasive nuclear medicine procedures (CDC, 1992f). Although these incidents occurred out of 38 million annual procedures, they have prompted guidelines and recommendations to reduce procedure-related risks. The most well known case of provider-to-patient HIV transmission occurred when a Florida dentist infected at least six patients with HIV (O'Brien et al., 1992). Genetic testing showed that all six patients were infected with a strain of HIV similar to that carried by the dentist, suggesting that the dentist was the source of the patient infections. The infections seemed to have occurred during procedures performed with instruments contaminated by previous use on the HIV-infected dentist himself (Gerberding, 1992), or through other means of improper infection control. Although this case is considered unique, and risk of dentist-to-patient exposure is extremely low, HIV-infection control standards for dental practice have been established (CDC, 1992j).

On the basis of these and other cases, the American Medical Association has recommended that any "physician who knows that he or she has an infectious disease should not engage in any activity that creates risk of transmission of the disease to others" (Gerberding, Littell, Brown, & Schecter, 1990). For all health-care providers, infection-control guidelines, or *universal precautions*, assure protection against exposure to HIV in either transmission direction (CDC, 1987b). In addition, protocols are established for administering anti-HIV drugs immediately after potential occupational exposure to prevent the onset of infection. Given concerns expressed by both patients and providers, some have called for mandatory testing of patients, and others have demanded that providers disclose their HIV serostatus to patients. However, such measures risk infringing on privacy rights and will require careful examination of their relative costs and benefits before they are instituted (Brennan, 1991). Again, it is important to emphasize that transmission from HIV-infected providers to patients is extremely rare. Illustrating this is a study of 19,036 persons treated by 57 HIV-infected health-care workers that failed to identify a single case of HIV transmission to patients (CDC, 1993c).

Transmission Through Casual Contact and Atypical Modes

Direct contact with the blood of a person with AIDS can result in HIV transmission, but even cases of transmission after household exposure to blood are rare (CDC, 1994a). Nonetheless, a great deal of speculation and fear exists concerning HIV transmission through a variety of nonspecific, casual contacts with infected persons and through mediating mechanisms of transmission. Numerous studies conducted with individuals who live with HIV-infected persons, who have daily household exposure to body fluids, and who share eating utensils and bathroom facilities, have consistently shown that people who do not engage in sexual acts with infected persons do not become infected. In one investigation, Freidland et al. (1986) studied 68 children and 33 adults who shared close quarters with 39 AIDS patients. The study failed to find any evidence of casual transmission of HIV. Likewise, no cases of HIV transmission are known to occur in schools or day-care settings (Rogers & Kilbourne, 1992).

Because HIV has been isolated in body secretions other than blood, semen, and vaginal fluids, it is commonly believed that contact with these other fluids carries risk for HIV infection. Although HIV is found in tears and urine, there is no evidence that contact with these fluids results in HIV infection. Even if infection from tears or urine were possible, it would require long and extensive exposure for transmission to occur (Lifson, 1988). Infection from saliva, on the other hand, has been more controversial, with studies yielding conflicting results. The consensus is that contact with the saliva of an infected person through kissing, cardiopulmonary resuscitation (CPR), or other such contacts carries no risk for infection, unless of course there is blood present in the saliva. Thus, aside from genital sexual contact, shared injection equipment, and freak accidents, close contact poses no risk for HIV transmission.

Other behaviors and mediating mechanisms once believed to present at least some risk for HIV infection have not been supported by epidemiological studies. For example, it was once believed that insects that first bite an infected person could transmit HIV to subsequent bite recipients. Studies have shown, however, that HIV does not replicate in arthropod cells, making insects an impossible host for HIV (Srinivasan, York, & Bohan, 1987). Furthermore, the amount of blood residue on an insect stinger would not be sufficient for HIV transmission because insects ingest blood; they do not inject it. Studies in areas with both high rates of AIDS cases and dense populations of mosquitoes have demonstrated that HIV infection is unrelated to mosquito exposure and that elderly persons and children do not show high rates of HIV infection, despite their higher rates of insect bites (Castro, Lifson, et al., 1988). Other theoretically possible modes of HIV transmission, such as tattooing, which involves needle puncture, and human bites, have not shown significant risks for HIV transmission (Castro, Lieb, et al., 1988; Lifson, 1988).

PATTERNS OF THE EPIDEMIC

The HIV–AIDS epidemic is monitored through two central systems. First, local health departments, the CDC, and the World Health Organization follow the number of people diagnosed with AIDS. Even the most accurate AIDS case monitoring, however, can only estimate the extent of the HIV epidemic as it existed 10 years earlier. A second source of information is collected through HIV-antibody testing. HIVsero-prevalence studies yield the rate of HIV infection in specific populations. The limitations of AIDS case reporting have led many states to require reporting new HIV infections to health departments. Seroprevalence surveys are also conducted on volunteers, but these methods underestimate the magnitude of the HIV epidemic because participants demonstrate lower rates of HIV seroprevalence than do people who refuse to participate (Karon, Dondero, & Curran, 1988).

HIV–AIDS is a pandemic affecting all continents and virtually every country of the world. Mathematical models show that the AIDS pandemic has a continuous expansion. It is estimated that 30.6 million people in the world were infected with HIV and 10.4 million have developed AIDS (Mann & Tarantola, 1996). The most heavily affected regions include sub-Saharan Africa, Southeast Asia, Latin America, and North America, with the highest prevalence occurring in developing countries. There are several explanations for why AIDS is more prevalent in developing as compared with industrialized countries, including co-epidemics of ulcerative sexually transmitted infections that facilitate HIV transmission, variations in strains of HIV that differ in their infectivity, access to HIV testing and treatment, culturally related sexual practices such as prostitution, resistance to condom use, and sexual networks that span across high-risk groups.

Cases of AIDS in North America and the Caribbean have increased substantially each year since 1980. For example, the first case of AIDS reported in Canada occurred in 1982, and 30,000 adult HIV infections were estimated in 1994 (Mann & Tarantola, 1996). In Canada, nearly 70% of all AIDS cases have occurred among men who have sex with men. In contrast, HIV infection in Puerto Rico has primarily resulted from heterosexual contact. Puerto Rico represents the second highest rate of AIDS among all U.S. cities and territories, claiming the majority of AIDS cases from U.S. territories. The annual rate of increase in AIDS cases is illustrated in Figure 1.6. While the first 100,000 cases of AIDS occurred in the first decade of the U.S. epidemic, the second 100,000 accumulated in just 2 years, and the third 100,000 in less than 2 years. Because the number of AIDS cases includes people infected with HIV over 10 years ago, it is impossible to know exactly how many people are HIV infected at any given time. Appendix A provides a summary of the U.S. HIV–AIDS epidemiology.

Seroprevalence studies show varying degrees of HIV infection across segments of the U.S. population. Studies of men who report having sex with other men consistently show that significant numbers test positive for HIV (Chmiel et al., 1987; Quinn, Groseclose, Spence, Provost, & Hook, 1992). Seroprevalence among injection-drug-using adults in Houston is 11% (M. L. Williams, 1990), whereas seroprevalence for treatment-seeking injection drug users in New York City is as high as 60% (Stoneburner, Chiasson, Weisfuse, & Thomas, 1990). Seroprevalence among sexually transmitted infection (STI) clinic patients ranges between 2% and 15%, depending on geographic region and when the study was conducted (Quinn et al., 1992). A national study of 40 metropolitan areas between 1988 and 1992 found that one third of STI clinic patients were HIV infected (Weinstock, Sidhu, Gwinn, Karon, & Peterson, 1995). As many as 70% of hemophiliacs who received blood components are HIV infected (Bartlett, 1993a). Other populations studied include homeless youth in New York City, of which 16% of 18- to 20-year-olds were HIV infected (Hein, 1990),

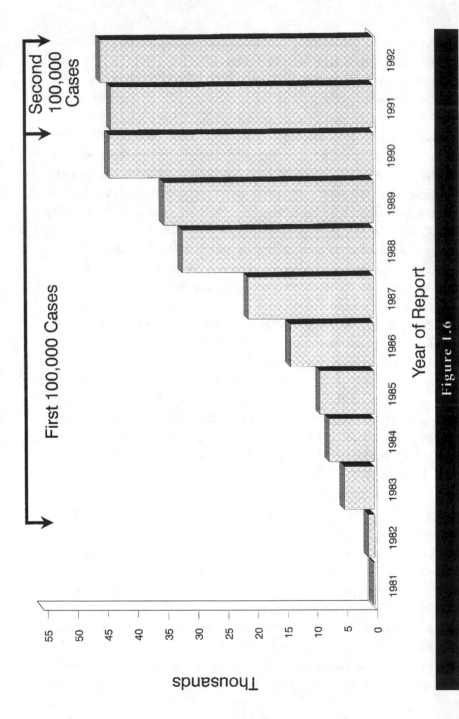

Figure 1.6

Expansion of the AIDS epidemic from 1981 to 1992.

and runaway adolescents in New York City, with 5% HIV infected (Stricof, Kennedy, Nattell, Weisfuse, & Novick, 1991). One in ten homeless adults in Miami are HIV seropositive (CDC, 1991a), and between 4% and 33% of adults with psychiatric disorders have HIV infection (M. P. Carey, Weinhardt, & Carey, 1995). High seroprevalence rates occur among prison inmates and commercial sex workers, with rates higher for minority than for nonminority people.

AIDS has been reported in every state in the United States, with the greatest number of cases in larger metropolitan areas. AIDS is among the leading causes of death for U.S. men and women aged 35 to 44. AIDS is particularly devastating in larger cities, with AIDS accounting for one third to one half of deaths of young men in cities such as Ft. Lauderdale, New Haven, Minneapolis, Seattle, and San Diego (Selik, Chu, & Buehler, 1993).

The disproportionate number of AIDS cases in urban centers has characterized the AIDS epidemic since its beginning. In New York state, AIDS has been the leading cause of death among men 25 to 44 years old and among women 20 to 39 years old (P. F. Smith, Mikl, Hyde, & Morse, 1991), and the vast majority of deaths because of AIDS in New York state have occurred in New York City (Selik et al., 1993). Among U.S. cases of AIDS, 85% occur in metropolitan areas. Thus, as in previous epidemics, cities carry the greatest burden in the AIDS crisis.

Inner cities, like underdeveloped countries, consist of highly mobile and rapidly changing populations, with transience, poverty, social injustices, prostitution, and illegal drug use facilitating the spread of infectious diseases (Morrow, Colebunders, & Chin, 1989). As HIV has spread, individuals have migrated to rural areas. Many rural towns have increased rates of AIDS that parallel patterns observed in U.S. epidemic centers a decade ago (Davis, Cameron, & Stapleton, 1992).

The spread of HIV in any given area is determined by four principal factors:

1. *seroprevalence;* rates of infection determine the probability that an uninfected person will encounter an infected partner.

2. *transmission efficiency;* HIV infection occurs with greatest efficiency through anal and vaginal intercourse and sharing drug-injection equipment.
3. *partner mixing;* the number of partners an individual has who are potentially infected contributes to the chances of infection.
4. *infectivity;* this is the degree and duration that an infected person can potentially infect others.

For HIV, infectivity varies with treatment status and disease state, but individuals are variably infectious for life.

Links within and between sexual and drug-using networks determine the pattern and rate of the HIV epidemic. For example, bisexual men who contract HIV from a male sex partner may spread the virus to female partners. Injection drug users spread HIV to non-injection-drug-using sex partners, and infected sex workers infect their sexual trade customers. Thus, there are numerous subepidemics of HIV emerging across several subpopulations. Because HIV is spread within sexual and drug-injecting networks, individuals who engage in risk behaviors in areas with high rates of AIDS experience relatively high levels of risk.

CHARACTERISTICS OF HIGHLY AFFECTED SUBPOPULATIONS

Although HIV infection occurs across all geographic areas and demographic groups, some subpopulations have been affected longest over the course of the epidemic. People at risk for HIV infection are defined on the basis of two necessary conditions: HIV prevalence rates and behavior risk. As described previously, prevalence of HIV in a population is important because it determines the probability that a risk behavior will result in exposure to HIV. The greater HIV seroprevalence in a subpopulation, the higher risk of infection. Behaviors that confer risk for HIV transmission are the means by which HIV is exposed to infectable cells. However, individuals with HIV infection often report multiple modes of possible exposure. Thus, although it has become less relevant to discuss traditional risk groups as the HIV epidemic amplifies, certain subpopulations continue to represent the greatest number of HIV infections and AIDS cases.

Men Who Have Sex With Men

Because the first and greatest numbers of AIDS cases in the United States have occurred among men who have sex with men, most attention regarding the AIDS epidemic has been given to this group. Although high HIV seroprevalence rates occur in gay communities, men who have sex with men are only at high risk for HIV infection when they practice unprotected anal intercourse. In one study of over 2,000 men sampled from gay bars in 16 cities across the United States, Kelly et al. (1992) found that 31% of men reported engaging in anal intercourse without condoms. Men who engaged in unprotected anal intercourse were younger and were less likely to perceive safer sex as the social norm than were men who did not engage in this highest-risk sexual behavior. Lemp et al. (1994) also found one third of young gay men had recently engaged in unprotected anal intercourse in the San Francisco Bay area. Condom use and safer sex practices are less prevalent among homosexually active men who do not identify as gay or bisexual. Homosexually active adolescent males may be at exceptionally high risk, with two thirds of gay and bisexual adolescent males reporting a lifetime history of anal intercourse (Rotheram-Borus, Rossario, Van Rossem, Reid, & Gillis, 1995). Still, there is considerable evidence that the HIV epidemic among homosexually active men in New York City has leveled off, that rates of HIV transmission among gay and bisexual men have decreased nationally since 1985, that HIV infections in San Francisco have been reduced, and that the number of AIDS cases among gay and bisexual men has declined. Changes in behavior observed among men who have sex with men in larger cities account for these declines in HIV and AIDS. Unfortunately, similar declines in AIDS have not been observed among gay and bisexual men outside of HIV epicenters, particularly among ethnic minority men. There is also evidence that a resurgence of HIV infections may occur in U.S. cities as suggested by trends in other sexually transmitted infections. Gonorrhea, for example, increased 24% between 1994 and 1995 in men who have sex with men in San Francisco, and Seattle saw a 125% increase in homosexually transmitted gonorrhea between 1994 and 1996 (CDC, 1997). The co-incidence of HIV and other STIs leads to the expectation that increases in HIV infections will follow these trends.

Injection Drug Users

Syringe and needle sharing, like sexual behaviors, occur within close, intimate, and private relationships as well as between anonymous partners. HIV transmission occurs when syringes are shared within a network of users, where an infected person contaminates injection equipment that is subsequently used by others. Injection drug users may congregate in shooting galleries, which are common in large cities, where HIV seroprevalence rates are highest (Chitwood et al., 1990). Sharing needles, renting injection equipment, and other practices common to shooting galleries increase the risks for contracting HIV. Researchers in one study of injection needles collected from shooting galleries in a high-AIDS-incidence area found that 10% were contaminated with HIV-infected blood (Chitwood et al., 1990).

Research in social networks of injection drug users has shown close linkages among injectors and their sex partners. Analyses demonstrate that HIV is spread within injecting networks and that linkages across networks facilitate further spread (S. R. Friedman et al., 1997). HIV transmission among injection drug users is complicated by several sociocultural factors. First, people infected with HIV may infect their non-injecting sex partners. Second, a close association exists between injection drug use and commercial sex work, with 30% of female injectors engaging in sexual commerce (Castro et al., 1988) and 76% of HIV-infected prostitutes using injection drugs (CDC, 1987a). Third, non-injected drugs are also closely connected to sexually transmitted infections (Chiasson et al., 1991). Injection drug users who smoke crack cocaine are at greater risk of contracting sexually transmitted HIV infection than are people who only inject drugs (R. E. Booth, Watters, &

Chitwood, 1993). Finally, it is common to exchange noninjected drugs for sex, particularly crack cocaine, further illustrating the complex link between drug use and HIV risk (Schoenbaum, Weber, Vermund, & Gayle, 1990).

Heterosexual Men and Women

Heterosexual transmission of HIV accounts for the greatest number of AIDS cases in the world. In Europe, AIDS resulting from heterosexual HIV transmission increased from 11% in 1990 to 16% in 1995, whereas cases that were due to injection drug use remained stable and homosexual transmission cases actually declined (Mann & Tarantola, 1996). Southeast Asia has experienced dramatic increases in HIV infections, with the majority of cases being due to heterosexual transmission. In 1995 in Southeast Asia, including India, Indonesia, and the Philippines, there were an estimated 2.5 million new HIV infections. Fueled by injection drug transmission of HIV, the epidemic in Asia has spread through commercial sex trade and into subsequent heterosexual relations. However, the heterosexual epidemic of AIDS is most well established in Africa, where in some regions nearly 25% of the population is HIV seropositive (Caldwell & Caldwell, 1996).

Throughout the United Sates, heterosexual adults demonstrate high rates of HIV-risk-related behaviors. In a random digit-dial telephone survey, Catania, Coates, et al. (1992) found that 15% to 31% of 10,630 adults were at behavioral risk for HIV infection. The study also found that 7% reported two or more sex partners in the previous year. Ericksen and Trocki (1992) reported that 22% of a nationally representative sample reported two to four sex partners in the previous 5 years. Other national surveys found similar rates of risk-related sexual behaviors practiced among heterosexuals (Billy et al., 1993). As HIV becomes more prevalent among heterosexuals in North America, substantial increases in HIV infection rates are expected.

Among heterosexuals, women are at particular risk for HIV infection. The number of women diagnosed with AIDS in the United States increased 15% between 1990 and 1991 and rose an additional 10% from 1991 to 1992, making AIDS the leading cause of death among young women in New York City and among the leading causes of death in young men and women nationally. The number of women with AIDS who were heterosexually infected surpassed the number infected by injecting drugs for the first time in 1992 (see Figure 1.7).

AIDS has thus far occurred disproportionately among women of color and women living in U.S. inner cities. Of HIV-infected newborns in New York City, 89% are born to women of color (Novick et al., 1991). About half of all HIV infections in women result from having an injection-drug-using or bisexual male sex partner. Women infected with HIV are also frequent users of noninjected drugs. For example, Lindsay et al. (1992) found that 25% of HIV-infected women use crack cocaine, and cocaine use has been tied to elevated risk for HIV infection (Booth et al., 1993; Chiasson et al., 1991). There are other factors that place women at elevated risk for HIV infection, including the large number of infected men with whom women become sexually involved, the high efficiency of male-to-female HIV transmission, and the many inequalities in heterosexual relationships in which women may be disadvantaged in negotiating condom use with sex partners.

People With Other Sexually Transmitted Infections

Women and men who contract sexually transmitted infections are at risk for HIV because the virus is transmitted through the same pathways as other STIs and because HIV and non-HIV infections frequently co-occur. STI patients are likely to maintain high rates of sexual risk behaviors after treatment, increasing the chance of spreading HIV (Hutchinson et al., 1991). A history of STI is a strong independent predictor of HIV infection, particularly when non-HIV infections involve genital ulcers, as is the case for nearly 25 million people with genital herpes in the United States (Aral & Holmes, 1991). Chlamydia and gonorrhea infections also facilitate HIV transmission because of inflammation of mucous membranes. Non-ulcerating diseases that form a discharge containing infected or susceptible cells also increase transmission risks (Royce et al., 1997). Among sexually transmitted infections, syphilis is the single best predictor of HIV infection (Castro

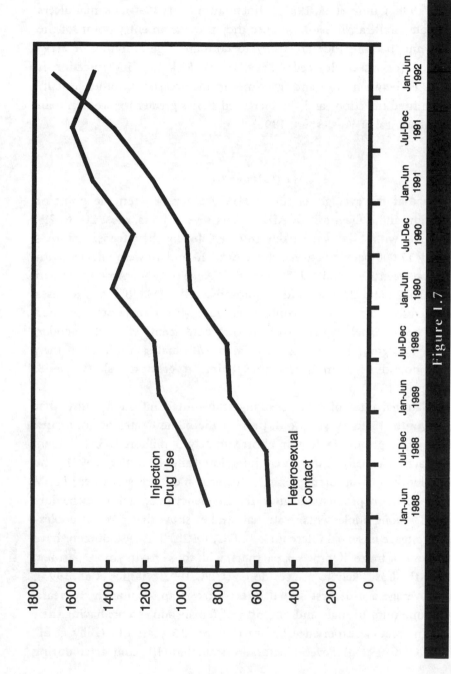

Figure 1.7

Rates of AIDS cases among women attributed to heterosexual and injection drug use transmission.

et al., 1988; Quinn et al., 1988; Schoenbaum et al., 1990). Genital ulcers facilitate viral transmission because they provide an entry point for the virus and because they are likely to contain large amounts of HIV-infected (or infectable) cells (Levy, 1992). Risk for HIV infection is increased between three and five times in the presence of other sexually transmitted infections and the increased risk is greater for women than for men (Aral & Wasserheit, 1996).

Adolescents

Given that the average length of HIV latency between the point of infection and a diagnosis of AIDS spans several years, most 20- to 29-year-olds with AIDS were likely infected during their teens. Approximately 17,000 people between the ages of 13 and 19 were infected with HIV between 1981 and 1987 (Gayle & D'Angelo, 1991). Among women between 20 and 24 years old diagnosed with AIDS, 48% of the cases resulted from heterosexual contact, whereas 64% of male cases resulted from homosexual contact. Risk among adolescents varies by gender, ethnic background, and geographic area, with males, ethnic minorities, and adolescents from inner cities being at greatest risk (Gayle & D'Angelo, 1991).

National rates of other sexually transmitted infections show that U.S. youth, 15 to 19 years old, present the highest rates of gonorrhea of any age group. Each year approximately 3 million U.S. teenagers contract a sexually transmitted infection (Eng & Butler, 1997). The prevalence of co-occurring sexual infections and increasing rates of HIV are particularly problematic given the frequency of sexual risk behaviors found among adolescents. National studies show that 54% of adolescents engage in sexual intercourse (CDC, 1992h) and 19% of teens have had four or more lifetime sex partners, with those having more partners being the least likely to use condoms (CDC 1992h; Tanfer et al., 1993). The average age of first sexual intercourse is approximately 16 years, with one third of male and one fifth of female adolescents having their first intercourse experience before they are 15 years old (Billy et al., 1993; CDC, 1992g). Several factors indicate that HIV contracted during adolescence will continue to rise, including high rates of unplanned pregnancies and substance use in association with sex (Hein, 1990), high rates of HIV infection among inner-city marginalized youth (Eng & Butler, 1997), and prevalent misinformation regarding risk (Gayle & D'Angelo, 1991; Quadrel, Fischhoff, & Davis, 1993).

Seriously Mentally Ill Adults

Individuals with serious and persistent mental illnesses in AIDS epicenters demonstrate alarming rates of HIV infection. M. P. Carey et al. (1995) conducted a comprehensive review of the epidemiological, medical, nursing, psychiatric, and psychological literatures to obtain estimates of the seroprevalence of HIV infection among seriously mentally ill adults. Evidence from nine independent studies showed that between 4% and 23% of the seriously mentally ill were HIV infected. Across studies, a total of 2,345 male and female patients were tested with an overall average HIV seroprevalence rate of 8%. An additional study subsequently reported that 6% of over 500 psychiatric patients were HIV infected (Stewart, Zuckerman, & Ingle, 1994). These rates of HIV infection exceed those in the general population and rival rates found in the highest risk groups, such as injection drug users and STI clinic patients.

Like other populations, HIV transmission risks among the seriously mentally ill are related to substance use, high rates of other STIs, failure to use condoms consistently, and relatively closed sexual networks. However, risks posed to the seriously mentally ill are also influenced by symptoms of mental illness and poor interpersonal social skills (Kalichman, Carey, & Carey, 1996). Cognitive disturbances, hypersexual behavior, and impaired judgment can impede risk reduction efforts. These characteristics of serious mental illness, combined with tendencies toward substance abuse and closed sexual networks, have created an alarming situation for this often neglected population.

The Homeless

HIV seroprevalence studies show that as many as one in five homeless men with serious mental illnesses in New York City may be infected with HIV (M. P. Carey et al., 1995). Homeless men of unknown mental health status in New York City shelters have also shown high rates of HIV infection (Torres, Mani, & Altholz, 1990), with similar findings reported among indigent women (Nyamathi, Bennett, Leake, Lewis, & Flaskerud, 1993) and runaway homeless adolescents (Athey, 1991; Rotheram-Borus & Koopman, 1991).

Homelessness itself may facilitate risks for HIV infection in several ways. First, the homeless tend to cluster in urban areas with high HIV incidence rates. Second, other STIs that may facilitate HIV transmission are also epidemic among the homeless. Third, high frequencies of sexual intercourse with multiple partners, and infrequent use of condoms characterize the sex lives of many homeless men and women. For example, a study of 145 homeless men surveyed in shelters in Milwaukee, Wisconsin, reported that one third had multiple sex partners in the past month and more than half had been treated for an STI (Kelly, Heckman, Helfrich, Mence, Adair, & Broyles, 1995). Similarly, St. Lawrence and Brasfield (1995) surveyed homeless men and women at a soup kitchen and found more than half had multiple sex partners and almost half had recently traded sex for money or drugs. Thus, high rates of sexual activity, partner mixing, co-occurrence of other STIs, and lack of condom use combine to recreate in U.S. inner cities many of the conditions believed to have facilitated heterosexually transmitted HIV in Africa (Inciardi, 1994). In a study of 330 homeless men, Kalichman, Belcher, Cherry, Williams, Sauders, and Allers (1998) found high rates of unprotected sex with multiple partners and sexual risk behavior was closely associated with crack cocaine use. Nearly half of homeless men in this study had been treated for an STI, and one in five reported having had sex with another man.

Incarcerated Populations

AIDS has become an increasingly important problem in U.S. prison systems. Compared with first-time blood donors, a proxy for the general public, rates of HIV infection are 50 times higher among prison males and 130 times higher for prison females. HIV seroprevalence can reach as high as 25% in U.S. prisons (Eng & Butler, 1997). HIV is most likely spread within prisons through injection drug use, sexual intercourse, and possibly tattooing. For women prisoners, the risk for HIV is greatest from injection drug use, both before arrest and during incarceration. HIV is prevalent in prisons throughout the world, with inmate seroprevalence rates commonly reaching 20% to 30%. HIV co-occurs with tuberculosis and hepatitis C in many prison systems, further complicating its management (Turnbull, 1997).

Other Populations at Risk

Several subpopulations that exhibit behavior patterns carrying significant risk for HIV transmission within closed sexual networks have been identified. Of particular interest are subgroups whose sexual behavior and relationships indicate that when HIV is introduced within a sexual network, the virus will rapidly spread. Individuals who exchange sex for money, drugs, or for survival are at considerable risk for HIV infection because of the interrelationships among substance use, injection drug use, and multiple sexual contacts. Commercial sex workers are at particularly high risk, with 16% to 55% of street prostitutes in U.S. cities testing HIV-seropositive (Campbell, 1990). Nearly 4 million U.S. migrant and seasonal workers are at risk because of living in closed and isolated communities with HIV seroprevalence rates over 5% (CDC, 1992c).

In contrast, groups that are at low risk for HIV infection have also been identified. Although there are isolated case reports of sexual HIV transmission between women (Chu, Buehler, Fleming, & Berkelman, 1990; Chu et al., 1994; Marmor et al., 1986; Monzon & Capellan, 1987; Rich, Buck, Tuomala, & Kazanjian, 1993), lesbians appear at low risk unless they inject drugs, have male sex partners, or come in contact with an infected female partner's blood. Although older adults tend to be sexually active as a group, persons over the age of 55 who did not receive a blood transfusion prior to 1985 are also at low risk for HIV infection (Catania et al., 1989). Thus, as the HIV epidemic expands, people at highest risk remain those who engage in behaviors that afford efficient HIV transmission within sexual and injection-drug-using networks with high rates of HIV infection.

GLOBAL PATTERNS OF AIDS

The spread of HIV varies greatly across geographic regions of the world. The World Health Organization estimates that nearly 23 million people in the world are living with HIV–AIDS, with 75% of people with AIDS living in Africa, 8% in North America, 7% in Latin America and the Caribbean, and 6% in Asia. Different epidemiologic patterns across continents are striking and lead to disparate rates of disease among men and women, heterosexuals and homosexuals, and infected children. In North America, Western Europe, Australia, New Zealand, and urban areas of Latin America, HIV has been primarily spread through male homosexual and bisexual contact and through contaminated injection equipment. In contrast, primarily heterosexual spread and transmission through contaminated blood products characterize HIV infection in sub-Saharan Africa and some Caribbean Islands. Other regions including North Africa, the Middle East, Eastern Europe, Asia, and the Pacific, are characterized by infection introduced by migration and transcontinental travel. New patterns emerge as the epidemic grows, and epidemics that were once driven by one mode of transmission shift to others.

The geographic diversity of the HIV pandemic is also the result of the distribution of various strains of HIV. HIV subtype E, for example, is more prominent than other strains in Asia and Africa where HIV is primarily heterosexually transmitted. This subtype is also markedly more efficient at infecting the Langerhans cells of the reproductive tract. Subtype C is also replicated more efficiently in Langerhans cells than other strains (Soto-Ramirez et al., 1996). On the other hand, HIV subtype B is more prevalent in North America and Western Europe, and occurs most often in homosexual and bisexual epidemics. Subtype B is also primarily responsible for the injection drug transmitted HIV epidemic in Thailand (Expert Group of the Joint United Nations Programme on HIV/AIDS, 1997). Thus, the HIV pandemic is actually a composite of numerous subepidemics in distinct geographic regions, with differing patterns of spread, modes of transmission, and biological, behavioral, and ecological cofactors.

AIDS AND POVERTY

Historically, epidemics ravage those living in poverty to a much greater extent than more affluent segments of societies. Poor sanitation, inadequate sewage treatment, poor access to medical care, nutrition, and other living conditions create an environment within which illness can spread. AIDS is no exception. Conditions such as co-occurring STI epidemics, contaminated blood supplies, and nonsterile medical facilities can facilitate the spread of HIV. People living in poverty may lack access to condoms, given that condoms are often made available through health care providers. Access to HIV antibody testing determines who is aware of his or her HIV infection status, and access to treatment may influence infectivity of those infected (Eng & Butler, 1997). Access to anti-HIV medications plays a particularly crucial role in preventing perinatal HIV transmission, as reflected in the drop in HIV infections among U.S. newborns from a peak of 1,800 to less than 500 perinatal infections per year. In contrast, about 1,000 babies in the world are born HIV infected each day, and this rate is relatively stable.

AIDS is most prevalent in the developing world. Countries with the greatest poverty have also experienced the most devastation from AIDS (Gillies, Tolley, & Wolstenholme, 1996). However, some of the most affluent nations, such as the United States, have also experienced significant loss from AIDS. Still, even within more affluent countries, AIDS is associated with poverty. Injection drug use and crack cocaine provide an escape from poverty, and these drugs drive a segment of the AIDS epidemic. Selling sex for survival, including to obtain money, food, shelter, or addictive drugs, promotes transmission in both developing and developed countries (Gillies et al., 1996). Impoverished areas also become closed subcultures, allowing for the rapid spread of HIV. Thus, poverty itself, independent of other social influences, creates communities vulnerable to AIDS.

CONCLUSION

An overwhelming amount of evidence shows that AIDS is the direct result of HIV infection. Although there are cases of HIV infection and

AIDS that remain unclassified with respect to mode of transmission, virtually all cases of AIDS are eventually linked to sexual behavior, injection drug use, or receiving blood or blood products. Despite the fact that HIV is controllable through behavior changes and that the vast majority of people who are at risk are also aware of how HIV is contracted, the AIDS epidemic is expanding at a rapid pace. Thus far, projections of the number of AIDS cases have been accurate within margins of error. Worldwide, the HIV epidemic doubles every 1 to 3 years among heterosexually active adults (Potts et al., 1991).

Given the amplification of the AIDS pandemic, the rapid increase in the number of infected persons, and the fact that people with HIV infection are living longer, an increasing percentage of the population will be HIV infected in coming years. The number of persons with HIV and AIDS who require care and treatment will therefore also increase. Many of the psychological issues faced by people living with HIV result from adjustment to a life-threatening illness. Aspects of the lengthy process of HIV infection itself pose enormous challenges. An understanding of the HIV–AIDS disease process is a necessary step to understanding the psychological ramifications of AIDS.

2

Clinical Course and Manifestations

AIDS emerged as a global health threat faster than any previous disease in history. AIDS is the first to establish itself as a leading cause of death within the same decade of its discovery and is now among the leading causes of death in young men and women. By 1986, AIDS was responsible for 38% of all deaths in San Francisco men ages 20 to 49 (Saunders, Rutherford, Lemp, & Barnhart, 1990), and this figure increased to 61% in 1990 (Selik et al., 1993). By midyear 1997, over 380,000 people had died of an AIDS-related condition in the United States. In contrast to other causes of death, which remain relatively stable, deaths that are due to AIDS steadily increase each year (see Figure 2.1). HIV infection is silent for most of its duration, only becoming overtly symptomatic at its later stages. The natural history of HIV infection is highly variable and has changed over the course of the epidemic. There is now considerable evidence that people infected with HIV will develop AIDS and will die of an AIDS-related illness. The length of time from infection to AIDS varies from as short as 1 year to as long as 15 years or more (Friedman, Franklin, Freels, & Weil, 1991; Schechter et al., 1990). Between 5% and 10% of HIV-infected people progress to AIDS within 4 years, and nearly 50% develop AIDS by 10

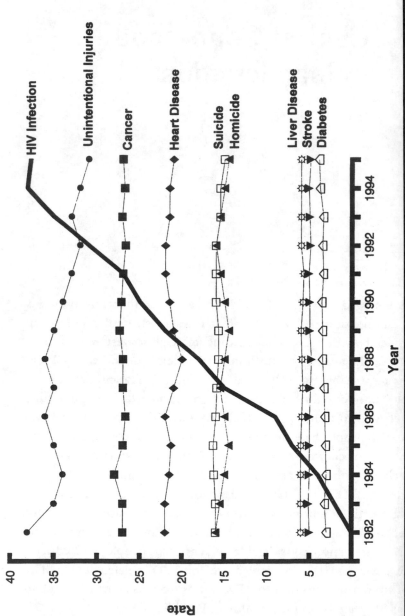

Figure 2.1

Death rates per 100,000 population from leading causes of death among persons aged 25 to 44 years by year in the United States, 1982–1995 (Centers for Disease Control and Prevention, 1997).

years after initial infection (Brettle & Leen, 1991; A. R. Moss & Bacchetti, 1989).

Advances in anti-HIV treatments have significantly altered the course of HIV infection and can delay the onset of AIDS, increasing the survival expectancies for people with HIV–AIDS (Enger et al., 1996). For the first time in the U.S. HIV epidemic, deaths that are due to AIDS declined 28% in 1996, compared with rates in 1995. Decreased AIDS deaths co-occurred with reduced AIDS-related illnesses. Again, these reductions in AIDS illnesses and deaths are attributed to accessing new treatments and not to reductions in new HIV infections, demonstrating a growing population of people living with HIV–AIDS.

Despite the importance of antiretroviral treatments in altering the course of HIV disease, no single factor or combination of factors accounts for variability in HIV progression. Differences in rates of decline occur among individuals who contract HIV through different modes of transmission. For example, the San Francisco City Cohort Study, primarily comprising men who have sex with men, found that 54% of HIV-seropositive men progress to AIDS within 11 years of being infected, whereas 49% of people infected through blood transfusions develop AIDS within 7 years (Clement & Hollander, 1992). Vella et al. (1995) found that HIV-infected men who contract HIV through homosexual contact progress faster to AIDS than do other people, and the difference was related to Kaposi's sarcoma. Other studies, however, have not found survival differences across transmission groups (von Overbeck et al., 1994). In the absence of treatment, most studies have found that the average duration from time of HIV infection to AIDS is between 7 and 10 years. The time between contracting HIV and developing AIDS is for the most part characterized by an absence of serious illness.

Several systems have been developed for describing and staging HIV infection. In an early classification scheme, the CDC proposed a four-stage model that included an acute infection syndrome, a long period of asymptomatic infection, the development of persistent generalized lymphadenopathy (enlarged lymph nodes), and later disease manifestations. A second staging system developed by the CDC included an expanded list of diseases associated with AIDS and an early symptomatic phase referred to as AIDS-related complex (ARC). In the 1987 CDC system, stages I and II consisted of asymptomatic periods, stage III was characterized by chronic lymphadenopathy, and the substages of stage IV represented later phases (see Table 2.1).

Most recent staging systems rely on tracking the number of T-helper lymphocyte cells over the course of infection. For example, Bartlett's (1993a) system classifies people with T-helper cell counts greater than 500 cells/mm^3 as asymptomatic, those with cell counts between 500 and 200 cells/mm^3 as usually asymptomatic, and individuals with T-helper counts below 200 as vulnerable to major complications of AIDS, with most AIDS conditions occurring at or below 100 cells/mm^3. Similarly, Clement and Hollander (1992) offered a system with three stages of infection: early-stage disease defined by T-helper cell counts greater than 500, a middle stage with counts between 500 and 200, and later-stage disease defined by T-helper counts less than 200.

HIV TESTING

Some diagnostic tests for HIV infection involve detecting HIV genetic material directly in blood, such as PCR amplification techniques, or actually culturing the virus from cells. However, the most common tests identify antibodies to the virus rather than the presence of HIV itself. Antibodies produced by the immune system provide immune footprints to viral infection. Antibody tests are easier, safer, and less expensive than are actual viral-detection procedures because antibody tests do not require direct contact with HIV.

The standard procedures for HIV antibody testing involve providing written informed consent and 20 to 30 minutes of pretest counseling that includes an explanation of the test, discussions of limited confidentiality when tests are not anonymous, personalized risk assessments, and exploration of individual concerns. The test procedure itself involves drawing blood and sending samples for laboratory analysis. Posttest result notification and counseling usually occurs about 2 weeks after the initial visit, although there are rapid tests that provide results in a single same-day visit.

Table 2.1
Centers for Disease Control (1987) Staging System for Human Immunodeficiency Virus Infection

Stage	Description
I	Acute HIV infection; asymptomatic or possible acute viral reaction
II	Latent infection
III	Chronic lymphadenopathy
IV-A	Constitutional symptoms; weight loss, fever, chronic diarrhea
IV-B	HIV-induced neuropathology; dementia, myelopathy, peripheral neuropathy
IV-C	Opportunistic infections
IV-D	HIV-associated tumors
IV-E	Other conditions

Although procedures may vary, blood collected for testing is first subjected to an *enzyme-linked immunosorbent assay* (ELISA or EIA) that tests for antibodies to HIV. EIA tests are performed first because they are highly sensitive to HIV antibodies. If an EIA test is negative, it is extremely unlikely that the person is HIV infected. In other words, false negative results from EIA tests are rare. However, positive EIA tests must be repeated because the procedure lacks specificity to HIV antibodies. Thus, a greater likelihood exists that an EIA result will be a false positive (Saag, 1997). For this reason, EIA tests are used for screening blood samples for HIV antibodies. After a blood specimen receives a repeated positive EIA, the test is confirmed using a *Western blot procedure* or immunofluorescence assay (IFA). Like EIA, Western blot techniques detect HIV antibodies, but a Western blot has greater specificity because it determines the exact antigens toward which antibodies are directed. A positive Western blot result means detection of two out of three precise antigen groups from components of HIV. This level of specificity reduces the chances of false positive results to an extremely low probability (Saag, 1997). Thus, both a positive repeated EIA screening test and a positive Western blot confirmatory test are required for diagnosis of HIV infection.

There are a number of situations in which a person can be tested for HIV. Most common are tests conducted in clinics and community settings, where blood is drawn and sent off for analysis. However, new testing technologies are revolutionizing the HIV testing experience. Home HIV testing, for example, became available in the early 1990s. The first home tests were not really home tests at all, but rather home collection kits, where small samples of blood were collected on absorbent paper and sent to a laboratory for analysis with results obtained by telephone. In contrast, true home tests will allow for home analysis, much like home pregnancy tests. In both home collection and home testing, the testing experience is altered, but the immune assays are the same as those used in laboratory analysis. Another testing advance has been rapid testing in clinical settings. The *Single Use Diagnostic System* (SUDS) is performed in an on-site laboratory and provides results in 10 to 15 minutes (Kassler, 1997). Tests for HIV antibodies are also available for use with saliva and urine, removing the need for drawing blood. Developments in HIV testing technologies have challenged testing counseling services but have also increased access to HIV testing.

HIV antibody testing is now among the most accurate diagnostic tools in medicine. HIV tests that indicate a false negative result (i.e., the person is not found infected when he or she really is infected) almost always caused by collecting the blood sample during the incubation window period before HIV antibodies are fully established. People may not, therefore, know they have HIV during the first month or two of infection, although HIV can be transmitted to others during this time. Because a false negative test result is possible, all people who receive this result should be tested again approximately 3 months later. People who test HIV seropositive and have no identifiable risk history should also be retested, although false positive test results only occur because of laboratory errors (Bartlett, 1993a).

In addition to receiving either a positive or a negative result, a third possible outcome is an indeterminate result, neither conclusively positive nor negative. Indeterminate HIV-test results usually occur when the EIA test is positive and only one of the two required specific antigens is detected by Western blot. Ambiguous results occur with respect to both HIV-1 and HIV-2 antibody tests and are most commonly found among individuals infected with HIV who are in the process of developing antibodies. It is also possible to have an indeterminate test result because of other infections or after receiving vaccinations for other illnesses. Indeterminate tests should be repeated 2 to 6 months later.

HIV testing is the only reliable means of determining HIV infection. Even after symptoms, many HIV-related illnesses can be caused by non-HIV immune-suppressing conditions. Thus, individuals with symptoms should be tested for HIV antibodies and should not assume they have HIV on the basis of illness alone.

PRIMARY HIV INFECTION

Following the introduction of HIV to infectable cells, the body mounts an immune response that, unfortunately, is ineffective at stopping HIV infection. In response to HIV, the body may react with a brief period of acute infection symptoms. The usual time that lapses between exposure and acute illness is about 2 to 4 weeks, with the duration of symptoms lasting only 1 to 2 weeks (A. Carr & Cooper, 1997). Acute retroviral illness, when it does occur, is the earliest clinically recognizable event in the natural history of early HIV infection. Response to retroviral infection is similar to the vague symptoms of mononucleosis and influenza. Primary HIV infection is often underdiagnosed in clinical settings (Schacker, Collier, Hughes, Shea, & Corey, 1996). However, retroviral infection is a distinct and recognizable clinical syndrome. Most typically, acute HIV-symptom illness, or primary HIV infection, presents with persistent fever, lethargy, malaise, muscle weakness, headache, pain in or around the eyes, sensitivity to bright light, sore throat, diarrhea, nausea, and skin rashes (Tindall, Carr, & Cooper, 1995; Tindall, Imrie, Donovan, Penny, & Cooper, 1992). In most cases, primary HIV infection symptoms resolve themselves and usually do not recur.

Not all people infected with HIV, however, develop symptoms of primary infection. Table 2.2 presents the frequencies of primary symptoms for persons experiencing acute HIV reactions. Studies find that between 53% and 93% of individuals experience an acute response to HIV infection (A. Carr & Cooper, 1997). Symptoms occur among people infected through each major route of HIV transmission, and, at present, there is no conclusive evidence that any particular group is more likely to develop symptomatic acute illness. In addition to the aforementioned early symptoms, HIV-seropositive people may develop persistent generalized lymphadenopathy, defined by enlarged lymph nodes that are detectable by touch and remain enlarged for a minimum of 3 months. Swollen lymph nodes in the armpits, neck, or groin are common in HIV infection, as well as in other viral infections, with 70% of HIV-seropositive individuals having swollen nodes within the first few weeks of infection (A. Carr & Cooper, 1997; Tindall et al., 1992).

Table 2.2

Symptoms of Acute Antiretroviral Illness With Their Expected Frequencies for Those Affected

Acute Symptom	Percent of People With Acute Symptoms
Fever	96
Lymphadenopathy	74
Pharyngitis	70
Rash	70
Myalgia	54
Diarrhea	32
Headache	32
Nausea and vomiting	27
Thrush	12
Neurologic symptoms	12

In the case of HIV infection, swollen lymph nodes are the result of disseminated HIV throughout the lymphatic system (Pantaleo, Graziosi, & Fauci, 1993). Most studies show that persistent lymphadenopathy does not have prognostic value for disease progression toward AIDS (A. R. Moss & Bacchetti, 1989; Schechter et al., 1990).

Following acute symptoms of HIV infection, although not dependent on the occurrence of such symptoms, antibodies are produced against HIV. Establishing HIV antibodies, or seroconversion to HIV, results after reaching a threshold of HIV replication and depends on the immune competency of the host to mount an antibody response (Imagawa et al., 1989). Viral load is high during acute infection, reaching as high as 10^6 virus copies per milliliter of plasma (A. Carr & Cooper, 1997). On average, HIV antibodies are detectable through serological testing slightly more than 2 months after viral transmission, and 95% of HIV-infected people develop antibodies within 3 months of becoming infected (Saag, 1995). However, the incubation period for HIV may last longer than 3 months, and in rare cases incubation may last 2 to 3 years (Glasner & Kaslow, 1990; Imagawa et al., 1989). Variability in establishing HIV antibodies can result from numerous factors, including the virulence of HIV strains, the dose of virus transmitted, frequency of exposure, and an individual's immune response. It is during the earliest days of acute HIV infection that anti-HIV drugs may avert infection. Zidovudine (AZT), for example, administered to humans and nonhuman animals exposed to HIV can reduce infection rates and otherwise reduce initial viral load, which can in turn have a positive effect on prognosis (A. Carr & Cooper, 1997; Gerberding, 1997).

ASYMPTOMATIC HIV INFECTION

During most of HIV infection, individuals appear, feel, and are otherwise healthy. As much as 50% to 80% of the time that a person has HIV, they are symptom free. The virus is actively depleting T-helper lymphocytes during clinically asymptomatic phases, and HIV is also transmittable to others during this time. In general, increases in viral burden in plasma and elevated HIV genetic material in blood cells correspond with a depletion of CD4 cells (Staprans & Feinberg, 1997). Thus, viral load tends to be low during asymptomatic phases, when CD4 cell counts tend to be high. It was once thought that HIV replicated less during asymptomatic periods, primarily because of low concentrations of virus in the bloodstream. Although considered a *latency period*, asymptomatic HIV infection does not constitute a time of microbiological inactivity (Pantaleo et al., 1993). In fact, HIV is quite productive in lymph nodes of symptom free patients (Temin & Bolognesi, 1993). Following years of destruction, the immune system slowly degenerates, increasing vulnerability to illness.

The primary target of HIV, T-helper lymphocytes, is one of three types of thymus-originating cells (T-cells) of the immune system. These cells function to distinguish self from nonself and rid the body of foreign agents (see Huston, 1997, for an overview of the immune system). Cytotoxic T-cells identify and destroy infectious agents, suppressor T-cells reduce immune responses, and T-helper cells induce responses from several branches of the immune system. T-helper lymphocytes have several functions, including the induction of non-T-helper cell activity. Cell-mediated immunity results from cytokines that guide multiple immune responses. For example, T-helper lymphocytes mediate through cytokines the activity of natural killer cells, which in turn destroy viral-infected and certain cancer cells. Impaired activity of natural killer cells is an outcome of T-helper cell dysfunction. Cytokines also direct proliferation and maturation of several immune cells (see Figure 2.2).

Decreased numbers of T-helper lymphocytes were among the first immune abnormalities described in patients with AIDS. Over the course of HIV infection, the average decline in T-helper lymphocytes ranges from 50 to 80 cells/mm^3 per year (Bartlett, 1993a). At this rate, over a 10-year period, T-helper cell counts drop to between 200 and 0 cells/mm^3, increasing vulnerability to infections and malignancies. The strongest predictors of developing AIDS are increases in viral load, declines in rates of CD4 cells, blood concentration of CD4 cells relative to other immune cells, and combinations of these indexes (Vlahov et al., 1998).

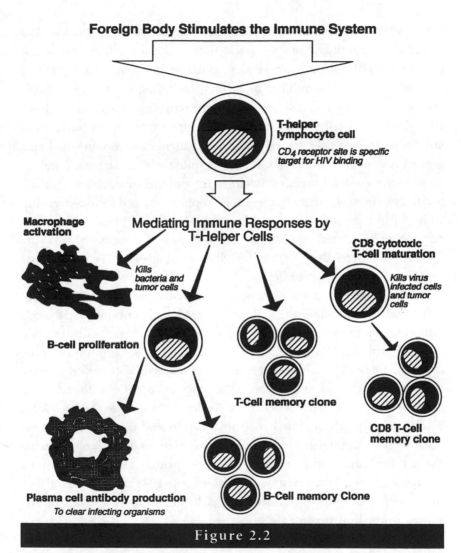

Foreign Body Stimulates the Immune System

T-helper lymphocyte cell

CD4 receptor site is specific target for HIV binding

Macrophage activation

Mediating Immune Responses by T-Helper Cells

CD8 cytotoxic T-cell maturation

Kills bacteria and tumor cells

Kills virus infected cells and tumor cells

B-cell proliferation

T-Cell memory clone

CD8 T-Cell memory clone

Plasma cell antibody production
To clear infecting organisms

B-Cell memory Clone

Figure 2.2

Functional roles of T-helper (CD4) lymphocytes in relation to other cells in the human immune system.

Because the number of T-helper cells is inversely related to HIV symptoms, low T-helper cell counts indicate impending illness (Hutchinson et al., 1991). During asymptomatic periods, T-helper cell counts are usually between 500 and 200 (Lifson, Hessol, Buchbinder, & Holmberg, 1991), although nearly half of individuals with counts below 200 are also asymptomatic at any given time. T-helper cell counts are a marker for HIV disease progression, but they are limited by extreme fluctuations due to a number of factors, including variability in laboratory procedures and changes in cell concentrations over diurnal cycles. Changes in cell counts are also difficult to interpret because there are no normative data for HIV-infected patients and noninfected risk groups (Clement & Hollander, 1992). Despite their limitations, T-helper lymphocyte counts have set guidelines for prognostic decisions, for initiating medications that suppress HIV replication, and for determining when to initiate prophylaxis against opportunistic illnesses. Thus, the risk for AIDS-related conditions increases over the course of HIV infection, and a reliable marker for disease progression is the loss of functional T-helper lymphocytes.

Vulnerability to disease increases as the immune system loses T-helper cells and therefore T-helper-cell-mediated immunity. Although immune-system suppression does not necessarily mean symptomatic illness, having an HIV-related illness does suggest severe immune suppression. Only 2% of HIV infections progress to AIDS within 2 years of infection, whereas as many as 10% progress to AIDS within 4 years (A. R. Moss & Bacchetti, 1989; J. M. Taylor, Schwartz, & Detels, 1986). The average length of time between infection and developing AIDS is 7 to 10 years among homosexually active men, and it is considerably shorter for adults who contracted HIV through blood transfusions (Laurence, 1992; Lui, Darrow, & Rutherford, 1988). The interval between infection and illness, however, is lengthening as a result of advances in medical treatments.

FACTORS ASSOCIATED WITH HIV PROGRESSION TO AIDS

There are several potential influences on the duration and course of most infectious diseases, including sociodemographic factors, general health status, nutrition, previous illness history, genetic-immune factors, variations in viral strains, and seasons of the year (S. Cohen & Williamson, 1991; Solomon, Kemeny, & Temoshok, 1991). Among sociode-mographic characteristics, age is consistently associated with HIV progression, with older people having more rapid rates of immune suppression. A. R. Moss and Bacchetti (1989) found that people over age 40 infected with HIV were more likely to become ill sooner than individuals infected at younger ages. Older adults progress faster to AIDS, and, once diagnosed with AIDS, older adults die sooner than do younger adults (Chaisson, Keruly, & Moore, 1995; Hogg et al., 1994). Clement and Hollander (1992) reported that being diagnosed with AIDS at age 35 and older is associated with a substantially poorer prognosis. Decreased survival times observed with advancing age, however, are not entirely understood. The accelerated rate of disease may involve a decreased ability to contend with opportunistic infections (Lemp, Payne, Neal, Temelso, & Rutherford, 1990).

Ethnic minorities demonstrate a more rapid decline in T-helper lymphocytes than do Whites, and there are ethnic differences in the relative frequency of AIDS-related illnesses (A. E. Greenberg et al., 1992). Sex differences in prognosis have also been suggested; the suggestion being that men live longer after an AIDS diagnosis than do women (e.g., Lemp et al., 1990; Melnick et al., 1994), even after accounting for differences in lag time to diagnosis and variations in AIDS definitions in women (Murrain, 1993). Disease progression also varies by primary route of HIV transmission. Individuals who become HIV infected through injection drug use survive longer compared with those infected through other modes of HIV transmission (Melnick et al., 1994), whereas contracting HIV by blood transfusion results in a rapid death following an AIDS diagnosis (Lemp et al., 1990; Myers, Prose, & Bartlett, 1993).

The route of contracting HIV is also related to relative frequencies of AIDS-related illnesses and probably accounts for other observed differences. Men who contract HIV sexually from other men are more likely to develop Kaposi's sarcoma, and injection drug users are more likely to develop *Pneumocystis carinii* pneumonia (PCP), recurrent bacterial pneumonia, and pulmonary tuberculosis (A. E. Greenberg et al., 1992). Differences in onset of AIDS are often attributed to relative risks for various opportunistic illnesses, such as Kaposi's sarcoma that most frequently occurs in men (Spijkerman et al., 1996). Differences in transmission routes may also account for most of the differences in opportunistic illnesses between men and women (Murrain, 1993). AIDS diagnoses in heterosexual men and women often result from PCP, wasting, and candidiasis, whereas Kaposi's sarcoma is far more common in men who have sex with men (Fleming, Ciesielski, Byers, Castro, & Berkelman, 1993). However, the associations between disease and HIV transmission routes are not well understood, with such factors as primary path of entry into the bloodstream, the volume of HIV transmitted, and number of exposures to the virus all potentially mediating HIV infection (Hamburg, Koenig, & Fauci, 1990).

In addition to demographic and transmission-associated factors, an infected person's health status influences the course of HIV infection. For example, some studies show that pregnancy may accelerate the loss of T-helper lymphocytes in HIV seropositive women (Biggar et al., 1989). However, other studies have failed to replicate these relationships, bringing the effects of pregnancy on HIV disease processes into question (Brettle & Leen, 1991; Carpenter et al., 1991). Cigarette smoking has also been associated with immune-system functioning (Royce & Winkelstein, 1990) and the progression of HIV infection to AIDS (Brettle & Leen, 1991). Ultraviolet light activates genetic expression of HIV (Morrey et al., 1991; Vogel, Cepeda, Tschachler, Napolitano, & Jay, 1992), suggesting that excessive exposure to the sun or tanning lights may promote HIV progression (Vogel et al., 1992; Wallace & Lasker, 1992). However, clinical studies have not supported an association between solar ultraviolet radiation and rapidity of HIV progression to AIDS (Saah et al., 1997). Exercise and nutrition, on the other hand, may slow HIV disease, although there is thus far little empirical support for direct relationships. There is also little evidence that alcohol and other psychoactive substance use play significant roles in HIV infection (Di Franco, Sheppard, Hunter, Tosteson, & Ascher, 1996; Dingle & Oei, 1997).

The most widely accepted cofactors for HIV infection, although not universally accepted, are infections with other pathogens (for a review, see Aral & Wasserheit, 1996). In particular, the interaction between HIV and other viruses (i.e., herpes viruses) is considered important in HIV progression. Sexually transmitted pathogens and infectious agents spread through nonsterile preparations of drug injecting equipment trigger immune responses that can stimulate HIV and activate HIV's replication cycle (Morrow, Colebunders, & Chin, 1989). Coinfection with other immune-suppressing viruses can also facilitate the progression of HIV (Brettle & Leen, 1991; Tindall et al., 1995). Even worse, multiple infections are synergistic and make prognosis dependent on a chain of unpredictable biomedical events. Repeated exposures to HIV complicate the picture further by multiple strains of the virus with varied properties. Variations in viral strain result from the drift in molecular composition demonstrated in HIV isolates both within and between infected individuals.

Potential cofactors of HIV infection tend to co-occur with cumulative effects. For example, findings regarding shorter survival times for women and ethnic minorities could be explained because women and minorities are often infected through injection drug use (Melnick et al., 1994; Murrain, 1993). In addition, exposure to infectious agents that may facilitate HIV disease occurs in different patterns among ethnic groups, sexes, and sexual-orientation subgroups (A. E. Greenberg et al., 1992). Associations between potential cofactors and disease progression are therefore open to multiple interpretations, including bidirectional causes and unidentified third variables. For example, early in the HIV epidemic it was observed that men who sexually contracted HIV from other men and who had a history of using nitrite inhalers (*poppers*) were at increased risk for developing Kaposi's sarcoma (e.g., Polk et al., 1987). Further support for linking nitrite inhaler use with HIV infection came from research showing short-term effects of nitrites on branches of the human immune system (Dax, Adler, Nagel, Lange, & Jaffe, 1991). Subsequent research, however, has shown that Kaposi's sarcoma in men who have sex with men is actually associated with sexual behaviors that afford direct contact with human feces (Beral et al., 1992). In fact, the relationship between fecal contact and developing Kaposi's sarcoma is linear, with higher rates of oral—anal sexual contact related to increased risk for Kaposi's sarcoma. As it turns out, Kaposi's sarcoma is associated with human herpes virus-8 that is likely transmitted through anal sex

(Ambroziak et al., 1995; Y. Chang et al., 1994; Serraino, Franceschi, Del Maso, & La Vecchia, 1995). Nitrites, therefore, may be a frequent substance used by men who engage in anal sex practices, which are in turn associated with Kaposi's sarcoma. This example illustrates the complex interplay among potential cofactors for HIV progression, AIDS-related conditions, and behavioral practices.

The only factors that are conclusively associated with progression of HIV infection are those related to accessing health care. Antiretroviral therapies slow the progress of HIV infection and can delay the development of AIDS. Early treatment with antiretrovirals reduces HIV genetic material in blood, increases CD4 cell counts, prolongs the time until HIV-related symptoms develop, and improves survival (Volberding, 1997). It is also apparent that early access to treatment of opportunistic illnesses plays a crucial role in AIDS survival. Thus, access to quality care may be the single most important factor in living with AIDS. Illustrating this point is a study of 403 men with HIV infection that found significant differences in survival among persons receiving treatment from primary care physicians with greater experience in treating HIV–AIDS cases (Kitahata et al., 1996). Access to care may, therefore, account for many of the differences in survival observed in men and women, African Americans and Whites, and individuals exposed to HIV through various modes of transmission.

LATER STAGE HIV INFECTION

Following long asymptomatic periods a number of diffuse and non-specific illnesses may develop. Symptoms of HIV infection include chronic low-grade fever, persistent fatigue, diarrhea lasting at least 2 weeks, rashes or other skin conditions, unintentional weight loss, night sweats, and mild infections of the mouth or throat. These symptoms were once referred to as AIDS-Related Complex (ARC) because it was thought that they signaled the imminent onset of AIDS. The term ARC has lost clinical meaningfulness, however, because symptoms do not necessarily occur before AIDS.

Severe depletion of T-helper lymphocytes, increased viral load, and the onset of specific illnesses characterize the later stages of HIV infection. Most clinical manifestations of HIV infection are evident relatively late in the course of disease, occurring only after significant immune impairment. Illnesses that occur late in HIV infection reflect the defective cell-mediated immunity caused by diminished numbers and functional disturbances of T-helper lymphocytes. Similar immune dysfunction commonly occurs in cancer chemotherapy, certain lymphomas and other malignancies, and organ transplants (Bartlett, 1993a). T-helper lymphocyte counts below 200 cells/mm^3 indicate an increased risk for significant weight loss, chronic diarrhea, new or persistent outbreaks of genital herpes, skin rashes, and infections of the mouth, esophagus, and vagina (Kaslow et al., 1987; Lifson et al., 1991). Over 35% of all HIV-related hospitalizations, 29% of hospital costs, and over 35% of HIV-seropositive hospital inpatient deaths occur among people who become systemically ill but have not yet been diagnosed with AIDS (Andrulis, Weslowski, Hintz, & Spolarich, 1992).

Cohorts followed before the widespread availability of antiretroviral medications showed that most people survive between 11 and 12 months after receiving an AIDS diagnosis, less than 11% survive 3 years, and yet others are known to have a slow-progressing disease, surviving 15 years and beyond (Bacchetti, Osmond, Chaisson, & Moss, 1988; Lemp et al., 1990; Pantaleo et al., 1995; Rothenberg et al., 1987). T-helper counts below 200 substantially increase risk for developing AIDS (Lifson et al., 1991; Masur et al., 1989; Phair et al., 1990), with 80% of people developing AIDS-related illness within 3 years of T-helper cell counts dropping below 200 (S. W. Chang, Katz, & Hernandez, 1992). The probability of serious illnesses increases as T-helper lymphocytes decline, with survival times for people with T-helper cell counts below 50 cells/mm^3 being generally less than 1 to 2 years (Clement & Hollander, 1992).

Several factors appear to predict survival following the onset of AIDS-related conditions. For example, the initial condition leading to an AIDS diagnosis predicts survival. Most consistently, individuals first diagnosed with Kaposi's sarcoma are more likely to survive longer than are people diagnosed with *Pneumocystis carinii* pneumonia, who in turn survive longer than those initially diagnosed with other AIDS-associated illnesses (Friedman et al., 1991; Luo, Kaldor, McDonald, & Cooper, 1995). Rothenberg et al. (1987) found that 72% of patients initially diagnosed with Kaposi's sarcoma survived 1 year, and 30% survived 5 years, a substantially greater survival time than is associated with other AIDS-related illnesses. Friedman et al. (1991) concluded that the role of initial AIDS diagnosis in survival may be attributed to the organ system involved, the degree of immune suppression that characterizes its onset, and the effectiveness of available treatments. Of course, early studies provide information about initial diagnoses before combination antiretroviral therapies became available. The role of initial diagnosis on AIDS progression must therefore be reconsidered in the context of new treatments.

Survival time is also associated with characteristics of individuals, among which the sex of the infected person is the most controversial. Friedman et al. (1991) found that women who received an AIDS diagnosis survived for significantly shorter time than men did. However, subsequent research has failed to show that nongynecologic manifestations of HIV infection differ among men and women, and there are no known sex differences in AIDS prognosis or in the rate of disease progression from HIV infection to AIDS (Brettle & Leen, 1991; Kloser & Craig, 1994; Melnick et al., 1994; Minkoff & DeHovitz, 1991). Thus, although early explanations for findings of women surviving shorter periods of time tended to stress potential biological cofactors, such as genetics and hormones, sociocultural factors, such as poverty and access to health care, now offer the best explanation for women surviving with AIDS for shorter times (Ickovics & Rodin, 1992). Men with HIV infection are diagnosed earlier, receive better medical care, and have stronger social support networks than do women, and those differences likely account for variations in survival (Carpenter et al., 1991; Melnick et al., 1994). A history of using injection drugs also contributes to an earlier death for women with AIDS (Melnick et al., 1994). Finally, sex differences in survival appear related to women historically having limited access to adequate health care (Brettle & Leen, 1991; Carpenter et al., 1991).

Ethnicity also predicts AIDS survival, with African Americans surviving a shorter time with AIDS than Whites (e.g., Lagakos, Fischl, Stein, Lim, & Volberding, 1991; Rothenberg et al., 1987). Differences in survival may be the result of several factors, including differences in immune functioning, prevalence of cofactors for disease progression, and differences in routes of contracting HIV. Consistent with mortality in general (Geronimus, Bound, Waidmann, Hillemeier, & Burns, 1996), AIDS survival is, however, best accounted for by sociodemographic differences between African Americans and Whites (Curtis & Patrick, 1993).

As the immune system becomes depleted, multiple opportunistic infections become more likely. Luo et al. (1995) reported that multiple combinations of illness result in different lengths of survival. Co-occurrence of Kaposi's sarcoma, PCP, candidiasis, and herpes simplex virus result in longer survival than combinations of other illnesses. It is also common for people to experience multiple opportunistic diseases prior to death. Chan, Neaton, Saravolatz, Crane, and Osterberger (1995) found that 47% of AIDS patients experience two or three AIDS-defining conditions before death and that 22% experience four or more illnesses.

In summary, later stages of HIV infection are the result of increased viral burden and a progressive depletion of the immune system. Loss of T-helper lymphocytes directly and indirectly impairs immune functioning over long clinically asymptomatic periods. Although studies show that some demographic and risk-related characteristics may be related to survival following an AIDS diagnosis, initial AIDS-defining illnesses have reliably predicted prognosis. Viral and host factors, such as virulence of HIV strains and coinfection with other viruses, as well as response to antiretroviral therapies have much to do with the duration of survival. Many differences in survival are also related to sociocultural factors, particularly access to quality medical care. Nearer to the end of the disease process, people with HIV infection face an array of serious health threats as their immune systems decline.

NONPROGRESSIVE HIV

Approximately 5% of people with HIV have nonprogressing infection, living 10 to 15 years in good health and with stable CD4 cell counts

(Staprans & Feinberg, 1997). Although nonprogressive HIV infection is probably the result of many factors, low viral load is a common characteristic in these individuals and is probably due to greater neutralizing antibodies against HIV (Haynes, Pantaleo, & Fauci, 1996; Pantaleo et al., 1995). In a study of ten people who survived between 12 and 15 years without symptoms and with stable CD4 counts, Cao, Qin, Zhang, Safrit, and Ho (1995) found low viral load and strong immune responses against the virus as their common denominators. Some nonprogressors also seem infected with a less virulent strain of HIV. Specifically, a strain of HIV with the deletions of the *nef* gene has been associated with nonprogressive HIV infection (Staprans & Feinberg, 1997). HIV-2 progresses slower than HIV-1 infection, and HIV-2 may offer some protective immunity against HIV-1 (Travers et al., 1995). HIV nonprogressors, therefore, may hold the key to understanding how the immune system can interact with the virus to suppress infection.

In a study of psychological characteristics of slow progressing illness, *non-progressive infection* was defined as living 8 or more years with a CD4 cell count over 500 and remaining relatively symptom free (Troop, Easterbrook, Thornton, Flynn, Gazzard, & Catalan, 1997). Nonprogressors attributed their good health to a number of factors including having a positive outlook, having a sense of control, accepting their HIV status, avoiding substance use and stress, and getting ample rest and sleep. Although the study design limited the ability to draw causal conclusions, nonprogressive HIV infection was believed to result from active coping, a finding that may offer insight into the psychological adaptation to HIV infection.

AIDS DIAGNOSIS

HIV directly causes a number of illnesses including HIV infection of the lymph nodes, brain, kidneys, abdominal cavity, and lungs. Most AIDS-defining conditions, however, result after damage to the immune system, including cancers and opportunistic infections that would otherwise be kept in check. The most common clinical presentations of

HIV infection are persistent lymphadenopathy, pulmonary symptoms suggestive of pneumonia, cytopenia (diminution of blood cells), fungal infections, constitutional symptoms such as persistent fever and diarrhea, weight loss, bacterial infections, tuberculosis, persistent symptoms of sexually transmitted infections, and nervous system disorders (Bartlett, 1993a).

The first formal diagnostic criteria for AIDS were established in 1982 as a result of early clinical experiences with men who contracted HIV infection through homosexual activity. The diagnosis was updated in 1985 and again in 1987 to include additional indicator diseases that characterized the diversity of HIV-infected individuals. The 1987 case definition for adults and adolescents consisted of 23 clinical conditions. The case definition for children differed from adults by including recurrent bacterial infections and pulmonary problems among indicator diseases and by not considering children under 15 months old with HIV antibodies as HIV infected because of passive perinatal transfer of maternal antibodies.

The CDC AIDS case definition was once again expanded in 1993 (see Figure 2.3). In reference to adding conditions in the diagnosis of AIDS, the CDC stated that "the objectives of these changes are to simplify the classification of HIV infection, to reflect current standards of medical care for HIV infected persons, and to categorize more accurately HIV-related morbidity" (CDC, 1992e, p. 2). The revised case definition also addresses several criticisms of previous diagnostic criteria, such as failure to include manifestations of HIV common in women (S. W. Chang et al., 1992; Kloser & Craig, 1994). The CDC definition continues to include the 23 original conditions and adds three new illnesses: pulmonary tuberculosis, recurrent pneumonia, and invasive cervical cancer. Pulmonary tuberculosis (TB) was added because HIV-induced immune suppression increases the likelihood of activating latent TB (Buehler & Ward, 1993). Recurrent pneumonia was added because of the prevalence of bacterial pneumonia, with as much as a fivefold increase in HIV-infected injection drug users compared with their non-HIV-infected counterparts (Hirschtick et al., 1995). Finally, invasive cervical cancer was added to the revised case definition because

AIDS-Defining Conditions

* Candidiasis infection of bronchi, trachea, or lungs
* Candidiasis infection of esophagus
* Invasive cervical cancer
* Coccidioidoidomycosis, disseminated or extrapulmonary
* Cryptococcosis, extrapulmonary
* Cryptosporidiosis, intestinal, > 1 month
* Cytomegalovirus retinitis with loss of vision
* Cytomegalovirus disease
* HIV-related encephalopathy
* Herpes simplex infection, > 1 month
* Histoplasmosis, disseminated or extrapulmonary
* Isosporiasis, intestinal, > 1 month
* Kaposi's sarcoma
* Burkitt's lymphoma
* Immunoblastic lymphoma
* Primary lymphoma of brain
* *Mycobacterium avium* complex
* *Mycobacterium tuberculosis*
* *Mycobacterium,* disseminated or extrapulmonary
* *Pneumocystis carinii* pneumonia
* Recurrent pneumonia
* Progressive multifocal leukoencephalopathy
* Recurrent salmonella septicemia
* Toxoplasmosis of the brain
* HIV wasting syndrome

Figure 2.3

AIDS conditions included in the 1993 Centers for Disease Control and Prevention case definition of AIDS.

as many as 22% of HIV-infected women experience signs of early cervical disease.

The most significant change in the 1993 AIDS case definition was the inclusion of immune diagnostic criteria. Unlike previous AIDS diagnoses, the definition specifies that individuals who are asymptomatic but receive an accurate, although not necessarily most recent, T-helper lymphocyte cell count below 200 cells/mm^3 in conjunction with HIV infection meet the criteria for AIDS. Immune status is included in the case definition because immune markers are associated with disease progression independent of illness. Another reason for considering immune markers is that T-helper cell counts carry similar meaning among subgroups of infected persons who may vary in illnesses, some of which may not yet be listed in the AIDS case definition. Finally, people with suppressed immune systems who did not yet have a case-defining illness can become eligible for disability benefits.

A substantial increase in the number of AIDS cases occurred in 1993 because of the inclusion of T-helper counts below 200 cells/mm^3 in the diagnostic criteria for AIDS. Figure 2.4 shows the first quarter of 1993 increase in AIDS resulting from the new definition over and above the cases fitting the 1987 definition. Of the 35,779 AIDS cases

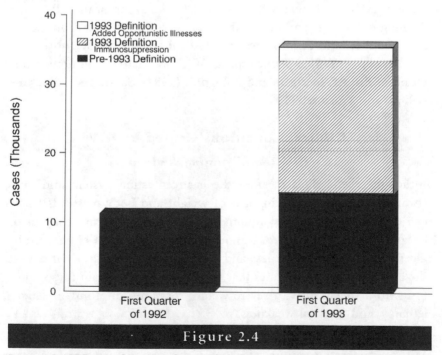

Figure 2.4

Increased AIDS cases because of expanded 1993 definition for both immune suppression and opportunistic illnesses.

reported in the first quarter of 1993, 60% were based on criteria from the expanded definition, the majority resulting from criteria related to suppressed T-helper lymphocyte counts. Nearly half of all AIDS cases in 1993 were attributed to the T-helper cell criteria. According to the CDC (1992e), if all of the estimated one million HIV-infected persons in the United States obtained T-helper cell counts, as many as 120,000 to 190,000 would have less than 200 cells/mm^3 but would not yet have developed AIDS-defining illnesses.

Each AIDS-defining condition entails its own disease processes and prognosis. Figure 2.5 illustrates the proportion of adolescent and adult AIDS cases initially diagnosed with various opportunistic conditions. As shown, the majority of AIDS cases are initially diagnosed with PCP. Numerous other AIDS-defining conditions are rare and do not typically occur as an initial diagnosis. The signs, symptoms, and complications of each condition pose substantially different challenges for people living with AIDS. The next section is a brief description of the AIDS case-defining conditions and other diseases that commonly confront people living with HIV infection. Greater detail concerning the diagnostic, disease process, and therapeutic aspects of AIDS-related conditions can be found in Broder, Merigan, and Bolognesi (1994), Sande and Volberding (1997), and Wormser (1992).

Clinical Conditions Caused by HIV

HIV-Related Wasting Syndrome

Although several diseases affect the gastrointestinal system and cause chronic, persistent, disabling loss of weight and body mass, HIV itself can directly cause these symptoms. Diagnosis is determined by involuntary loss of at least 10% of body weight along with either chronic diarrhea or chronic weakness and fever over the course of 30 days in the absence of other illnesses that could otherwise explain these symptoms. In association with severe weight loss are symptoms of fatigue, lethargy, and physical weakness.

HIV-Related Neurological Disease

Mild to moderate cognitive, affective, and motor disturbances can occur in HIV infection, with individuals at later stages of AIDS experiencing

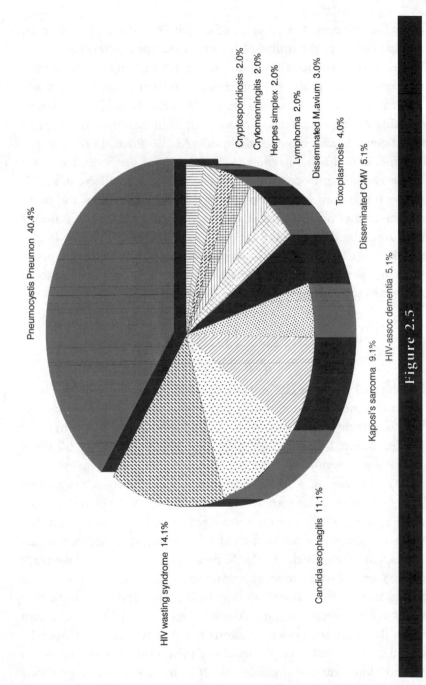

Figure 2.5

Initial AIDS defining diagnoses for adults in the United States.

more such symptoms. Subtle signs of cognitive dysfunction, however, can appear earlier in the course of infection (Koppel, 1992). Early signs of HIV-related neurological disease include difficulty maintaining concentration, memory problems, and motor disturbances including slowing of arm, leg, and eye movements (R. W. Price & Sidtis, 1992). Demyelinating neuropathologies also occur early in infection, resulting in impaired sensory and motor functioning (R. W. Price, 1997). Neurological disease is usually diagnosed when symptoms become moderate to severe and disrupt occupational, basic self-care, intellectual, social, or motor functioning. The toxic effects of HIV infection of the brain cause a cascade of neurological problems. Clinical symptoms are almost always caused by diffuse brain damage rather than focal lesions (R. W. Price, 1997). At least some neurological effects of HIV infection occur in as many as 90% of HIV-infected individuals, although functional impairment ranges from none to profound.

AIDS-Related Malignancies

Kaposi's Sarcoma

Although rare before the HIV epidemic, Kaposi's sarcoma (KS) has been the most common malignancy in people with AIDS, with the majority of cases occurring among men who sexually contracted HIV from other men. Men infected through sex with men are 20,000 to 40,000 times more likely to develop KS than are same-age HIV seronegative men. Relatively few cases of KS have occurred among injection drug users, and only 2% of cases have an initial diagnosis of KS (Kaplan & Northfelt, 1997; Wofsy, 1992). For the relatively few women who develop KS, they most commonly have contracted HIV through sex with a bisexual man (Kaplan & Northfelt, 1992). Kaposi's sarcoma typically develops as a mass on the skin, mucous membranes, or internal organs. The disease is usually first noticed as skin lesions that appear as dark red-to-violet colored areas on light-skinned persons, and black or brown areas on dark-skinned persons. Lesions commonly first occur near the head and neck, as well as on the inside of the mouth. It is also common for KS to afflict internal organs, with 20% to 50% of cases involving the lungs (A. Levine, Gill, & Salahuddin, 1992). Thus, the lethality of KS is entirely dependent on the site of disease. In most cases, however, KS has an aggressive and unpredictable course.

Kaposi's sarcoma is caused by human herpes virus-8 (HHV-8), which seems to be transmitted through contact with human feces (Beral et al., 1992; Y. Chang et al., 1994). As many as one third of HIV seropositive gay men are infected with HHV-8, compared to 3% of HIV seropositive women (Kedes, Ganem, Ameli, Bacchetti, & Greenblatt, 1997). When KS develops in the absence of other HIV-related diseases, it usually occurs early in immune suppression. There has, however, been a steady decline in the number of KS cases observed in recent years among people with AIDS (Taylor et al., 1991).

In addition to being an AIDS-defining condition and a life-threatening malignancy, KS carries additional psychological burden because of its skin lesions. Symptoms of KS are disfiguring, and their appearance will frequently mark a person as being seriously ill and can lead to identifying a person as having AIDS. The result of KS symptoms, therefore, can interfere with privacy rights and add a stigmatizing dimension to an already stigmatized disease.

Invasive Cervical Cancer

Cervical abnormalities, particularly cervical dysplasia, are common precursors to cervical cancer. Several studies have shown that HIV-infected women frequently develop cervical dysplasia, with prevalence rates as high as 10 times greater than those found in non-HIV-infected women (CDC, 1992e). Cervical dysplasia in women with HIV infection is related to advanced immune suppression. Studies of women who receive organ transplants, however, suggest that progression of cervical dysplasia to cervical cancer may require prolonged periods of immune suppression. Therefore, relatively few cases of invasive cervical cancer have been reported among HIV-infected women (Kaplan & Northfelt, 1992). However, women with HIV who do develop cervical cancer have more advanced disease than HIV seronegative women (Kaplan & Northfelt, 1997). Invasive cervical cancer was added to the 1993 AIDS case definition following controversy about previous exclusion of conditions related to AIDS in women (Buehler & Ward, 1993). Inclusion of invasive cervical cancer as an AIDS-defining condition was also meant to emphasize "the importance of integrating gynecologic care into medical services for HIV infected women" (CDC, 1992e, p. 8). Early detection of cervical cancer is possible with pap exams, which should be a regular part of health care for HIV seropositive women.

HIV-Related Lymphomas

Non-Hodgkin's lymphomas were among the earliest recognized manifestations of HIV infection. Unlike other lymphomas, those related to HIV infection tend to progress rapidly and have extremely poor prognoses (Naficy & Soave, 1992). There have been substantial increases in lymphomas among gay and bisexual men as a result of HIV infection (Koblin et al., 1996). Although most non-HIV-associated lymphomas involve disease contained to the lymph nodes, HIV lymphomas are distinguished by their widespread involvement of vital organs. Approximately 26% of HIV-related lymphomas involve the gastrointestinal system, 25% bone marrow, 12% liver, 9% kidneys, and 9% lungs (Naficy & Soave, 1992). Most common, however, is central nervous system involvement, occurring in 25% to 32% of HIV-related cases of lymphoma (Herndier, Kaplan, & McGrath, 1994). Symptoms of central nervous system lymphoma include seizures, localized neurologic dysfunction, and headache. HIV-related lymphoma usually occurs late in infection, after other AIDS-related conditions have occurred and when T-helper lymphocyte counts drop below 50 cells/mm^3 (Kaplan & Northfelt, 1997). Lymphomas pose a considerable threat to people with HIV infection, resulting in relatively short survival following diagnosis (Luo et al., 1995).

Fungal Infections

Pneumocystis Carinii Pneumonia

Pneumocystis carinii pneumonia (PCP) is the most frequently diagnosed AIDS-defining condition in the U.S. epidemic. Prior to the wide-scale use of prophylactic medications, active PCP occurred in as many as 80% of advanced cases (Bartlett, 1993a). First classified as a protozoan, most authorities now agree *Pneumocystis carinii* is a fungus (Decker &

Masur, 1997; Hopewell, 1992; Stansell & Huang, 1997), although the exact taxonomy remains debated. *Pneumocystis carinii* exists in the environment and is nearly universally contracted at young ages through inhalation of fungus particles (Hopewell, 1992). However, *Pneumocystis carinii* is only clinically expressed under severe immune suppression, particularly when T-helper lymphocyte cell counts drop below 200. However, children infected with HIV develop PCP at earlier stages of infection. Thus, because almost everyone is exposed to *Pneumocystis carinii*, and because the organism is suppressed by cellular immunity mediated by T-helper lymphocytes, it has been the predominant manifestation of AIDS in the United States.

Pneumocystis carinii pneumonia can have early and diffuse symptoms, including mild tightness of the chest, chronic fever, fatigue, and weight loss. Respiratory symptoms usually include dry and nonproductive cough and progressive shortness of breath. As the pneumonia progresses, tasks with even limited demands become taxing. *Pneumocystis carinii* can, although it rarely does, infect the skin, central nervous system, eyes, abdominal walls, lymph nodes, kidneys, liver, and several other organ systems. Thus, although *Pneumocystis carinii* is usually limited to the respiratory system, it can become widely disseminated. Fortunately, fewer people with AIDS are developing PCP because of prophylactic medications, but PCP remains a significant threat to people at advanced stages of AIDS (Saah et al., 1995; Stansell & Huang, 1997).

Candidiasis

Candida is a fungus that is normally found in the mouth and esophagus (Finley, Joshi, & Neill, 1992). With immune suppression, however, candida progresses to active disease. Oral infection with candidiasis is commonly called *thrush*, and it usually forms removable white plaques on the surface of the tongue and oral cavity (Greenspan, Greenspan, & Winkler, 1992). Plaques may be small or large and local or widespread, and they can alternatively appear as small red areas rather than white patches. Thrush is found in later stages of HIV disease and was described in the first U.S. cases of AIDS. Localized candida infection is related to declining numbers of T-helper lymphocytes and is often the first indicator of advanced immune suppression (Bartlett, 1993a; Finley et al., 1992). Although for an AIDS diagnosis candidiasis must involve the esophagus, bronchi, trachea, or lungs, infection may also occur in other organ systems, including the gastrointestinal system and the vaginal tract. Vaginal candidiasis is one of the earliest signs of immune suppression for women with HIV infection, causing discomfort and discharge and often occurring when T-helper cell counts are still relatively high (Kloser & Craig, 1994; Wofsy, 1992).

Coccidioidomycosis

An infection that occurs after fungus particles are inhaled into the lungs (Sarosi, 1992), coccidioidomycosis is among the least frequent AIDS-defining conditions. Suppressed T-helper lymphocyte mediated immunity allows for progressive coccidioidomycosis of both the inside and outside lung (Sarosi, 1992). Risk for coccidioidomycosis is greatest in areas where the fungus is endemic, including the southwestern United States. Risk increases in direct proportion to declining T-helper lymphocytes, particularly when cell counts drop below 250. There are two general forms of coccidioidomycosis, primary and chronic. The primary form is an acute self-limiting condition involving only the respiratory system. On the other hand, the chronic form of the disease may involve several organ systems. People with severely impaired immune systems are most likely to develop pulmonary disease followed by widespread dissemination (Finley et al., 1992). For coccidioidomycosis to allow an AIDS diagnosis, the disease must become disseminated to nonpulmonary organs.

Cryptococcoses

Advanced HIV infection increases susceptibility to cryptococcal infections, affecting as many as 6% to 9% of people with AIDS (Masci, Poon, Wormser, & Bottone, 1992; Stansell & Sande, 1992). Although the disease may occur in any organ system and often affects the respiratory system, the most common form is cryptococcal meningitis, with symptoms of headache, stiff neck, nausea, vomiting, malaise, and possible seizures (Saag, 1997). Other common symptoms include hypersensitivity to light and marked changes in mental status.

Histoplasmosis

Like other fungal infections, exposure to histoplasmosis occurs through inhaling fungus particles, with infection potentially disseminating to other organ systems. Clinical manifestations of infection include fever, skin rashes, anemia, lymphadenopathy, and involvement of vital organs (Finley et al., 1992). Histoplasmosis occurs at varying rates across regions of North America, with the greatest concentrations occurring in the central and south-central United States and in the Ontario and Quebec Canadian provinces (Sarosi, 1992). As many as 27% of AIDS patients in these areas develop histoplasmosis, as compared with regions where infection is virtually nonexistent (Finley et al., 1992).

Viral Infections

Cytomegalovirus

Cytomegalovirus (CMV) is a herpes virus common in people with HIV infection, with a majority of people with AIDS developing some form of active CMV infection (Drew, Buhles, & Erlich, 1992). Cytomegalovirus can cause pneumonia, vaginal infection, hepatitis, encephalitis, and colitis. However, the most common manifestations are CMV retinitis, CMV esophagitis, and CMV colitis. Among the most distressing manifestations of CMV is retinitis, which threatens the vision of as many as 40% of people with AIDS (Drew, Stempien, & Erlich, 1997). Irreversible loss of visual acuity and blindness often result from untreated CMV retinitis. Almost all patients who develop CMV retinitis have T-helper lymphocyte counts below 50 cells/mm^3 (Drew et al., 1992), making it one of the later manifestations of HIV infection. In addition to symptomatic illness, CMV also has immune-suppressing effects of its own, potentially complicating the course of HIV infection (Yarrish, 1992). Although CMV infection is difficult to treat, advances in antiviral medications have been effective in helping to manage this condition.

Herpes Simplex Virus

Because more than 25 million people in the United States are infected with herpes simplex virus (HSV; Aral & Holmes, 1991), and because

HIV infection is often associated with other sexually transmitted infections, people with HIV are frequently co-infected with HSV. In fact, as many as 95% of gay men with AIDS and 77% of all HIV-infected people were previously infected with HSV (Drew et al., 1992). Symptoms of HSV include small, painful, erupting blisters. When outbreaks of herpes lesions persist for at least 1 month, they constitute an AIDS-defining condition. HSV causes ulcers of the oral, genital, and anal mucous linings (Finley et al., 1992). In non-immune-suppressed persons, herpes blisters heal within 2 to 4 weeks of their onset. People with compromised immune systems, however, may have chronic lesions lasting months when untreated or unresponsive to treatment (Drew et al., 1997; Minkoff & DeHovitz, 1991). Herpes simplex lesions may occur in the esophagus, causing pain that interferes with swallowing. Pneumonitis pulmonary infection, and encephalitis are also possible although relatively rare manifestations. Finally, like CMV, HSV is a potential cofactor in the progression of HIV infection (Brettle & Leen, 1991).

Epstein–Barr Virus and Hairy Leukoplakia

Epstein–Barr virus is associated with infectious mononucleosis. In people with HIV infection, Epstein-Barr virus also involves hairy leukoplakia, an AIDS-defining condition with white lesions on the mouth and tongue (Greenspan et al., 1992). Hairy leukoplakia occurs in 19% of individuals with otherwise asymptomatic HIV infection, and more frequently among people with advanced immune suppression (Greenspan et al., 1992). Although hairy leukoplakia may resolve on its own, symptoms are relieved by a number of treatments, including antiviral medications.

Progressive Multifocal Leukoencephalopathy

Caused by a human papovavirus, progressive multifocal leukoencephalopathy (PML) occurs in approximately 2% to 4% of AIDS cases (Bacellar et al., 1994; Worley & Price, 1992). The papovavirus infects the oligodendrocytes of the brain, cells that are responsible for producing the myelin sheath that coats and insulates neurons (Krupp, Belman, & Shneidman, 1992). The neurologic symptoms of PML are usually rapid, progressive, and fatal, with the majority of afflicted people dying within months (Krupp et al., 1992). Symptoms of PML include changes in mental status, memory, and language; headache; seizure; loss of coordinated movements; and other motor disturbances (Krupp et al., 1992; Worley & Price, 1992). Neurological deficits are focal, affecting specific functions, in contrast to the diffuse and generalized symptoms of HIV encephalopathy (R. W. Price, 1997).

Protozoan Infections

Toxoplasmosis

The intracellular protozoan *Toxoplasma gondii* causes toxoplasmosis, the most common infection of the human central nervous system (Mariuz & Luft, 1992; Wong, Israelski, & Remington, 1995). Exposure to *Toxoplasma gondii* occurs principally through contact with cat feces (Mariuz & Luft, 1992). Between 20% and 47% of people with AIDS who carry *Toxoplasma gondii* eventually develop toxoplasmosis encephalitis (Israelski & Remington, 1992). Manifestations are often insidious and usually include a mixture of focal and generalized neurological symptoms, including thought disturbances, lethargy, confusion, memory and language deficits, and motor disturbances. Relapse to active illness is also common following apparently successful treatment (Kovacs, 1995).

Cryptosporidiosis

Infection with cryptosporidiosis occurs after spores of the microorganism are either inhaled or ingested (Naficy & Soave, 1992). Cryptosporidia causes chronic diarrhea and is responsible for about 4% of all diarrhea-related illnesses in U.S. AIDS cases (Finley et al., 1992). Infection can involve any area of the gastrointestinal tract, but the usual site is the small intestine. The AIDS case definition requires that symptoms of chronic diarrhea caused by cryptosporidia persist for a minimum of one month. Cryptosporidiosis also causes gallbladder disease in up to 10% of U.S. AIDS cases (Finley et al., 1992). Treatment for this infection is extremely limited, and symptoms, therefore, are chronic, debilitating, and often lethal. Outbreaks in cities where drinking water or swimming pools have been contaminated by cryptosporidiosis have resulted in several deaths among people with suppressed immune systems. For example, a 1993 outbreak of waterborne cryptosporidiosis in Milwaukee, Wisconsin, caused over 400,000 people to become ill, including countless people with HIV–AIDS (Vakil et al., 1996). People with HIV infection are therefore advised to routinely boil their drinking water or use only bottled water.

Isosporiasis

Isosporiasis is reported in less than 1% of U.S. AIDS cases but in more than 15% of people with AIDS in Haiti (Naficy & Soave, 1992). Like cryptosporidiosis, this infection strikes the gastrointestinal tract, causing diarrhea, abdominal cramping, and weight loss. However, unlike other protozoan infections, effective treatments are available for isosporiasis (Cello, 1992).

Bacterial Infections

Mycobacterium Diseases

Mycobacterial infections include mycobacterium TB, mycobacterium avium complex, and other disseminated mycobacteria. Following a long period of decline in incidence, mycobacterium TB has reclaimed its place among global health threats (Mann & Tarantola, 1996; Raviglione, Snider, & Kochi, 1995) and as a major U.S. epidemic (Pitchenik & Fertel, 1992). An estimated 4% to 40% of people with AIDS in the United States have active TB, and 40% of individuals with active TB may be HIV infected. The scenario is even worse in developing countries, where TB in sub-Saharan Africa has doubled in recent years (Mann & Tarantola, 1996). In some African countries, nearly one third of people with HIV–AIDS present clinically with TB as their first manifestation of HIV infection. Mycobacterial TB is contracted person to person through respiratory routes, posing an alarming situation. Active mycobacterial TB occurs relatively early in HIV infection, usually with T-helper lymphocyte cell counts between 500 and 200.

Tuberculosis can become disseminated to a number of organ systems, with less than half of all TB cases in AIDS being confined to the lungs (Jacobson, 1992). The course of TB in people with AIDS is typically aggressive, particularly when untreated. Symptoms may include fever, night sweats, fatigue, malaise, and weight loss. When TB is pulmonary, symptoms will usually include persistent cough, production of sputum, and chest pain. Pulmonary disease occurs in 70% to 90% of HIV-infected individuals with TB (Pitchenik & Fertel, 1992). However, antituberculosis drugs are highly effective when used properly (Jacobson, 1992). Unfortunately, as the TB epidemic has escalated, several multiple-drug-resistant strains of mycobacterium TB have emerged (Gordin et al., 1996; Telzak et al., 1995). Thus, HIV and TB reciprocally complicate each other's courses. People with HIV are at greater risk of developing TB, standard medical interventions for TB are less effective in HIV-infected individuals, and TB may be more infectious in people with HIV infection.

In addition to mycobacterium TB, mycobacterium avium complex (MAC) occurs in HIV infection. Although discussed as a single disease, MAC consists of two closely related organisms, *mycobacterium avium* and *mycobacterium intracellular*, with mycobacterium avium occurring more frequently. MAC is contracted through contaminated soil, food, water, and airborne water droplets. Although affecting as many as 40% of AIDS cases in the United States, disseminated MAC is virtually nonexistent in non-HIV-infected people (Pitchenik & Fertel, 1992). MAC has increased each year of the HIV epidemic. Disseminated MAC usually occurs late in HIV infection, typically in people with T-helper lymphocyte counts below 100 (Jacobson, 1992). Clinically, MAC has diffuse symptoms that include fever, weight loss, malaise, severe anemia, anorexia, and a number of gastrointestinal symptoms, including chronic diarrhea, abdominal pain, and malabsorption (CDC, 1993a; Horsburgh, 1991; Jacobson, 1992). Disseminated MAC is often lethal in people with AIDS. Because MAC occurs late in HIV infection, other opportunistic illnesses commonly precede MAC (Horsburgh, 1991; Pitchenik & Fertel, 1992). Unfortunately, there are few effective treatments for MAC, although there have been advances in preventive medications (Jacobson, 1997).

Recurrent Bacterial Pneumonia

Pneumonia caused by any one of nine different bacteria frequently occurs in people with HIV infection (Chaisson, 1992; A. E. Greenberg et al., 1992). Bacterial pneumonia was observed early in the HIV epidemic, and pulmonary infections have contributed substantially to HIV-related deaths. Community-acquired pneumonia occurs more frequently in people with HIV than people not infected with HIV, and bacterial pneumonia is associated with diminished CD4 cell counts (Hirschtick et al., 1995). The onset of bacterial pneumonia is typically abrupt and can last several days, making it distinguishable from the insidious onset and persistent symptoms of PCP (Chaisson, 1992). Bacterial pneumonia in HIV-infected individuals has a course similar to that found in immune-competent individuals, including persistent fever, productive cough, dyspnea (labored or difficult breathing), and chest pain (Chaisson, 1992). However, unlike people with healthy immune systems, symptoms of pneumonia in HIV infection persist for long periods of time.

Nonpneumonia-Causing Bacterial Infections

People with compromised immune systems are vulnerable to a wide range of bacterial infections. Most infections associated with HIV involve the gastrointestinal system, skin, meninges, and sinuses (Chaisson, 1992). Bacterial infections tend to occur early in immune suppression, reflecting the aggressive disease-causing capabilities of bacteria in even relatively healthy people.

Recurrent salmonella infection frequently occurs early in HIV infection and is an AIDS-defining condition (Simberkoff & Leaf, 1992). More than 50% of salmonella infections cause severe diarrhea (Scrager, 1988), and nearly half involve febrile illness (high fevers that can lead to seizures; Chaisson, 1992). Salmonella infection in people with HIV is most likely to recur because of incomplete elimination of the disease during what would usually be adequate treatment. Salmonella is also likely to become resistant to treatments following their recurrent use (Chaisson, 1992).

Sinusitis is another common bacterial infection that is persistent when it occurs in HIV-infected persons. Caused by as many as four different bacteria, symptoms of sinusitis include fever, headache, and upper respiratory distress (Scrager, 1988). Symptoms are most chronic for people with T-helper lymphocyte counts below 200 cells/mm³ (Chaisson, 1992). Additional bacterial infections common to HIV infection include oral infections such as gingivitis and periodontitis, both of which can be progressive and painful. *Staphylococcus* infection of soft tissues is also more serious with compromised immunity (Jacobson, 1997).

Pelvic inflammatory disease resulting from gonorrhea becomes persistent and aggressive in HIV-infected women (Minkoff & DeHovitz, 1991). Syphilis also takes an aggressive course in immune suppression and includes an increased risk of neurosyphilis (Minkoff & DeHovitz, 1991). HIV infection further complicates syphilis by speeding up its course and reducing the effectiveness of antibiotic treatments (Bolan, 1992). Thus, similar to other bacterial infections, co-infection of HIV and sexually transmitted bacteria poses specific problems not encountered when bacterial infections occur in people with functional immune systems.

Other Conditions Not Yet Included in the AIDS Case Definition

Virtually any infection or malignancy can become a complication of HIV infection. For example, although only three cancers are included as AIDS case-defining conditions (non-Hodgkin's lymphoma, KS, and invasive cervical cancer), HIV infection is associated with Hodgkin's disease, melanoma, and cancers of the colon, lung, and testes (Kaplan & Northfelt, 1997). Numerous viral, protozoan, fungal, and bacterial infections that are usually managed by immune responses frequently cause serious illness. For example, varicella-zoster virus causes chicken pox in childhood and usually remains inactive throughout adulthood. When reactivated in adulthood, varicella-zoster virus causes shingles, painful skin eruptions in association with nerve endings. However, shingles are common in early and late HIV infection and usually take an aggressive course (Cockerell, 1992).

Although not always life threatening, many conditions that coincide with HIV can cause discomfort, disfigurement, and reduce quality of life. Bacterial, viral, and parasitic infections of the skin can be difficult to treat (Berger, 1997). Immune suppression can lead to adverse reactions to drugs and insect bites, also causing dermatologic complications. Oral infections can cause discomfort and interfere with appetite and ability to eat. Risk for cancers of the mouth and throat also increase with declines in immunity (Greenspan & Greenspan, 1992). A whole array of gastrointestinal manifestations arises with advancing HIV infection, including parasites contracted from drinking water and recreational activities. Outbreaks of *Giardia lambia* and *Shigella sonnei* are commonplace and can cause significant disease in people with AIDS. HIV infection therefore brings a myriad of illnesses, all of which are more difficult to treat and more problematic as immune suppression advances.

In summary, manifestations of HIV infection result from interactions between several defects in the protective immune system because of interference with and destruction of T-helper lymphocytes (Bollinger & Siliciano, 1992). Thus, as HIV infection progresses, disease-causing agents that are usually either completely suppressed or easily managed become potentially lethal. Serious immune suppression is also likely to result in simultaneous infections and malignancies that require multiple medical interventions. For these reasons, medical treatments that slow the loss of T-helper lymphocytes, prevent malignancies, or protect against opportunistic infections have been the principal means of combating AIDS.

REVERSALS OF AIDS DIAGNOSES

As a result of effective combinations of anti-HIV medications, an AIDS diagnosis is no longer the marker for an irreversible decline that it once was. People are diagnosed with AIDS when their T-helper cell count drops below 200 cells/mm^3. However, it is now common for combination therapies to rebound T-helper cells in conjunction with reductions in viral load, and these changes can remain stable for some time. People with an AIDS diagnosis who may even be disabled can find themselves with elevated T-helper cells and improved health. Although the clinical diagnosis of AIDS is unlikely removed in such cases, the personal and social experience of AIDS will undoubtedly change. People with asymptomatic late stage HIV infection will become increasingly more common, suggesting a redefinition of the meaning of AIDS and its course. For example, many people with AIDS may become re-employed, go back to school, and restart their lives in other ways. The psychological aspects of reversing the course of AIDS, as well as the likely setbacks and cycles between reversals and setbacks as of yet are unknown.

PEDIATRIC AIDS

For some children in U.S. inner cities, AIDS has become the leading cause of death as is the case for Hispanic and African American children 1 to 4 years old in New York City. By midyear 1997, nearly 8,000 children with AIDS were reported in the United States, with 400 to 500 U.S. children dying of AIDS complications each year since 1991. Unlike the early days of the epidemic before blood transfusions were safe, 99% of children with HIV infection now acquire the virus from an HIV infected mother. Recent years have seen significant advances in pre-venting mother to fetus or infant HIV transmission. Administering AZT to mothers and infants decreases transmission risks by as much as 67%. Another factor reducing the number of HIV infected children in the United States is the successful prevention of injection drug related HIV transmission in women. In 1990, the number of children born to HIV seropositive women infected through injection drugs declined to a rate lower than for women infected through heterosexual contact. Never-theless, sexually transmitted HIV continues to escalate and children born to infected mothers remain at high risk.

Infants born to HIV-seropositive women will test HIV seropositive on standard antibody tests because the mother's antibodies pass the placenta. Infants are therefore tested using virus cultures and PCR tech-niques to provide direct evidence for infection. These tests are repeated several times during the first 3 years of life to confirm the child's HIV-infection status. Most truly negative infants will test HIV antibody neg-ative by 18 months.

Table 2.3

Frequencies of AIDS-Defining Conditions in U.S. Children Under Age 13 Through December, 1995

Pediatric Condition	Percent of AIDS Cases
PCP	34
Lymphoid interstitial pneumonitis	24
Recurrent bacterial infections	20
HIV wasting syndrome	17
Candida esophagitis	15
HIV encephalopathy	15
CMV disease	8
Mycobacterium avium infection	7
Severe herpes infection	5
Pulmonary candidiasis	4
Cryptosporidiosis	4
Other opportunistic infections	6
Cancers	2

NOTE: Data from Centers for Disease Control and Prevention, 1997.

HIV manifests differently in children compared with adults. Table 2.3 presents the frequencies of AIDS-defining conditions in U.S. children. Like adults, PCP is the most common AIDS-related condition in children. However, other conditions such as lymphoid interstitial pneumonitis (a slow progressing condition caused by a buildup of cells in the lungs) and recurrent bacterial infections are more common in children with AIDS. HIV infection generally progresses more rapidly in children than adults. However, some infants develop AIDS very early in life, whereas others show a slower progression of disease (Wara & Dorenbaum, 1997). The differences in progression appear closely related to the loss of T-helper lymphocyte cells (Kourtis et al., 1996). For the most part, HIV-infected children develop AIDS by age 5, and most have AIDS by age 10.

Children with AIDS are particularly susceptible to disorders of the central nervous system (CNS). HIV-related CNS disease may progress rapidly and can cause the loss of developmental milestones. Children can experience any number of opportunistic illnesses of the CNS and peripheral nervous system. In some cases, cortical atrophy and calcification with diffuse and or focal lesions can occur.

The diagnostic classification of AIDS for children also differs from adults. Children may be diagnosed as asymptomatic, moderately symptomatic, and severely symptomatic. Moderate symptoms include a variety of conditions, such as anemia, bacterial infections, candidiasis, cardiomyopathy, HSV and CMV infections, recurrent diarrhea, and others. Severe symptoms generally reflect the AIDS-defining conditions of adults. In addition, medical treatments for children differ from adults in terms of dosing, multiple drug interactions, and toxicity.

Another problem associated with pediatric AIDS is the growing number of orphans. A child born with HIV, by definition, is the child of an HIV-infected mother. In most cases, fathers of children with HIV are also HIV infected. Thus, being born to parents with life-threatening illnesses obviously creates a risk for becoming an orphan. The stigmas and ignorance that impede foster care and other means of providing for these children exacerbate the problem. The number of orphans because of AIDS, both infected and uninfected, will continue to grow as more women become infected with HIV and develop AIDS.

CONCLUSION

The costs of AIDS in terms of lives and human resources are immeasurable. The majority of people with AIDS are in the most productive years of their lives. Potential years of life lost because of AIDS are disproportionate among subgroups, particularly ethnic minorities. As early as 1987, AIDS deaths in New York and New Jersey among African American women were comparable to rates reported for women in South Africa (Chu, Buehler, & Berkelman, 1990). HIV infection has widened the mortality gap between ethnic groups in the United States, further decreasing the life expectancies for minorities.

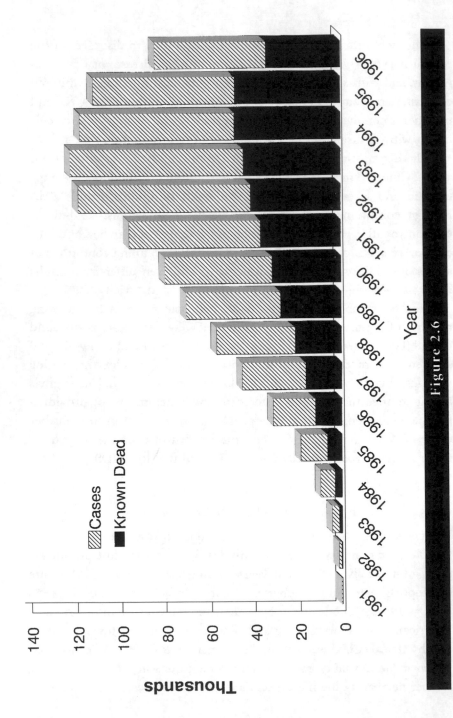

Figure 2.6

Rates of U.S. AIDS diagnoses and AIDS-related deaths, 1981–1996.

AIDS also directly strains the infrastructure of cities because of health care costs, demands placed on social services, lost work force, and so forth. From AIDS diagnosis to death, the cost of care falls between $62,000 and $73,000, and the estimated lifetime cost of HIV infection to death is well over $100,000 per person (Hellinger, 1993). Broadened criteria for an AIDS diagnosis places an even greater burden on services. Inner cities hit hardest by AIDS are even further depleted of their health and social service resources (Ozawa, Auslander, & Slonim-Nevo, 1993).

Individually, the cost of care for HIV infection is catastrophic. Using 15 months as a survival time following an AIDS diagnosis, the lifetime cost of AZT is over $2,200. Aerosol pentamidine, a PCP prophylactic, costs over $2,000 per year (Hellinger, 1990). These costs increased further as antiretroviral drug combinations became the standard of care. Although some people with HIV infection have private health insurance, the majority relies on public assistance. People with HIV infection will increasingly need public funds as insurance companies require HIV testing prior to accepting applicants. As the number of HIV infections increases, and as people with HIV continue to live longer, there will be increasingly more HIV seropositive patients in need of care. These two patterns, more people becoming HIV infected and infected individuals living longer, promise to continue over the next several years. As shown in Figure 2.6, new cases of AIDS have increased each year of the U.S. epidemic, whereas the number of deaths because of AIDS has decreased. This picture tells a story of how the growing number of AIDS cases will translate to an even larger population of people living longer with HIV–AIDS. Advances in treatments for HIV infection and its opportunistic illnesses, therefore, bring hope for longer survival and improved quality of life.

3

Medical Treatments

People living with HIV infection in industrialized countries are surviving longer today than at any other time in the history of AIDS, with nearly a doubling of life expectancy in the past decade. Rapid advances in the medical management of HIV disease have improved both the quantity and quality of life for countless people who have access to care. Advances have occurred for both treating HIV infection and preventing opportunistic illnesses. In addition to traditional medicine, a wide range of complimentary therapies is available. This chapter reviews current approaches to combating HIV infection and its associated illnesses. First, drugs that target HIV infection itself, antiretrovirals, are discussed, highlighting both their promises and challenges. Next, an overview of treatments for opportunistic illnesses and complementary therapies is presented. Finally, the chapter concludes with a discussion of issues related to medication adherence.

ANTIRETROVIRAL THERAPIES

For most viral infections, immune system responses are intact and antiviral medications work in concert with the body's natural immunity to effectively fight infection. However, because HIV selectively targets the branch of the immune system that recognizes disease-causing antigens and coordinates immune responses, antiretroviral treatments must act on their own to suppress HIV. Medications that directly inhibit the virus offer the greatest hope in treating HIV infection. Antiretrovirals work through several mechanisms. The HIV replication cycle provides points of potential attack on HIV. For example, *tat*, one of HIV's regulatory genes, is essential for the synthesis of proteins used for HIV production. A drug that inhibits the activity of the *tat* gene will disrupt the HIV replication cycle and stop production of HIV in chronically infected as well as newly infected cells.

Antiretrovirals can also work by disrupting the protective outer envelope of the virus, interrupting the ability of HIV to bind with infectable cells, or by interfering with the viral replication cycle (Lipsky, 1996). Exhibit 3.1 summarizes the opportunities for anti-HIV drug actions, and Table 3.1 lists the available antiretroviral medications. Most approaches to HIV treatment have relied on disrupting the viral replication cycle by interfering with key enzymes in this process. The first generation of antiretroviral medications consisted of a class of drugs

Exhibit 3.1

Opportunities for Anti-HIV Drug Actions

Binding of HIV to the membrane of target cells.

Inhibiting reverse transcriptase that converts HIV RNA to DNA

Inhibiting the enzyme Rnase H that degrades HIV RNA after conversion to DNA.

Inhibiting the actions of HIV integrase that integrates HIV DNA into host cells.

Inhibiting the expression of HIV genetic material once integrated into the host cell.

Inhibiting protease that splices proteins for assembling new virus particles.

Table 3.1	
Medications used in treating HIV infection	
Drug Type	Drug Name
Nucleoside reverse-transcriptase inhibitors	Zidovudine (AZT, Retrovir)
	Didanosine (ddI, Videx)
	Zalcitabine (ddC, Hivid)
	Stavudine (D4T, Zerit)
	Lamivudine (3TC, Epivir)
	Lamivudine/zidovudine (Combivir)
Non-nucleoside reverse transcriptase inhibitors	Delavirdine (Rescriptor)
	Nevirapine (Viramune)
Protease inhibitors	Saquinavir (Invirase)
	Fortovase—Saquinavir in Soft Gel Formulation
	Ritonavir (Norvir)
	Indinavir (Crixivan)
	Nelfinavir (Viracept)

that targets the enzyme reverse transcriptase, the first of which was zidovudine (AZT). The second major class of antiretrovirals is the protease inhibitors. The following sections describe drugs with principal actions of inhibiting reverse transcriptase and protease.

First Generation Anti-HIV Drugs: Reverse Transcriptase Inhibitors

Reverse transcriptase inhibitors are the most well developed and widely studied antiretroviral medications (Myers, Prose, & Bartlett, 1993). Reverse transcriptase is necessary for the replication of HIV and is not found in non-HIV-infected cells. Thus, inhibiting reverse transcriptase does not interfere with normal cell functioning. Viral replication is interrupted at the point where RNA is transcribed to DNA. A nucleic acid from the antiretroviral drug is incorporated into the RNA–DNA transcription process, causing a termination in the chain of nucleic acids. Reverse transcriptase inhibitors, however, can only suppress HIV replication in newly infected cells. Once HIV is established in a cell, the effects of reverse transcriptase inhibitors are limited.

The first approved and most widely used reverse transcriptase inhibitor is zidovudine (AZT), a drug developed in the 1960s to treat nonhuman retroviruses. Numerous studies have shown that in most cases AZT is effective in slowing HIV progression. Results from AZT treatment include increased numbers of T-helper lymphocytes, decreased HIV activity, reduced frequency and severity of opportunistic illnesses, improved general health status, and increased survival time (Enger et al., 1996; Volberding, 1997), with further evidence showing that AIDS is delayed by AZT (Schecter et al., 1990). Lemp, Payne, Neal, Temelso, and Rutherford (1990) found that patients receiving AZT had increased survival times across subgroups of people infected through various modes of HIV transmission. In addition, Moore, Hidalgo, Sugland, and Chaisson (1991) showed that survival with AIDS has increased substantially since 1987 and that AZT therapy is attributed with much of this improvement. AZT is effective in the early phases of infection. Kinloch-de Loes et al. (1995) showed that AZT used during primary infection, the earliest weeks of infection, may result in an improved clinical course and higher T-helper cell counts. People with AIDS treated with AZT also demonstrate greater longevity than those who, for whatever reason, do not receive treatment. When started within one year of receiving an AIDS diagnosis, AZT has also shown promising results (Lundgren et al., 1994).

AZT is often initiated when T-helper lymphocyte counts fall below 500 (Saag, 1992; Schooley, 1992) but are over 300 (Bartlett, 1993b). Early treatment with AZT, before the onset of overt immune suppression or opportunistic illnesses, has been the standard of care in HIV infection (Clement & Hollander, 1992). Treatment with AZT early in HIV infection is correlated with longer survival times (Jacobson et al., 1991). People treated before the onset of AIDS survive longer after an AIDS diagnosis when compared to people not treated early (Graham et al., 1992). Antiretroviral therapy is tolerated best when a person is generally healthy because AZT is highly toxic when given at advanced stages of immune suppression. However, results from clinical trials show that the maximum benefits of AZT are time limited, and there is disagreement about exactly when treatment should be initiated.

There are a number of problems associated with AZT monotherapy. AZT may slow the dissemination of HIV but will not prevent persistent infection (Tindall, Imrie, Donovan, Penny, & Cooper, 1992). In addition, people treated with AZT are vulnerable to early side effects that result from its toxicity including headache, insomnia, nausea, vomiting, abdominal pain, diarrhea, fatigue, rash, muscle pain, and fever (Fischl, 1992), although most side effects do resolve within weeks (Bartlett, 1993a). The most threatening adverse effect of AZT is bone marrow suppression, causing anemia and other potentially more serious conditions. Bone marrow suppression, therefore, leads to immediate discontinuation of AZT treatment.

Prolonged use of AZT, particularly when started early in HIV infection, can result in long-term, often irreversible, side effects (Clement & Hollander, 1992). AZT toxicity is directly related to dose, with adjustments frequently relieving adverse symptoms. Related to the toxicity of this drug are the possible teratogenic effects on pregnancy, although they have not yet been fully determined. Expectations for adverse effects of AZT are among the most common reasons for refusing antiretroviral treatment (Perry, Ryan, Ashman, & Jacobsberg, 1992).

Additional reverse transcriptase inhibiting drugs are available, including Dideoxycytidine (ddC), Dideoxyinosine (ddI), Lamivudine (3TC), and 3'-Deoxythymidine-2'-ene (d4T). Each of these drugs functions similarly to AZT by inhibiting the action of reverse transcriptase, and therefore interfering with HIV replication. A combination of antiretrovirals is now the standard of care in HIV treatment. For example, the antiretroviral actions of ddC are increased when taken in combination with AZT (Schooley, 1992). Unfortunately, ddC also has toxic side effects, including peripheral neuropathy (numbness, tingling, or pain in the hands and feet), oral ulcerations, and skin rashes. Similarly, ddI can cause peripheral neuropathy, diarrhea, and pancreatitis. In addition, d4T and 3TC interfere with HIV's integration into host cells, although they too have their share of side effects. Nevertheless, combinations of nucleoside analog reverse transcriptase inhibitors slow the progress of HIV infection and improve survival time (Hammer et al., 1997). The nucleoside reverse transcriptase inhibitors differ slightly in their chemistry but are grouped together because they share similar molecular structures and share common mechanisms against the virus.

A more recent class of drugs has been developed to provide a second tier of reverse transcriptase inhibitors. Non-nucleoside reverse transcriptase inhibitors (NN-RTIs) function similarly as the nucleoside agents, terminating the nucleic acid chain at an earlier site. These drugs are used in combination with other reverse transcriptase inhibitors to slow HIV infection. Two NN-RTIs that have been approved for use in combination with nucleoside RTIs are delavidine and nevirapine.

Concurrent use of two or more treatments, or convergent combination therapy, may increase effectiveness and prevent developing multiple drug resistance. For example, the synergistic reverse transcriptase inhibitory effects of AZT and ddI were well-established early in AIDS treatment (Bartlett, 1993a; Fischl, 1992; Schooley, 1992). AZT in combination with ddC, d4T, and 3TC has also shown more potent effects in slowing HIV infection. Non-nucleoside reverse transcriptase inhibitors are among the drugs approved for use only in combination with other antiretrovirals. The genetic mutation rate of HIV gives the virus a significant advantage in developing drug resistance, particularly when single treatments are used in monotherapy.

Second Generation Anti-HIV Drugs: Protease Inhibitors

Protease inhibitors are another class of available antiretroviral medications. Protease inhibitors, the first of which was approved in the United States by the FDA in December 1995, are used in combination with reverse transcriptase inhibitors. For example, the so-called "AIDS cocktail" or triple combination therapy, consists of a protease inhibitor and two reverse transcriptase inhibitors (J. Cohen, 1997), although treatment with two protease inhibitors is becoming increasingly more common (Deeks, 1997). Similar to reverse transcriptase inhibitors, pro-

tease inhibitors work by disrupting the HIV replication cycle. HIV protease is another enzyme essential to the replication of the virus. Rather
than acting on the process of RNA–DNA transcription as does reverse
transcriptase, protease is necessary for breaking down viral proteins into
their proper components for the maturation of new virus particles (see
Figure 3.1). Without protease, the structural formation and organization
of viral proteins remain incomplete, rendering inactive virus particles.
Therefore, complementing the actions of reverse transcriptase inhibitors
that have their effects in the early stages of HIV replication, protease
inhibitors interrupt processes in the final stages of viral production (see
Figure 3.2). The promising combination of both reverse transcriptase
inhibitors and protease inhibitors comes from delivering a double

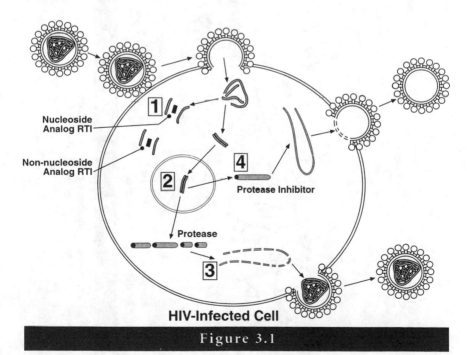

HIV-Infected Cell

Figure 3.1

Protease inhibitor effects on HIV cycle: (1) HIV RNA is reverse transcribed to
DNA, (2) Viral DNA is integrated with cell DNA to direct protein synthesis, (3)
Protease splices proteins for assembling new virus particles, (4) Protease inhibitors
interfere with viral assembly.

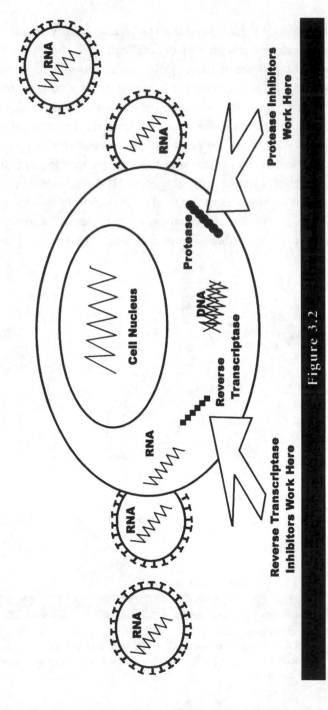

Figure 3.2

Reverse transcriptase and protease inhibitor points of action.

punch, hitting HIV early and late in its replication cycle (Ho, 1996; Lipsky, 1996).

Early results from clinical trials on combination therapies that included protease inhibitors were very encouraging (Danner et al., 1995; Gulick et al., 1997; Hammer et al., 1997). Assisted by advances in newly developed methods for monitoring viral load (Katzenstein et al., 1996), clinical trials of combination treatments, or highly active antiretroviral therapy (HAART), showed dramatic declines in the amount of HIV present in blood soon after initiating combination therapies. Within 2 weeks of starting treatment, patients showed a 100-fold reduction in the amount of HIV in their blood (Ho, 1996), with HIV in the blood becoming undetectable (fewer than 400 copies of HIV RNA per ml) in some cases (Markowitz et al., 1995). In conjunction with reductions in viral load, increases in CD4 cells were also observed, indicating improvement in immune system functioning. Although only demonstrating a relatively short-term effectiveness of protease inhibitors, clinical trials of combining protease inhibitors with reverse transcriptase inhibitors have given hope to many people living with HIV infection.

Protease inhibitors are not, however, universally effective, and there is evidence that HIV may evade long-term use of HAART. First, although viral load may be reduced to undetectable levels, reservoirs of HIV have been found outside of blood in individuals apparently successfully treated on HAART (Chun et al., 1997). HIV has also been found to remain capable of replication after being suppressed for long periods of time (Wong, Hezareh, Gunthard, Havlir, Ignacio, et al., 1997). In addition, the outcome of protease inhibitors for those not enrolled in clinical trials may not be so dramatic. For example, Fatkenheurer et al. (1997) found an unexpectedly high rate of failure for people taking protease inhibitors outside of clinical trials. The study showed that people who had previously taken antiretroviral medications experienced the least benefit of protease inhibitors, suggesting that viral resistance may have been at play in some treatment failures. It is also possible that treatment failure occurred for people who were not adherent to treatment regimens, a more likely occurrence in real clinical settings compared with highly selected cohorts in clinical trials. In a study conducted at San Francisco General Hospital, approximately 50% of patients failed on treatment with indinavir and ritanovir (Deeks, 1997). Treatment failure was associated with having a CD4 count below 200 cells/mm³, prior antiretroviral therapy, and evidence of treatment nonadherence.

Psychological Aspects of HAART

History has shown that news about advances and setbacks in HIV treatments influences treatment seeking behaviors (Schroder & Barton, 1994). Along with their promise for extending lives and improving quality of life, HAART also poses several behavioral and psychosocial challenges. Protease inhibitors add to the already cumbersome treatment demands placed on people living with HIV infection and AIDS. Some protease inhibitors also have interactive effects with drugs used to treat mental-health problems. Another issue is the cost of protease inhibitors, particularly for the uninsured, underinsured, and people living in developing countries. These drugs are expensive and are unlikely to be available to the poor. Finally, the hope that fills today's renewed optimism for treating HIV and AIDS could give rise to AIDS complacency, and there is great potential for misuse of these drugs as an unproved chemoprophylactic against HIV transmission.

Interactions With Psychiatric Medications

The metabolic pathways of protease inhibitors are shared with several psychoactive medications used to treat mental health problems (Shader, von Moltke, Schmider, Harmatz, & Greenblatt, 1996). The liver cytochrome P450 oxidase system metabolizes protease inhibitors. The potential for drug interactions was illustrated by a study showing that between 30% and 77% of candidates for HAART may be taking drugs that carry risks for interactions with protease inhibitors (Van Cleef, Fisher, & Polk, 1997). Table 3.2 lists drugs that are contraindicated for co-administration with protease inhibitors.

Co-administration of protease inhibitors with potentially interactive psychoactive drugs may change the metabolism of drug substrates, risking accumulations of toxic substances. For example, administering ritonavir and diazepam (Valium) can cause excessive sedation and pos-

Table 3.2
Psychoactive Medications Contraindicated for Co-administration With HIV Protease Inhibitors

Drug Class	Indinavir	Ritonavir	Saquinavir	Nelfinavir
Antidepressants	None	bupropion (Wellbutrin, Zyban)	None	None
Neuroleptics	None	clozapine (Clozaril)	None	None
		pimozide (Orap)		
Psychotropics	midazolam (Versed)	clorazepate (Tranxene)	None	midazolam (Versed)
	triazolam (Halcion)	diazepam (Valium, Diastat)		triazolam (Halcion)
		estazolam (ProSom)		
		flurazepam (Dalmane)		
		midazolam (Versed)		
		triazolam (Halcion)		
		zolpidem (Ambien)		

sibly respiratory depression (Chuck & Rodvold, in press). Ritonavir is a particularly problematic protease inhibitor, potentially interacting with analgesics (e.g., meperidine), antiemetics (e.g., cisapride), neuroleptics (e.g., clozapine, pimozide), and hypnotics (e.g., alprazolam, diazepam; Deeks, Smith, Holodnly, & Kahn, 1997). Co-administration of ritonavir and pimozide (Orap), alprazolam (Xanax), midazolam (Versed), triazolam (Halcion), diazepam (Valium), or zolpidem (Ambien) can result in increased bioavailability of these drugs (Chuck & Rodvold, in press; Shader et al., 1996).

Psychopharmacological research has shown relatively specific interactions of various protease inhibitors with psychoactive drugs (von Moltke et al., in press). Clinically meaningful interactions result from four possibilities: (a) protease inhibitors can slow the metabolism of the psychoactive drug (e.g., benzodiazepines, methadone, and MDMA) causing accumulations of serum concentrations and therefore toxic effects; (b) protease inhibitors induce the metabolism of psychotropic drugs (e.g., lorazepam [Ativan], valproate [Depacon]) reducing their therapeutic benefits and possibly causing withdrawal symptoms; (c) psychotropic drugs (e.g., nefazodone hydrochloride [Serzone]) slow the metabolism of the protease inhibitor, the result of which could be increased side effects of the protease inhibitor, potentially affecting dosing and adherence; and (d) psychotropic drugs can induce the metabolism of protease inhibitors (e.g., phenobarbitol, carbamazepine [Tegretol]) therefore increasing the clearance of the protease inhibitor and reducing its therapeutic benefits (Chuck & Rodvold, in press; Rabkin & Ferrando, 1997). Treatment decisions involving co-administration of protease inhibitors, particularly ritonavir, with psychoactive drugs must therefore be informed by potential interactions. Alternative drugs and dosing adjustments can avoid such complications.

Economics of Treatment

Protease inhibitors and the drugs that must be taken with them cost between $10,000 and $15,000 per year (between $6,000 and $8,000 per year for the protease inhibitor alone), plus lab costs and doctor visits. Because combination therapies are being recommended for people as soon as they learn of being HIV infected, with or without symptoms or immune suppression, the cost per person will add billions of dollars to an already expensive illness. The lifetime treatment of a person with HIV infection was over $120,000 from time of infection to death, with most of the costs incurred later in the disease process (Hellinger, 1993). Protease inhibitors may delay the onset of symptomatic illness, however, potentially reducing the costs of terminal care while greatly increasing the costs and length of early treatment. In addition, successful treatment will reduce hospitalizations, also cutting the costs of HIV infection. Early reports suggest that combination therapies can lead to a 36% reduction in AIDS diagnoses and an over 33% reduction in hospitalizations (J. Cohen, 1997). Hospitals have started downsizing or closing inpatient services dedicated to AIDS while outpatient facilities have required expansion. Nevertheless, it remains to be seen what the true costs of protease inhibitors are in the scope of long-term care for HIV.

Like many other treatments that have been available much longer, protease inhibitors will probably not be accessible to the majority of people in the world who are living with HIV infection, both in developing countries and in poverty stricken areas of developed countries. Thus, in an atmosphere of hope there could be a widening gap in treatment between the haves and have nots in the AIDS epidemic. Although access to care is not a new issue in AIDS treatment, it will be exacerbated by the costs of HAART.

Treatment Outcome Expectancies

The increased optimism that comes with new HIV treatments can have widespread implications; revitalization of hope that protease inhibitors offer might itself have health-promoting benefits. Hope and optimism are common characteristics of long-term survivors with HIV–AIDS (Rabkin, Remien, Katoff, & Williams, 1993), and research has suggested that positive attitudes about one's prognosis may increase survival time (G. M. Reed, Kemeny, Taylor, Wang, & Visscher, 1994). People living with HIV–AIDS, many of whom had contemplated their own death, may suddenly start contemplating their survival. People who had worked their way through bureaucracies to access disability benefits may suddenly consider reemployment, a return to school, career changes, and other life redefining decisions. Relationships are also re-evaluated in the context of living longer than one was planning (Rabkin & Ferrando, 1997). Relationship partners who had been caregivers may no longer be needed in the same way, and people may end relationships because they are no longer dependent on a partner. Family relations and social networks may also be rebuilt as ones health improves. Unfortunately, it is unknown how people adjust to these changing roles. Decisions regarding geographic relocation will also occur, as people feel healthier and less tied to particular medical providers. Regrouping to start a second life occurs with great uncertainty, particularly for people who have experienced past promises and treatment failures.

Existential issues of a second life agenda are fruitful grounds for psychotherapy (Rabkin & Ferrando, 1997). Goals for the future are almost always set with great uncertainty. Considering the possibility of setbacks can be demoralizing and dampen the enthusiasm that comes with improved health. People starting HAART have survived to a time with greater treatment options—a goal that many of their friends were not so fortunate to realize. Although survivor guilt was common to AIDS before the advent of HAART, it will likely intensify in eras of new treatments.

When Promising Treatments Fail

Breakthroughs in HIV treatments bring great expectations. Many people with HIV–AIDS subject themselves to treatments with unpleasant side effects in the hope of living to the next treatment advance, with the ultimate goal of controlling the progression of HIV. The success of HAART is defined by achieving and sustaining clinically meaningful suppression of viral load (Deeks, 1997). However, not everyone responds positively to even the most promising treatment regimens. Failure can occur when viral load is not reduced after initiating HAART, or when side effects from treatment are intolerable, or when treatment that was at first successful loses its effect.

Rabkin and Ferrando (1997) described the potential emotional reactions to different reasons for treatment failure. Antiretroviral resistant strains of HIV, individual differences in immune system functioning, exposure to coinfecting pathogens, and general health status, are just some of the factors that likely account for why some people respond better to treatments than others. People who fail to respond to anti-HIV treatments will likely respond with anger and despair, much in the same way that people respond to failed attempts to treat other life threatening illnesses. Guilt is another emotional response to treatment failure; guilt perhaps for not adhering perfectly to the regimen, guilt for starting treatment too late or too early, and for having bought into unrealistic expectations for treatment success. Friends who are more successful in treatments can exacerbate the distress of treatment failure. A sense of helplessness and hopelessness can give rise to treatment inertia, a reluctance to try future treatments as they become available. The emotional loss of diminishing treatment effects can therefore pose more generalized adverse health consequences.

DRUG RESISTANCE AND TOXICITY

The necessity of using combinations of antiretroviral medications to combat HIV is driven by the diversity of HIV itself. HIV rapidly replicates and adapts well to pressures posed by treatments. Over the course of 10 years, the average duration of an individual's HIV infection, the virus replicates itself thousands of times, resulting in the production of as many as 10 trillion virus particles (Ho, 1995, 1996). The reverse transcription of genetic material, specifically forming DNA from viral RNA, is prone to error. In addition to viral mutation that occurs in the typical replication cycle of HIV, mutations also occur in response to antiretroviral treatments. Drug resistance occurs more readily when drug dosing is low (low potency), drugs are taken inconsistently (intermittent use), and when drugs are taken as monotherapy (Kuritzkes, 1996). Drug resistance is also associated with more rapid disease progression and increased risk of early death (Lipsky, 1996).

It has long been known that the use of any single drug in treating HIV infection will be of limited success, with an abundance of evidence to support the use of combinations of antiretrovirals for treating HIV (Ezzell, 1996; Hammer et al., 1996). Resistance can develop to AZT within months, and the risk for resistance increases over time, with as many as 50% of treated persons developing highly resistant strains within 2 years (Mayer, in press). Resistance also develops in response to other antiretrovirals, with the potential for cross-resistance to multiple drugs. Drug-resistant strains of HIV can be transmitted to sex and drug using partners, threatening the future use of antiretroviral treatments. However, viral DNA that includes resistant mutations becomes integrated with cell DNA, likely making the resistance permanent (Deeks et al., 1997). The use of drugs that target HIV at different stages of its replication cycle, particularly early and late in the course of HIV infection, decreases the ability of HIV to develop drug resistance (Cooper, 1994; Ho, 1995, 1996; Kuritzkes, 1996).

Another significant factor in antiretroviral therapies is their potential toxicity and adverse interactions. Antiretrovirals in general are highly toxic drugs. Most of these agents pose a variety of side effects that can range from uncomfortable to life threatening. Table 3.3 summarizes the side effects associated with antiretroviral drugs. The multitude of drugs taken by people living with HIV creates additional hazards through multiple drug interactions (Lee, 1997). For example, ganciclovir, an antiviral medication commonly used for preventing and treating CMV infection, can interact with AZT to cause hematologic toxicity. As another example, methadone, whether used in or out of substance abuse treatment, decreases AZT metabolism and interacts with some protease inhibitors. Aside from their direct impact on health, drug toxicity and adverse interactions play important roles in medication regimen adherence and in delays in seeking treatment.

DELAYING TREATMENT

When to initiate HAART is a point of controversy. Starting treatment early may suppress the propagation of mutant strains of HIV that would ultimately undermine treatment. HIV also disseminates rapidly throughout the body, so slowing the early progress of the virus may alter the course of infection. On the other hand, the effects of HAART can diminish over time, with the risks for nonadherence and treatment resistance increasing and potentially restricting later treatment options.

Table 3.3

Antiretroviral Medications and Approximate Percent of Patients Experiencing Side Effects

Drug Name	Head-ache	Fever	Malaise	Nausea	Diarrhea	Neurop-athy
Nucleoside reverse-transcriptase in-hibitors						
Zidovudine (AZT, Retrovir)[a]	42%	16%	8%	46%	12%	N/R
Didanosine (ddI, Videx)[b]	7%	12%	N/R	7%	28%	20%
Zalcitabine (ddC, Hivid)	2%	2%	4%	3%	2%	28%
Stavudine (D4T, Zerit)[c]	54%	50%	N/R	38%	50%	N/R
Lamivudine (3TC, Epivir)[d]	35%	10%	27%	33%	18%	12%
Lamivudine/zidovudine (Combivir)[e]	35%	10%	27%	33%	18%	12%
Non-nucleoside reverse transcriptase inhibitors						
Delavirdine (Rescriptor)[f]	5%	N/R	3%	5%	4%	N/R
Nevirapine (Viramune)[g]	3%	3%	N/R	5%	2%	0%
Protease inhibitors						
Saquinavir (Invirase)	2%	N/R	N/R	1%	5%	3%
Ritonavir (Norvir)[h]	8%	1%	4%	46%	21%	N/R
Indinavir (Crixivan)[i]	11%	N/R	2%	32%	4%	N/R
Nelfinavir (Viracept)[j]	N/R	N/R	N/R	3%	14%	N/R

NOTE: Data from Physicians' Desk Reference, 1998.
N/R = Not reported; Patients with advanced HIV [a]disease; ACTG 116B and [b]177; 40 mg [b]bid; 150 mg bid + [d]Retrovir; 300 mg Epivir plus 600 mg [e]Retrovir; 400 mg tid + Didanosine 200 mg [f]bid; ACTG [g]241; + [g]zidovudine; + [h]zidovudine; 500 mg tid + zidovudine + [j]lamivudine

The possibility of developing cross-resistant strains of HIV threatens losing sensitivity to an entire class of these agents, resulting in some people waiting to start HAART in an uncertain effort to optimize its potential benefits.

Decisions of when to start and when to delay HAART can be a source of stress for people living with HIV–AIDS. Similarly, changing drugs after having started one regimen can also be stressful given the risks for cross-resistance and reduced treatment potency. These decisions are influenced by the way that people perceive the relative success of others on similar treatments. In addition, people may be more or less active in treatment decision making and therefore have varying perceptions of internal and external control over HIV.

ANTI-HIV DRUGS AND PREVENTION

Despite the numerous cautions against overoptimism, people looking for an end to AIDS responded with jubilation to the early results from clinical trials of combination therapies. The prospect of "When AIDS Ends" has been proclaimed in news headlines and cover stories. It is unknown what the behavioral effects are when men and women hear that "the cure for AIDS is here." As mentioned earlier, thinking of AIDS as a manageable chronic condition may lead to a sense of complacency that can have dangerous repercussions. AIDS complacency may lower vigilance against the disease and undermine prevention efforts.

There has been much concern that talk of a cure could give rise to a heightened denial of risk that may unleash reckless behavior. Effective HIV treatments may become factors in individual decisions to engage in risk practices. There is also the risk that some could misuse these drugs in efforts to lower their infectivity by bringing down their viral load. A survey of gay and bisexual men found that those who engaged in unprotected anal intercourse as the receptive partner were significantly more likely to believe that new treatments for HIV infection reduce their risks for becoming infected; 23% of men who practice this single highest-risk behavior believed that it is safe to have unprotected receptive intercourse with an HIV-seropositive man who has an undetectable viral load, and 23% stated that new treatments for HIV relieve their worries about unsafe sex (Kalichman, Nachimson, Cherry, & Williams, in press). In a related study of 54 men who have sex with men, Dilley, Woods, and McFarland (1997) found that 26% of men were less concerned about becoming HIV infected because of new treatments. In addition, 15% of men indicated that they were more willing to take sexual risks because of the advent of new therapies.

Antiretroviral medications are also used to avert the onset of HIV infection following potential exposure. Research has suggested that antiretrovirals such as AZT used following occupational exposure to HIV, particularly needle-stick injuries, can prevent HIV infection. A case control study of health professionals showed that administration of AZT after needle-stick injury exposure to HIV reduced transmission risks by nearly 80% (Gerberding, 1997). Protocols for postexposure prophylaxis (PEP) for occupational exposure to HIV are available and include administering combinations of antiretrovirals, which usually include AZT and 3TC, within 1 to 2 hours following, or as soon after as possible, the potential exposure.

Another example of postexposure use of antiretrovirals is administering AZT to prevent perinatal HIV transmission. Administering combinations of reverse transcriptase inhibitors to pregnant women likely lowers their infectivity by reducing viral load. There are, however, additional mechanisms that are likely important in preventing perinatal transmission. In addition, administering treatment to newborns is a form of PEP and is an important aspect of preventing perinatal transmission. Thus, the idea behind postexposure prevention is to hit HIV hard during a window of opportunity between exposure and onset of infection.

The use of antiretrovirals for chemoprophylaxis in occupational and perinatal settings has led to a call for postexposure treatments following sexual transmission risks (Katz & Gerberding, 1997). The potential for a so-called "morning-after-pill" for HIV prevention (although the course of chemoprophylaxis takes weeks) drew considerable attention when combination therapies were shown to reduce viral load in lymphatic tissue and semen. If PEP can at best prevent infection and at least improve prognosis, the argument for its wide-scale use is obvious. Unfortunately, there are several concerns about using antiretroviral drugs for postsexual exposure risks. There is reason to believe that administering drugs after sex to prevent HIV infection may lead to complacency about AIDS and counter efforts to support safer sex. People are much more inclined to accept the quick fix of a pill in place of changing sexual behaviors.

Despite the cautions against PEP as a prevention strategy, many people at risk for HIV are likely to seek PEP as it becomes available. A survey of gay and bisexual men attending a gay pride festival found that 26% planned to use PEP to prevent themselves from becoming HIV infected (Kalichman, in press). The study also showed that men who planned to use PEP were younger, less well educated, more likely to have recently used marijuana, nitrite inhalants, and cocaine, and were more likely to have a history of injection drug use. Men intending to use PEP were also more likely to have practiced unprotected anal and oral intercourse as the receptive partner and were more likely to have multiple anal intercourse partners with whom they were receptive. Thus, gay and bisexual men are generally supportive of the immediate use of PEP and a significant number of men are planning to use PEP, particularly younger men who use multiple substances and who are at greatest risk for HIV infection. These results suggest that men who are at greatest risk are likely to seek PEP. In addition, behavioral histories of some men suggests that they may be at risk for nonadherence to strict PEP regimens and may seek multiple administrations of PEP.

STANDARDS OF CARE FOR ANTIRETROVIRAL THERAPY

The rapid development of new drugs to treat HIV and the accumulation of clinical experience treating people with HIV—AIDS lead to an ever-changing landscape of AIDS treatments. People living with HIV—AIDS are therefore bombarded with new treatment information. Just keeping up with new treatment options and changes in treatment protocols can become a major source of stress. With advances in treatment and increasingly sensitive tests for monitoring HIV infection status, standards of care are regularly updated and general principles of treatment are becoming available (Carpenter et al., 1997). Panels have been convened by the National Institutes of Health Office of AIDS Research, the Department of Health and Human Services, and the Henry J. Kaiser Family Foundation to determine principles of therapy for HIV infection. Together, these panels offer the following principles of therapy for HIV infection:

- Ongoing HIV replication leads to damage of the immune system and progression to AIDS. It is unusual for there to be long-term survival with HIV free of clinically significant immune dysfunction. Antiretroviral treatments are therefore aimed at improving such outcomes.
- Plasma HIV RNA levels (viral load) indicate the magnitude of HIV replication and its associated rate of immune system decline. On the other hand, the extent of HIV-induced immune damage already suffered is indicated by CD4 cell counts. Regular monitoring of both viral load and CD4 cell counts are therefore necessary to determine risks for disease progression and to indicate when to initiate or modify antiretroviral therapy.
- As rates of disease progression differ among individuals, treatment decisions should be individualized.
- Use of potent combinations of antiretroviral therapy suppress HIV replication to below levels of detection by sensitive tests of viral load, limiting the potential for the natural selection of antiretroviral-resistant HIV strains. Maximum achievable suppression of HIV replication should be the goal of therapy.
- The most effective means to accomplishing HIV suppression is the simultaneous initiation of combinations of effective anti-HIV drugs with which the patient has not been previously treated and that are not cross-resistant with antiretroviral agents with which the patient has been previously treated.

- Antiretroviral drugs used in combination therapy should always be used according to optimum schedules and dosages.
- Available antiretroviral drugs are limited in number, and cross-resistance between drugs is well documented. Therefore, any changes in antiretroviral therapy increase future limits in treatment effectiveness.
- Women should receive optimal antiretroviral therapy regardless of pregnancy status.
- The same treatment considerations apply to children as they do adults, although children pose unique pharmacologic, virologic, and immunologic considerations.
- Persons with acute primary HIV infection should be treated with combination antiretroviral therapy to suppress virus replication to achieve viral loads below detectable levels.
- HIV-infected persons, even those with viral loads below detectable levels, should be considered infectious and should be counseled to avoid sexual and drug use behaviors that are associated with HIV transmission.

(Panel on Clinical Practices for Treatment of HIV Infection, 1997; Volberding, 1997)

Another set of treatment guidelines more specific to when treatment should be started has been offered by Volberding (1997, p. 117),

- Initiate treatment before the onset of HIV-related symptoms.
- In general, treatment should be initiated when CD4 cell counts drop below 500/mm^3.
- Treatment should be considered when HIV RNA (viral load) is above 5,000 copies/mm^3 and recommended when HIV RNA is greater than 30,000 to 50,000 copies/ml^3 or if CD4 cell counts are rapidly declining.
- Treat HIV infected pregnant women and those with recent HIV exposures.

■ Therapy should be considered for primary HIV infection.

These and other treatment guidelines offer providers and patients a sense for how best to approach treating HIV infection. As understanding HIV and its mechanisms continues there will be continued developments and revisions of guidelines for treating HIV infection.

ANTI-HIV TREATMENTS ON THE HORIZON

Advances in antiretroviral therapy have revitalized hope for combating HIV infection. The powerful combination of reverse transcriptase inhibitors and protease inhibitors have stimulated testing drugs that interfere with other elements of the HIV replication cycle. For example, disulfide-substituted benzamide (DIBA) compounds have been developed as zinc-finger inhibitors; zinc-finger proteins are contained in the HIV nuclear capsid protein and are necessary for HIV replication and assembly (Lipsky, 1996). DIBA compounds inactivate HIV in vitro, and there is evidence that they may be less prone to resistance problems compared with other antiretrovirals. Zinc-finger inhibitors may therefore serve as a third point in the HIV replication cycle to target in conjunction with reverse transcriptase and protease inhibitors. Another crucial enzyme that is being targeted in treatment is integrase, an enzyme necessary for HIV to integrate its genetic material with that of the host cell (Ezzell, 1996). Impeding multiple steps in the replication cycle reduces HIV's ability to develop resistance and increases the possibility for long-term control over the virus.

Another advance in antiretroviral therapy is the combination of drugs into a single medication. For example, AZT and 3TC (lamivudine) have been combined into a single drug, Combivir, making it possible to take two antiretrovirals in one pill. Joining drugs reduces the complexity of combination therapy, with the potential benefit of increasing adherence. Of course, Combivir is produced by Glaxo Wellcome, which manufactures AZT and 3TC. Thus, the stiff competition among drug companies was not an issue in developing Combivir but will likely limit developing combined drugs that require joint ventures.

Treatments targeted to points of intervention outside of the HIV replication cycle have been less successful at slowing down HIV infection, unfortunately. For example, an avenue that has been less successful involves interfering with HIV's binding with CD4 receptor molecules (Myers et al., 1993). Receptor-based therapy is geared toward blocking HIV from attaching to the surface of and entering T-helper lymphocytes. Because HIV has such a strong affinity for CD4 surface molecules, infusion of soluble CD4 molecules into the bloodstream of infected persons could theoretically allow HIV to bind directly with free CD4 molecules, preventing the virus from subsequently binding with T-helper lymphocyte cells (McCutchan, 1990). Unfortunately, HIV is substantially less sensitive to recombinant, or free, CD4 than to CD4 surface receptors (Schooley, 1992). However, there are new approaches underway to interfere with HIV binding properties. Advances in understanding HIV's affinity for CD4 led to the discovery of chemokine receptors (CCR5 and CXCR4), that serve as coreceptors for binding HIV to targeted cells (J. Cohen, 1996a). The therapeutic value of chemokine receptors was apparent when it was discovered that some long-term nonprogressors have a mutant deletion gene for CCR5 that seems related to resisting infection. Chemokines are therefore a promising avenue for future treatments.

Gene therapy research is also well underway, focusing on the viability of implanting altered genes into HIV infected cells that will disable the virus. Using other viruses as a delivery system for altered genetic material, gene therapy has already shown promise in the laboratory. For example, M. J. Schnell, Johnson, Buonocore, and Rose (1997) showed that a genetically altered virus was able to infect and kill cells selectively that had been previously infected by HIV and spare those cells that were not yet infected. The protective virus then replicated in cells and acted as watchguards against the further spread of HIV. Other manipulated viruses have shown promise in stopping HIV replication and interfering with HIV binding to CD4 cells (Mebatsion, Finke, Weiland, & Conzelmann, 1997; Nolan, 1997). Gene transfer and other forms of gene therapy are therefore a likely part of future treatment efforts.

PROPHYLAXIS AND TREATMENTS FOR OPPORTUNISTIC ILLNESSES

Most manifestations of HIV infection involve opportunistic infections and malignancies that are usually protected by T-helper lymphocyte mediated immunity. Prevention of opportunistic illnesses results in sustained illness free periods for people with HIV infection. Because many opportunistic illnesses were rare before the era of AIDS, there has been a lot of work to establish prophylactic and treatment guidelines for opportunistic illnesses. For example, guidelines for prophylaxis against PCP include actions to prevent an initial episode of pneumonia called primary prophylaxis, in which people with suppressed immune systems routinely begin treatment with PCP prophylaxis. Dapsone and aerosolized pentamidine are two drugs that are effective in preventing primary and secondary episodes of PCP (Bozzette et al., 1995). These drugs are also effective in preventing PCP in HIV-infected children (Simonds et al., 1995). Prophylaxis is credited with reductions in cases of PCP over the course of the epidemic. Prophylactic treatments against PCP have extended the longevity of many HIV-infected individuals (Friedman, Franklin, Freels, & Weil, 1991; Hoover et al., 1993; Osmond, Charlebois, Lang, Shiboski, & Moss, 1994; Rothenberg et al., 1987).

Prophylaxis has also been established for toxoplasmosis encephalitis and mycobacterial infections. Antiviral drugs are also used widely to control recurrent symptoms of herpes viruses, Epstein-Barr, and members of other virus families. Some prophylactic agents offer additional advantages because they frequently guard against multiple opportunistic illnesses. For example, TMP–SMX, used as a PCP preventive, also helps protect against several other diseases (Bartlett, 1993a). Advances have also been made in preventing fungal infections (Powderly et al., 1995), and HIV-related malignancies (Kaplan & Northfelt, 1997).

In addition to prevention, numerous treatments are available to manage opportunistic illnesses once they occur. Most treatments effective in dealing with diseases in the context of a functional immune system do so in conjunction with cell-mediated immunity. Unfortunately, as the immune system deteriorates treatments for opportunistic illnesses require greater doses and more time to achieve equal effectiveness. This is problematic in and of itself because many treatments have adverse side effects with prolonged use, particularly when used by people with compromised immune systems. Another limitation is the potential for resistance to treatments over time as has been the case for tuberculosis and a variety of other bacterial and viral infections.

It is important to note that advances in the treatment of HIV-related diseases, like antiretroviral drugs, develop rapidly. New treatments are the product of converging areas of medicine, including but not limited to infectious diseases, immunology, oncology, hematology, neurology, and pharmacology. For example, oncology suggested that bone marrow transplantation may be of value in treating non-Hodgkin's lymphomas in AIDS patients (H. K. Holland et al., 1989). Similarly, clinical immunology has experimented with transplanting thymus gland tissue in AIDS patients with limited results that warrant further testing (Dwyer, Wood, McNamara, & Kinder, 1987). In addition, the use of testosterone for managing HIV wasting is grounded in endocrinology. As treatment approaches from various disciplines emerge they will likely be combined into promising new therapeutic avenues.

AIDS CLINICAL TRIALS

An important element of AIDS treatment is the network of drug studies for testing new therapies. The AIDS Clinical Trials Group (ACTG) is a federally funded structure that supports clinical studies testing the efficacy of HIV–AIDS treatments. Many of the major advances in HIV treatment have come from the ACTGs, including breakthroughs in using AZT to prevent perinatal HIV transmission and advances in protease inhibitors and HAART. Participants in ACTG studies often represent a highly selected population, particularly with respect to their potential to adhere to clinical study protocols. Participation in a clinical trial offers the opportunity to potentially benefit from a medical advance well ahead of others. Participants may also experience a sense of empowerment, involvement, and control, as well as the altruism that comes from helping to advance treatments for others.

COMPLEMENTARY TREATMENTS

People with HIV–AIDS often seek treatments that have not yet gone through rigorous approval processes. Searching for unconventional therapies when faced with a chronic, life-threatening disease can be a part of active involvement in one's treatment or can be motivated by disillusionment with traditional medicine. General population surveys conducted in the United States show that as many as one third of respondents use nontraditional therapies for medical ailments (Abrams, 1997). Although initially considered alternatives to standard medical care, unapproved treatments are more commonly used because they are not necessarily replacements as much as they are adjuncts to mainstream treatments.

The demand for complementary therapies for HIV–AIDS grew out of social activism in communities most affected by AIDS that were receiving too few drugs, far too slowly. People who seek complementary treatments are likely to be empowered and may gain a sense of control over their health. There are now established routes for disseminating complementary therapies, the most important of which are *buyers' clubs* that serve as distribution centers for otherwise unavailable treatments. Several newsletters inform people of the progress and development of traditional and complementary treatments. The demand and accessibility of complementary therapies has increased such that many primary care physicians routinely discuss these options with their patients (Abrams, 1997). A study of HIV seropositive men receiving treatment from an AIDS clinic in San Francisco found that 40% had received a prescription medication from someone other than their primary care provider and that 11% received treatment from an unorthodox provider (Greenblatt, Hollander, McMaster, & Henke, 1991).

Like traditional medicine, complementary therapies intervene at various points along the HIV replication cycle. Among the more common complementary therapies are megadoses of vitamin C, which has been shown to have antiviral activity (Abrams, 1997). Other antioxidants, such as betacarotene, are also used as antivirals in complementary therapy. In addition, complementary therapies can indirectly target HIV, such as those that modulate the immune system (e.g., naltrexone, disulfiram, and oral alpha interferon). Other complementary treatments include Chinese herbs used in combinations for controlling a variety of symptoms. Most of these products showed early promise but have not stood up to rigorous scientific testing. In a rare example of a randomized placebo controlled double blind clinical trial, Chinese herbal therapy for HIV infection showed no evidence for significant health impacts. However, participants in the study who believed they were being treated with herbal therapy showed improved life satisfaction (Abrams, 1997). Thus, a potential benefit of even ineffective treatments comes in the form of a placebo effect. Other treatment modalities have been suggested, such as chiropractic medicine, acupuncture, multiple vitamins, and mental imagery. Complementary treatments are acceptable to traditionalists to the extent that they do not interfere with standard medical care.

Although complementary treatments can involve holistic and naturalistic approaches, invasive procedures have also been sought. Two examples are passive hyperimmune therapy and ozone treatments. In passive hyperimmune therapy, or passive immunotherapy, unusually healthy HIV seropositive persons—who are probably HIV nonprogressors—donated blood plasma, which was then pooled for antibodies against multiple strains of HIV. The treated plasma was transfused into HIV-infected recipients, usually people with advanced HIV disease or AIDS. The idea behind the treatment was that antibodies from healthy patients might suppress HIV in others. The process was similar to that used in intravenous immune globin treatment, which is a general approach to building immunities in immune suppressed patients. Passive hyperimmune therapy for HIV infection differs because it attempts to concentrate antibodies against HIV (Jackson et al., 1988). In the second example, ozone therapy involved removing the blood of an HIV infected person over a series of transfusions, treating it with heat and exposing the blood to ultraviolet light, or ozone, or both. The entire process was intended to inactivate HIV and return the treated blood to the original patient. Unfortunately, there is little support for either passive hyperimmune or ozone therapies, with some evidence against their effectiveness (Garber, Cameron, Hawley-Foss, Greenway, & Shannon, 1991).

Several additional noteworthy complementary therapies are in current use. First, testosterone replacement therapy has received a considerable amount of attention because many men with advanced HIV disease are testosterone deficient. Usually treated with DHEA, a precursor to testosterone, this therapy is intended to increase body mass after being decimated by HIV wasting. There may also be an antiretroviral effect from DHEA. In addition, testosterone replacement is used in treating lethargy, depression, and loss of sexual interest (Rabkin, Rabkin, & Wagner, 1995; Wagner, Rabkin, & Rabkin, 1995). Another drug being used for treating HIV wasting is thalidomide, the infamous sedative that caused countless birth defects when it was first introduced. It is therefore feared that increased use of this drug will see the catastrophic effects of its teratogenicity.

Complementary therapies pose several challenges to HIV treatment. Many complementary approaches have serious adverse effects, including treatments that appear as benign as megadoses of vitamin C. It is also possible that complementary treatments will adversely interact with traditional medications. Many of these agents result in immune stimulation or immune suppression, either of which can interact in unpredictable and dangerous ways with HIV infection and traditional medications. The use of complementary therapies may interfere with individuals participating in standard medical care and AIDS clinical trials (Abrams, 1997). Deciding whether to use complementary treatments can also create tension between patients and their providers when there is disagreement concerning their use. People with HIV infection who are considering complementary treatments should be advised by a physician with experience in treating HIV infection.

TREATMENT ADHERENCE

Antiretroviral drugs, as well as many treatments for opportunistic illnesses, require careful adherence to complex treatment regimens. Treatment adherence is essential to reaching and maintaining therapeutic levels, a crucial aspect of preventing the development of drug resistant strains that ultimately render treatments ineffective. Strict adherence to treatment is essential in combination antiretroviral therapies, particularly those that include protease inhibitors. However, protease inhibitors can be among the most challenging drugs to adhere to, even when persons are highly motivated and capable of following complicated regimens. Optimal therapeutic effects of indinavir, for example, require that the drug be taken every 8 hours, not simply three times a day. Indinavir must also be taken on an empty stomach, at least 2 hours after and 1 hour before meals. In contrast, saquinavir must be taken with meals. Protease inhibitors are always taken with several other drugs in highly active antiretroviral therapy, plus any drugs for preventing and treating opportunistic illnesses. The necessity of treatment adherence often occurs in the wake of side effects common to these drug regimens (Deeks et al., 1997). As is the case with many treatments for chronic illnesses, adverse side effects, even when temporary, interfere with adherence (Rabkin & Chesney, 1998).

Several factors related to adherence with reverse transcriptase inhibitors have been identified. Poor adherence with antiretrovirals is associated with beliefs and perceptions about treatment efficacy (Mehta, Moore, & Graham, 1997). As many as one third of people taking reverse transcriptase inhibitors may discontinue their use (Samet et al., 1992), and an additional one third may intentionally alter their prescribed use (Aversa & Kimberlin, 1996). Failing to adhere with treatment can be the result of forgetting, lack of motivation, and intolerance of side effects. Treatment nonadherence can also be a response to the burdens of complicated drug regimens that can disrupt one's daily routines (Morse et al., 1991). Among people studied in an AIDS clinical trial, missed doses of antiretrovirals were most likely due to forgetting (43%), sleeping through a dose (36%), being away from home (32%), changing routine (27%), being too busy to take the dose (22%), feeling sick (11%), and being depressed (9%; Hecht, 1997). Added burdens in HIV treatment are particularly troublesome because of the often complicated, hectic, and unpredictable lives of many people affected by AIDS

(Besch, 1995). For example, homeless people living with HIV infection have been discussed as particularly high risk for antiretroviral non-adherence. The simple basic resources required to store multiple drugs, some of which require refrigeration and keeping track of doses and frequencies, pose enormous challenges to the homeless (Bangsberg, Tulsky, Hecht, & Moss, 1997; Lyman, 1997). Another key factor in medication adherence is the relationship between patient and provider. Patients who trust their provider and are more satisfied with their quality of care are more likely to adhere with treatment regimens (Ickovics & Meisler, in press; Stall et al., 1996). People who refuse to take anti-retrovirals commonly state that they believe the drugs are ineffective and toxic (Perry, Ryan, Ashman, & Jacobsberg, 1992). On the other hand, adherent use of antiretrovirals is related to optimistic beliefs and perceived benefits of taking anti-HIV drugs (Samet et al., 1992).

Substance abuse also raises specific concerns about treatment adherence because nonadherence is associated with cognitive and behavioral disturbances common to substance-abusing populations. For example, Singh et al. (1996) found that HIV-seropositive patients with a history of injection drug use were more likely to be antiretroviral non-adherent than those who had not used injection drugs. It was also found that nonadherent patients were more likely to experience symptoms of depression and lacked adaptive coping strategies. O'Connor and Samet (1996) also suggested that substance abusing patients present considerable challenges to medical management of HIV infection because of a host of problems, including resistance to comply with instructions, potential drug interactions, and conditions of living in poverty.

Adherence to anti-HIV treatments can therefore be placed in a larger context of behavioral adherence. For example, younger age, use of psychoactive substances, impoverished living conditions, and maladaptive coping are factors associated with both treatment nonadherence and continued unsafe sexual practices in persons living with HIV–AIDS. Depression and pessimistic thinking are also common to both treatment nonadherence and continued sexual risk behaviors. More serious mental illnesses that include paranoia, hostility, and grandiosity can impede treatment adherence (Mehta et al., 1997). Literacy and cognitive capacity to manage complex instructions play critical roles in treatment adherence. As many as 20% of people do not comprehend instructions for taking antiretroviral therapies in AIDS clinical trials (Chesney, 1997). Declining immune system markers, increased viral load, or onset of HIV symptoms can send a signal that treatment is not working and can undermine the perceived benefits of drugs. Although not yet empirically validated in a single predictive study, a set of risk factors appears associated with anti-HIV medication nonadherence (see Table 3.4).

Implications of Nonadherence

Among the greatest threats of nonadherence with treatments for infectious diseases is the potential risk for developing treatment resistant strains of disease causing agents. For example, multiple drug resistant

Table 3.4
Risk Factors Associated With Nonadherence With Antiretroviral Medications

Risk Factor	Probable Link to Nonadherence
Younger age	Lack of motivation, denial, resistance to comply, anger at diagnosis
Adverse side effects	Intolerance of drug toxicities, perceived costs outweigh benefits
Alcohol and other drugs	Cognitive impairment, adverse interactions
Poor relationship with physician	Lack of trust, anger
Economically disadvantaged	Access to care, multiple competing needs, low literacy, capacity to follow complex regimens
Transience	Stability of care, chaotic life stressors
Declining health	Undermined perceived benefits, panic, battle fatigue

tuberculosis has become a significant global health threat. Although multiple drug resistant tuberculosis resulted from a complex interaction of several factors, a lack of prompt and consistent treatment likely contributed to the severity of this problem (Hopewell, 1997). Incomplete courses of antibiotics in treating other bacterial infections as well as possibly antiviral drugs for viral infections potentially lead to the development of drug resistance.

Failure to adhere to treatment schedules is particularly troublesome with protease inhibitors because of HIV's ability to rapidly develop resistance to these drugs. The high rate of genetic mutations that occur in the context of rapid rates of viral replication accounts for HIV's ability to develop drug resistance. Risks for resistance are reduced with combination therapies because HIV is genetically limited in its ability to mutate simultaneously at multiple, coordinated genetic sites (Ho, 1996). Nonadherence with schedules for taking treatments affords HIV the opportunity to mutate and increases the likelihood of developing resistance to protease inhibitors as well as other anti-HIV medications. Once resistance to one particular antiretroviral drug has occurred, a strain of HIV may be resistant to the other treatments. The potential for cross-resistance may cause some people to wait before starting on a particular regimen.

Interventions for Nonadherence

Interventions to assist people in adhering to antiretroviral schedules have been adapted from behavioral medicine applications for other chronic illnesses. Table 3.5 summarizes factors to include in interventions for enhancing adherence to antiretroviral therapies as adapted from Hecht (1997). Daily calendars, for example, can be used to outline optimal meal schedules, dietary considerations, and dosing schedules for various combinations of drugs. Structuring daily activities around treatment can help establish treatment plans to assure that work schedules, vacations, travel, and time zone changes do not interfere with treatment. Planning ahead for possible interruptions to treatment can head off lapses in dosing. Devices such as timers and alarms also increase adherence with antiretroviral medications (Besch, 1995). A tech-

Table 3.5

Elements to Include in Medication Adherence Interventions

Risk Factor	Intervention
Patient motivation	Formulate realistic treatment goals
	Emphasize importance of adherence in achieving goals
Clarify instructions	Write instructions
	List names of drugs with instructions
	Structure doses and times with special instructions
Anticipate side effects	Prepare patient for side effects
	Develop strategies to manage side effects ahead of time
Lifestyle tailoring	Select a regimen that fits the patient—times, meals, and so forth
	Establish environmental cues for doses
	Integrate doses into daily routines
	Specify a place for keeping medications
	Develop patient-centered systems for medications
Prepare for changes in routine	Educate about how doses are linked to routines
	Plan ahead for vacations, weekends, life changes
	Problem solve changes in routines to not interfere with adherence
Simplify the regimen	Decrease numbers of pills and numbers of doses as much as possible
	Eliminate any unnecessary medications
	Reduce complexity of dosing and times
Address indirect problems	Treat depression and substance abuse
	Bolster realistic optimism
	Build positive relationships with providers

NOTE: Data is from Hecht (1997).

nology is evolving around adherence-enhancing devices, with drug bottle caps that beep or vibrate becoming widely available. Incorporating medications into daily routines and activities can also enhance adherence. Morse et al. (1991) found that nonadherence was greatest when anti-HIV therapies interfered with the daily lives of patients. Mapping medication schedules onto daily routines can be accomplished through the use of diaries, self-monitoring techniques, and calendars. Self-generated cues from one's daily life can be used for linking medication schedules to routine activities, creating a structure and system to support medication adherence.

Other interventions can also help people cope with the side effects that can lead to nonadherence with antiretrovirals. In particular, counseling may have added benefits of reducing risks for missing treatment dosing. Cognitive restructuring, relaxation training, and other techniques that have been useful in helping people adjust to medications can be useful for people taking antiretroviral drugs. Behavioral interventions for reducing nausea and vomiting that have been shown effective with cancer chemotherapy patients may be particularly important for gastrointestinal symptoms because some protease inhibitors interact with antiemetic medications. Among the cognitive and behavioral techniques that have been most widely used with cancer chemotherapy patients, progressive muscle-relaxation training combined with guided imagery seem most promising for reducing anxiety associated with treatment and the onset of side effects. Instructions for taking antiretrovirals can include practicing relaxation techniques before and after administering medications to gain a sense of control and distract attention away from potential side effects.

Because positive outcome expectancies are closely associated with treatment adherence, cognitive therapy and psychoeducational interventions can help bolster optimistic beliefs about treatment that are required of any long-term medical treatment. Cognitive restructuring to address negative thoughts about treatment can help keep the focus on treatment promises and reinforce adherence. Counseling and psychotherapy can improve the relationship between clients and medical providers. Developing a coparticipant role in one's own care is one of the most effective means of achieving consistent adherence to treatment (Sikkema & Kelly, 1996). Such techniques as discussing ways to become involved in one's own treatment and using role plays to help gain experience and confidence in being assertive with providers can also help improve adherence (Besch, 1995).

Finally, improving treatment adherence often requires building social supports for adhering to medication schedules. Nonadherence with anti-HIV treatments often occurs in the context of poor social support and social isolation (Besch, 1995). Family members, friends, and other significant people can be integrated into treatment regimens, helping to establish treatment routines and encouraging individuals to take their medications. Support groups can also reinforce medication adherence and provide feedback from peers regarding strategies for improving adherence. Many AIDS service organizations and infectious disease clinics offer buddy programs, where peers are assigned to provide check-ins and even daily reminders for taking medications, preventing lapses in treatment and providing ongoing support for resolving barriers to maintaining treatment adherence.

CONCLUSION

The short history of AIDS has seen many hopes and disappointments. The discovery of HIV as the cause of AIDS, for example, led many people to believe that a cure was surely near. Another example of renewed hope was when studies showed that AZT could slow the progression of HIV infection to AIDS. In each case, the evasive nature of HIV has become more apparent. The luxury of early optimism has been replaced by the cynicism that AIDS will likely get much worse before it gets any better. Although new treatments continue to bring renewed hope, the word *cure* is no longer in the AIDS lexicon. Instead of cure, the greatest hope is for *control*: both control over the spread of HIV and control over damage to the immune system that HIV causes.

The promise of treatment advances can only be kept when people who could most benefit from the drugs can actually access them. The vast majority of people in the world with AIDS do not in fact have access to even the most basic AIDS care. Relatively inexpensive pro-phylaxis against common opportunistic illnesses such as TB and PCP are unavailable in many countries with the greatest numbers of AIDS cases. Even worse is access to antiretroviral medications. An inability to access treatments creates inequities among people with HIV–AIDS—the source of resentment, anger, and despair. Thus, in concert with a deteriorating immune system and advancing stages of illness, there are numerous psychological and social manifestations of HIV–AIDS.

PART TWO

Psychological, Neuropsychological, and Social Sequelae

Ivan Illyich saw that he was dying, and he was in a constant state of despair. In the depth of his heart he knew he was dying, but not only was he unaccustomed to such an idea, he simply could not grasp it at all.

(Leo Tolstoy, 1886/1981, p. 93)

It was difficult, at times, for me to handle, but I tried to ignore the injustice, because I know the people were wrong. My family and I held no hatred for these people because we realized they were the victims of their own injustice. We had great faith that, with patience, understanding, and education, that my family and I could be helpful in changing their minds and attitudes around.

(Ryan White, Testimony before the President's Commission on AIDS 1987)

4

Psychological Sequelae

The threats of HIV infection to mental health, social relationships, and quality of life were well recognized early in the AIDS epidemic (Coates, Temoshok, & Mandel, 1984; Morin & Batchelor, 1984). The first studies of psychological adjustment to HIV infection found that HIV infected individuals experience significant emotional distress in response to testing HIV positive (e.g., Dilley, Ochitill, Perl, & Volberding, 1985; Donlou, Wolcott, Gottlieb, & Landsverk, 1985; Perry & Tross, 1984). The range of psychological aftermath of HIV infection is as broad as the HIV disease spectrum itself. Even acute psychotic reactions are among the most extreme responses to having HIV (Halstead, Riccio, Harlow, Oretti, & Thompson, 1988; Sewell et al., 1994). Factors such as stress, psychological disturbances predating HIV infection, comorbid substance abuse, and social displacement increase the psychological vulnerability that often occurs with any life-threatening illness.

This chapter focuses on the emotional reactions and behavioral responses that are common to HIV infection. First, stress is discussed as a contributing factor in emotionally adjusting to HIV. Second, emotional reactions related to HIV infection are reviewed at each phase of the disease. Third, the psychological sequelae of HIV infection are discussed, highlighting findings from empirical studies. Finally, an overview of the relationship between emotional distress and physical health is presented, focusing on interactions between stress, emotional responses, and the immune system.

THE STRESS CONTEXT OF HIV–AIDS

Stress occurs at multiple points of the HIV spectrum. The stress of having HIV is embedded in a context of preexisting stressors. As illustrated in Figure 4.1, people at risk for HIV may experience stress by

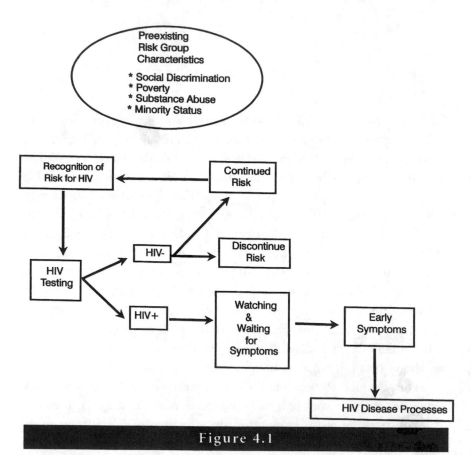

Figure 4.1

Conceptual framework of stressors related to HIV–AIDS.

virtue of recognizing their potential for becoming HIV infected. HIV testing itself is experienced as a significant stressor, particularly during the 2 to 3 weeks of waiting for test results. Upon testing HIV seropositive, individuals must face being diagnosed with a life threatening, stigmatized chronic illness. The course of HIV disease is cluttered with stressors that include symptoms, medical decision making, disclosure of HIV status, and the challenges of managing a life with HIV. However, the effects of stress on emotional well-being are complex and potentially mediated by psychosocial resources. Of particular importance are individual differences in coping styles and cognitive attribution processes.

AIDS affects people from diverse ethnic, socioeconomic, and sociocultural backgrounds. It is therefore meaningful to discuss HIV-related stressors with respect to specific communities and subpopulations. The sections below review the preexisting social contexts relevant to men who have sex with men, people living in urban environments, women, and adults with preexisting mental illness.

Men Who Have Sex With Men

Men who have sex with men have long been recognized as a socially stigmatized sexual minority (Solomon et al., 1991). It is common for families to reject homosexual members and for gay men to experience harassment and violence. Homophobia has subsequently been amplified by the AIDS crisis, both from outside and within gay communities. Among gay and bisexual men, it is common to assume personal responsibility for AIDS. However, finger pointing and condemnation, such as when people are labeled *hustlers, cruisers,* or *tricks,* fragment communities. Thus, blaming gay men for AIDS originates from outsiders and can become internalized.

HIV is a major source of stress for gay men living in most urban areas (Noh, Chandarana, Field, & Posthuma, 1990). Folkman, Chesney, Pollack, and Phillips (1992) found that the top five most stressful life domains for homosexual and bisexual men included illness of close friends and monitoring personal health. HIV-seropositive African American men who have sex with men report multiple stressful events, with most occurring in relation to work, family, finances, and friendships (Peterson, Folkman, & Bakeman, 1996). In a large study of self-identified gay men, D. Martin (1993) also observed five dimensions using a factor analysis of a threat-perception questionnaire: threats to personal goals and aspirations for the future, personal appearance, integrity, health, and the health of friends and partners. Although many sources of stress identified by Folkman et al. and Martin are not caused directly by HIV, the epidemic has created a new context for events that were previously stressful.

Cultural and ethnic differences within gay communities may lead to additional stress for gay men of color. Homophobia is more open among some ethnic minorities, fostering overt rejection. It is therefore common for ethnic minority men to report stress related to accepting their own sexual orientation (Ceballos-Capitaine et al., 1990). A large number of ethnic minority men who have sex with men do not label themselves as gay and thereby remain disconnected from gay social networks, limiting their ability to access information available through gay newspapers, brochures, and outreach to gay bars and organizations. Cultural differences, prejudices, and an absence of well-organized ethnic minority gay communities leads to social isolation of many gay men of color.

The Urban Environment

The majority of U.S. AIDS cases have been diagnosed in large urban centers. That urban areas are most affected by HIV is not unique to this epidemic. Congested living conditions, poor health resources, poverty, and relatively closed social and sexual networks all increase the potential for rapid spread of disease. Inner cities have been particularly vulnerable to AIDS because injection drug use and gay and bisexual men are concentrated in urban centers. A combination of factors has therefore brought the AIDS crisis to urban centers.

People with injection-drug-using addictions are well recognized as a socially marginalized group. Injection drug users are generally rejected and mistrusted on the basis of their drug use alone (Des Jarlais, Friedman, & Stoneburner, 1988). Socioeconomic stressors that coexist with injection drug use, social stigmas associated with drug addiction, and addiction to drugs itself complicate living with HIV–AIDS (Des Jarlais, Friedman, & Casriel, 1990; D. Miller & Pinching, 1989). As a group, injection drug users live generally chaotic, impoverished lives (D. Miller & Pinching, 1989). Drug use is therefore often a means of psychological escape from the inner city and poverty.

Women and men living in inner cities often lack access to resources that facilitate coping with HIV infection including access to health care (Jillson-Boostrom, 1992). Even when health care is available, services may not reach the inner-city poor. Sociopolitical abuses of the past have created barriers for many disadvantaged groups. For example, the Tuskegee Syphilis Study, which observed the natural history of untreated syphilis in a cohort of African Americans, has left many scars on the relationship between minorities and public health services. The remnants of Tuskegee deter African Americans from seeking public health services (Thomas & Quinn, 1991). Moreover, because of such events as the Tuskegee Study, ethnic minorities frequently express the belief that HIV is a means of oppression, as well as a form of genocide (Thomas & Quinn, 1991).

The social context of AIDS, particularly in urban areas, forms a complex hierarchy of competing life stressors and survival needs, of which AIDS is one of several. In a study of women living in Chicago, Kalichman, Hunter, and Kelly (1992) examined the relationships among stress-related social problems facing urban women. Several life stressors were perceived as more immediately pressing than AIDS, including employment, child care, and crime. Kalichman et al. also found that each social problem was perceived as a more serious concern for minorities than for nonminorities.

In a follow-up study, Kalichman, Somlai, Adair, and Weir (1996) conducted a similar survey of men and women receiving treatment for sexually transmitted diseases, 78% of whom were African American and 74% of whom were living in poverty. Because the sample was drawn from a clinic, it was thought that the participants would be more sensitized to AIDS than a general community sample. Men and women rated 11 social problems along dimensions of perceived seriousness. Results replicated the Kalichman et al. (1992) findings by showing that

AIDS was perceived as a greater concern than housing, alcoholism, and child care, but less of a problem than employment, crime, discrimination, drug abuse, and teen pregnancy. Using factor analyses, Kalichman et al. showed that perceptions of AIDS as a social problem were closely associated with other social problems. AIDS is therefore inextricably intertwined with a myriad of social problems plaguing inner cities, factors that will complicate adjusting to an HIV diagnosis.

Women

Women constitute another special population within the AIDS epidemic. Injection drug use has infected nearly half of women with HIV, and one in five women with AIDS contracted the virus by having sex with an injection-drug-using partner. Women infected with HIV are predominantly ethnic minorities and therefore face prejudices and discriminations placed on members of all three subgroups: minorities, women, and people with HIV (Minkoff & DeHovitz, 1991). Women with HIV often have multiple preexisting psychological and social problems that become compounded by their diagnosis of HIV infection (Catalan et al., 1996). Women who use injection drugs, both HIV seropositive and HIV seronegative, experience greater psychological distress than men (Rabkin, Johnson, Lin, et al., 1997). Women may experience stress from verbal and physical abuse as a result of initiating safer sexual practices (Wingood & DiClemente, 1997). HIV-seropositive women may have limited access to health care and may be unable to obtain treatment for HIV infection in a timely manner (Ickovics & Rodin, 1992). Another major source of stress among HIV-infected women is the possibility of becoming pregnant after infection or dealing with an existing pregnancy. For many women, the connection between HIV infection and pregnancy is immediate because prenatal clinics routinely conduct HIV screening.

Women are unlikely to have prior experience discussing HIV testing with a health-care provider and may be offered testing only after they are already pregnant (Minkoff & DeHovitz, 1991). Women who learn they are HIV seropositive early in a pregnancy must decide whether they should terminate the pregnancy. HIV-seropositive women often experience feeling guilty because of the potential harm caused to their unborn. HIV-seropositive pregnant women must also face several complicated treatment decisions, particularly those involving antiretroviral therapies to prevent perinatal HIV transmission.

Women with HIV infection who already have families face several stressful decisions. Studies of families with injection drug users have shown that women are most often the primary caregiver (Carr, 1975; Michaels & Levine, 1992). Women may be caregivers in families where their spouse is also HIV infected, and they may have an HIV-seropositive child, necessitating women to balance their own care with the needs of their family (Minkoff & DeHovitz, 1991). HIV-seropositive women with uninfected partners may be rejected, emotionally isolated, and financially disconnected. Many women with HIV infection are single parents and must plan for the long-term safety, shelter, and care of their children. The number of children and adolescents orphaned by AIDS is growing at a rapid pace, with over 45,000 orphans estimated at the end of 1995 (Michaels & Levine, 1992). Concerns for the future of their children are among the most pressing issues for HIV-seropositive mothers (Hackl et al., 1997).

The Seriously Mentally Ill

In a prospective study conducted among persons at risk for HIV infection, Perry, Jacobsberg, Fishman, Frances, et al. (1990) found high rates of psychological disturbances among HIV risk groups prior to receiving their HIV test results. Lifetime rates of psychiatric syndromes were roughly two times that of epidemiologic studies. Among those who tested HIV seropositive, the rates were nearly seven times as high as epidemiologic studies. High rates of psychological problems suggest substantial vulnerability to psychological distress and maladjustment for many people with HIV infection (Perry, Jacobsberg, Fishman, Frances, et al.).

There is also considerable overlap between characteristics of HIV risk groups and mental disorders. In particular, injection drug use is closely associated with antisocial personality disorder (Brooner, Greenfield, Schmidt, & Bigelow, 1993). Studies also suggest higher rates of bipolar affective and substance-abuse disorders among homosexually active men at risk for HIV infection (Perry, Jacobsberg, Fishman, Frances, et al., 1990; Pillard, 1988). Nearly one third of HIV-seropositive gay men in one study had a personality disorder diagnosis, a significantly higher rate than HIV-seronegative gay men (Perkins, Davidson, Leserman, Liao, & Evans, 1993). A study of volunteers for HIV antibody testing found that one third of people who tested HIV seropositive had preexisting personality disorders, compared to one in five who tested seronegative (Jacobsberg, Frances, & Perry, 1995). Of those who tested HIV seropositive, antisocial personality was the most frequently diagnosed disorder. Comorbidity of psychiatric history and HIV infection can complicate the course of illness by disrupting treatment and increasing the need for hospitalization (Uldall et al., 1994).

Recent research has focused on the HIV risk of persistently mentally ill adults. A majority of mentally ill adults are sexually active, frequently contract sexually transmitted infections, and often exhibit other HIV risk behaviors (Kalichman, Kelly, Johnson, & Bulto, 1994). Patterns of HIV risk among seriously mentally ill adults are particularly alarming because they occur in the context of high rates of HIV infection, with HIV seroprevalence as high as 7% for psychiatric inpatients, between 6% and 19% in homeless adults with psychiatric disorders, and 10% among alcohol-rehabilitation patients (M. P. Carey, Weinhardt, & Carey, 1995).

Several factors contribute to HIV risk among seriously mentally ill adults, including a lack of accurate information about HIV transmission, misperceptions of personal risk, failure to recognize risk-producing situations, and difficulty communicating assertively in sexual relationships (Carey, Carey, & Kalichman, 1997; Hanson et al., 1992). In addition, seriously mentally ill adults may be particularly vulnerable to contracting HIV because of impulsive sexual behaviors, relationships characterized by turmoil and transience, and the overlap among risk taking, psychopathology, and cognitive disturbances that leads to poor judgment (Carmen & Brady, 1990; Lyketsos, Hanson, et al., 1993). In summary, a large number of people at risk for HIV infection have preexisting mental health problems, and many of the stressors known to exist in inner cities, including poverty, substance abuse, and multiple competing survival needs, apply to persistently mentally ill adults. However, limited cognitive functions and coping resources among people with histories of serious mental illness will exacerbate the stress of HIV infection.

RECEIVING A POSITIVE HIV TEST RESULT

Initial reactions to receiving a positive HIV test result are characterized by shock and denial. Receiving a positive result can be so traumatic that it is nearly impossible for people to retain information provided to them during posttest counseling (D. Grant & Anns, 1988; Perry & Markowitz, 1988; Perry et al., 1993). Shortly after the immediate shock, people who test HIV positive experience anger, reactive depression, obsessive concerns about health, and generalized anxiety (Huggins, Elman, Baker, Forrester, & Lyter, 1991).

Following initial reactions to testing positive begins the process of adjusting to a life with HIV infection. In a prospective study of people at risk for HIV infection, Perry, Jacobsberg, Fishman, Weiler, et al. (1990) assessed emotional distress before, immediately after, and at 2 weeks and 10 weeks following receipt of test results. Using visual analogue scales of affective disturbances where participants reported anxiety and fears along a continuum, the study showed that people who tested HIV seropositive were distressed immediately before and immediately after receiving their test results. However, distress significantly decreased 2 weeks and 10 weeks later. Concerns of having infected others and fears of developing AIDS, which were both high when receiving test results, decreased at the follow-up assessments. Ironson et al. (1990) reported similar findings in a prospective study of gay men who suffered substantial distress upon learning they were HIV seropositive, with emotional states normalizing within 5 weeks after notification. In a study of women in the U.S. military, G. Brown and Rundell (1990) found a similar pattern of adjustment after testing HIV positive. In summary, testing HIV seropositive is a traumatic event, but most who test positive show evidence of adapting to their condition within weeks following test result notification.

Reactions to testing positive are influenced by the manner in which results are delivered. One study found that 23% of people who test HIV positive view the delivery of results as unclear, insensitive, and unkind (McCann & Wadsworth, 1991). The psychological effects of testing HIV seropositive also depend on where a person is in the HIV disease spectrum. People who test HIV seropositive early in the disease and in the absence of clinical symptoms become concerned about the possibility of developing symptoms and of someday having AIDS. The situation, however, is quite different for people who wait to get tested until they have symptoms. Beevor and Catalan (1993) found that, although women who test HIV seronegative are most likely motivated to get tested by their past behaviors, many women who test positive are motivated to get tested by developing symptoms. News of being infected with HIV when already symptomatic shortens the timeline for developing AIDS, and notification of HIV infection can occur simultaneously with an AIDS diagnosis.

HIV-RELATED STRESSORS

HIV infection is a lifelong condition that results in physical decline and has a very high mortality rate. Upon testing HIV positive, people must face threats to their long-term survival, the necessity of making immediate lifestyle changes, fears of potentially infecting others, health concerns, access to treatment, changes in appearance, and declining quality of life. HIV infection invariably involves a pervasive uncertainty about when opportunistic illnesses will strike. These uncertainties are exacerbated by long asymptomatic periods permeated by illnesses. Symptoms appear and disappear, keeping patients on a constant watch. Coupled with uncertainties about disease progression is the loss of control over directing one's own future. People who test HIV positive know that they may have a debilitating and life-threatening illness at any time.

Long asymptomatic periods are ultimately followed by symptomatic illnesses. During symptomatic HIV infection, almost any sign of illness can elevate anxiety. Distress, however, depends on where an individual is located in the spectrum of HIV disease. It is common for people to closely monitor their CD4 cell counts and viral load. Early symptoms serve as reminders that HIV is degrading the immune system and that the virus is becoming an increased threat. For women and men with children, becoming ill has the added burden of demanding assistance with childcare and anticipating their children's future.

The first signs of developing an opportunistic illness can cause acute distress, reminiscent of when one first tests HIV positive. For example, a 7-year longitudinal study of gay and bisexual men in New York City found that knowledge of HIV seropositivity and developing symptoms were associated with depression, traumatic stress reactions, suicidal ideations, and increased use of sedatives (J. L. Martin & Dean, 1993). These findings suggest that HIV-related illnesses contribute to maladjustment, including depression, anxiety, and preoccupations with AIDS (Mulder & Antoni, 1992).

HIV-related psychological distress also occurs in response to concerns over medical treatments aimed at controlling HIV infection. Multiple hospitalizations, intrusive treatments, side effects, and uncertainty over treatment effectiveness are common sources of stress (Solomon et al., 1991). The need to take medications, usually in large amounts taken several times a day, can continually disrupt efforts to cope (D. Miller & Pinching, 1989). Contributing further to distress associated with treatments is that they are taken with uncertainty and without potential to cure.

THE HIV DISEASE TRAJECTORY

AIDS is like cancer with respect to its life-threatening nature, lifelong duration, illness concerns, and existential issues (Chuang, Devins, Hunsley, & Gill, 1989; Faulstich, 1987). Like cancer, HIV infection is related to physical decline, bodily disfigurement, loss of physical functioning, emotional anguish, financial crisis, pain, and death; both cancer and AIDS are catastrophic (McCorkle & Quint-Benoliel, 1983). The course of cancer and many other life-threatening diseases, however, includes the availability of multiple curative treatments. J. Holland (1982) discussed four possible clinical courses of cancer: (a) a successful curative attempt that results in no recurrent disease, (b) a curative attempt with response but with later recurrence of disease, (c) a curative attempt and no effective response, and (d) no curative attempt (see Figure 4.2). The chance for a cure in three of the four courses offers hope. Thus, psychological adjustment to a life-threatening disease is influenced by the degree to which there are real possibilities for cure.

In contrast to cancer, it is not possible to offer curative attempts for HIV infection. The clinical course of HIV infection is therefore significantly different from that of other diseases. Although HIV-related illnesses are treated, and lives are extended, illnesses signify the underlying HIV disease process. At best, people can receive HIV–AIDS treatment in hope that they will live to the next generation of drugs and perhaps a cure. Symptomatic illness can be treated until, ultimately, there are no treatment responses and death ensues (see Figure 4.3). The prospect of persistent opportunistic illnesses in the midst of a degenerating immune system, therefore, poses a relentless succession of challenges over the course of HIV infection.

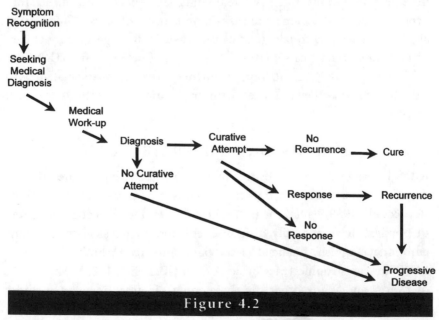

Figure 4.2

J. Holland's (1982) descriptive model of possible clinical courses of cancer.

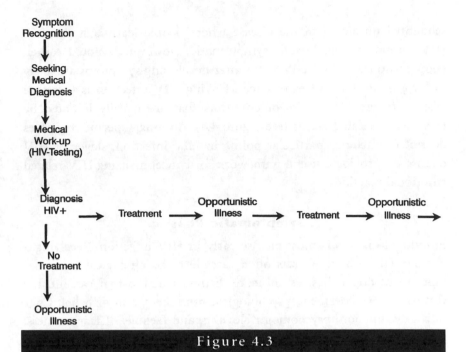

Figure 4.3

Descriptive model of possible clinical courses of HIV infection adapted from J. Holland (1982).

EMOTIONAL REACTIONS AT EACH PHASE OF HIV INFECTION

The psychological dimensions of HIV infection occur in the context of phases of HIV disease progression. Although there are several cohort studies of HIV-seropositive people, only a few have reported changes in psychological functioning over the natural history of HIV infection and none have done so for women. Psychological reactions are usually reported at one point in time, such as notification of HIV test results, asymptomatic periods, the onset of early symptoms, or during AIDS. An approximate chronological representation of emotional well being therefore follows the three major phases of HIV infection: absence of detectable symptoms, onset of early symptoms, and late illness. A framework for the psychological sequelae of HIV infection assumes a sequential unfolding of the disease where people learn that they are HIV seropositive while still asymptomatic. However, as noted earlier, people who learn their HIV status after developing symptoms are likely to have quite different experiences. Having HIV infection is therefore best represented by cycles of emotions that are usually initiated by HIV–AIDS-related events (see Figure 4.4). Although specific responses do not characterize particular points in HIV infection, stages of HIV disease do provide a useful framework for conceptualizing HIV-related emotional reactions.

Asymptomatic Phases

Emotional distress is most intense early in HIV infection. Receiving a positive HIV test result sets off a cascade of psychological responses that are described best as an acute distress reaction that can include confusion, bewilderment, psychological numbness, and disbelief. Cognitive dysfunction, psychomotor slowing, and feelings of fear, sadness, guilt, and anger are also common (Catalan, 1988; Ostrow, 1989). Atkinson et al. (1988) reported that most people with HIV infection who develop generalized anxiety disorder report the onset of symptoms at the time of HIV serologic testing. Similarly, Maj (1990) reported that as many as 90% of people recently diagnosed with HIV infection experience an acute distress reaction.

Acute distress following an HIV seropositive test result frequently includes symptoms of depression. Perry, Fishman, Jacobsberg, and Frances (1992) found that more than one third of people with early HIV infection showed signs of immediate emotional distress. Similarly, Cleary, Van Devanter, et al. (1993) reported that 31% of HIV-seropositive blood donors are clinically depressed at the time that they received their test results and remain depressed for at least 2 weeks. Hopelessness, maladaptive coping behaviors, health-compromising behaviors, and increased potential for suicide have all been observed early in the course of HIV infection (Glass, 1988; Ostrow, 1990).

Prospective research has shown that emotional distress declines over the course of HIV infection. Rabkin et al. (1991) found that symptoms of depression and generalized anxiety significantly declined over a 6-

month period. Cleary, Van Devanter, et al. (1993) also reported reduced depression shortly following HIV test result notification, with similar declines in distress following HIV diagnosis reported by other investigators (e.g., Kessler et al., 1988). Most compelling, however, was Perry et al.'s (1993) longitudinal study in New York City that showed severity of depression in HIV-seropositive individuals significantly declined 6 months after testing positive. In this study, emotional distress 1 year after receiving HIV-positive results did not significantly differ from HIV-seronegative individuals. In another study, Hintz, Kuck, Peterkin, Volk, and Zisook (1990) reported that people who were HIV seropositive and asymptomatic responded more favorably to antide-

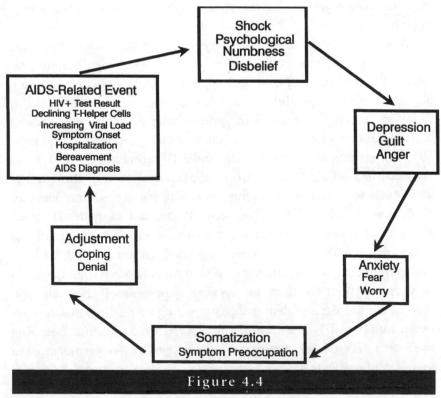

Figure 4.4

Emotional reaction cycles over the course of HIV disease.

pressant medications than did people with early and late symptomatic HIV disease.

Early Symptomatic Phases

The onset of HIV-related symptoms brings a new meaning and urgency to being HIV seropositive. The first signs of illness can cause a resurgence of depression, anxiety, somatization, and other mood disturbances. Early symptoms of HIV can lead to generalized anxiety, despair, and physical preoccupation (Hinkin et al., 1992; J. L. Martin & Dean, 1993). The first signs of illness signal the progression of HIV infection and, therefore, stimulate thoughts of soon developing AIDS. Symptoms may also fuel beliefs that medications and other treatments have not impeded the progression of the virus and may undermine adherence to treatment.

In addition to the first onset of symptoms, frequencies of illnesses elicit emotional reactions. Symptoms of HIV–AIDS significantly correlate with emotional distress and subjective impressions of declining physical health (Hays, Turner, & Coates, 1992; Kelly, Murphy, Bahr, Koob, et al., 1993). People with symptomatic HIV infection present more symptoms of depression and anxiety than both people who were HIV seropositive and asymptomatic and HIV seronegative (E. M. Martin, Robertson, et al., 1992). Ostrow, Monjan, et al. (1989) reported that individuals with HIV-related symptoms were five times more likely to be depressed. Belkin, Fleishman, Stein, Piette, and Mor (1992) found that 35% of people experiencing between four and eight constitutional symptoms of HIV infection were depressed, compared with 24% of those with three or less symptoms. Belkin et al. also reported that 64% of people with more than 14 physical symptoms of HIV infection showed clinical signs of depression, suggesting a linear relationship between number of HIV symptoms and levels of depression. Detecting one's own HIV-related symptoms such as swollen lymph nodes, skin lesions, and oral patches can lead directly to emotional turmoil (Kessler et al., 1988; Ostrow et al., 1986). Nevertheless, perceptions of symptoms alone do not explain dysphoria with advancing HIV disease, suggesting that multiple factors contribute to the association between illness and distress.

Later Symptomatic Phases and AIDS

Following an initial brief traumatic reaction to an AIDS diagnosis, many people living with AIDS are actually less distressed than people at both asymptomatic and early symptomatic phases of infection (Chuang et al., 1989; O'Dowd, Biderman, & McKegney, 1993), representing a different pattern than other chronic illnesses, where severity of depression usually increases with illness progression (e.g., Koenig, Meador, Cohen, & Blazer, 1988; Rodin & Voshart, 1986). Depression in other terminal illnesses increases over time because the course of disease tends to be persistently debilitating. In contrast, HIV infection cycles over long asymptomatic and then symptomatic periods. With a diagnosis of AIDS may come a sense of relief from now knowing the extent to which HIV has progressed (McKegney & O'Dowd, 1992). People with AIDS usually have had time to adjust to earlier diagnoses and symptoms. The distress of earlier HIV symptoms may build resiliency for subsequent diagnoses. Because HIV infection has long asymptomatic periods, people have often aged several years once they have AIDS, and older people tend to adjust better to chronic illness (Cassileth et al., 1984). Additional evidence that psychological distress does not increase over the course of HIV infection is offered by a prospective study of HIV seropositive men (Rabkin, Goetz, et al., 1997). Over the course of nine semiannual assessments, Rabkin et al. failed to show any increased rates of depressive symptoms or other distress over time. These results occurred despite significant progression of HIV illness. Seropositive men did increase their sense of hopelessness as illness progressed, demonstrating a reality-based perception of advancing HIV–AIDS.

Although many people with AIDS show extraordinary resilience to stress and adapt well to advancing HIV disease, many others are not free from significant emotional distress. Longitudinal research shows that physical symptoms and number of hospital days predict depressive symptoms in HIV-seropositive gay men (Siegel, Karus, & Raveis, 1997). Lyketsos et al. (1996) reported that depressive symptoms, both somatic and cognitive–affective symptoms, as well as syndromally diagnosed depression can develop approximately 1.5 years before diagnosis with AIDS and persist beyond receiving an AIDS diagnosis. This study concluded that depression clearly increases in frequency and severity as HIV–AIDS progresses. Belkin et al. (1992) found significant correlations between functional limitations, such as fatigue and loss of mobility, and both cognitive and affective symptoms of depression. Long-term survivors with AIDS indicate that the most intolerable aspects of HIV disease include the prospects of protracted pain, declining mental abilities, loss of vision, urinary incontinence, and loss of privacy and personal control (Rabkin, Wilson, & Kimpton, 1993). Cognitive disturbances from late-stage involvement of HIV in the central nervous system, potentially resulting in delirium and dementia, further complicate emotional health in later phases of HIV infection.

EMOTIONAL DISTRESS

Emotional reactions to HIV infection are as diverse as the epidemic itself. As discussed in the sections above, HIV-related events occur over the course of infection that serve as markers for vulnerability to emotional distress. People who receive HIV seropositive antibody test results undergo repeated medical examinations, must make critical treatment decisions, and are bombarded with information about health and illness. Thus, emotional turmoil can occur at any time, such as with the initiation of treatment, the development of symptoms, increases in viral load, the onset of opportunistic illnesses, hospitalizations, first AIDS-defining conditions, and declines in immunologic markers.

Simultaneous HIV-related events can be particularly emotionally devastating. People who seek HIV antibody testing after developing symptoms learn they have advanced HIV disease or AIDS. Advanced immune suppression will mean that a newly diagnosed person will simultaneously suffer opportunistic illnesses, exacerbating the already catastrophic event of testing HIV seropositive. Pregnant women who test HIV positive must face their own illness while managing the potential risks posed to their unborn. In contrast, when events of HIV infection occur sequentially over a longer period of time, distress reactions may be of less clinical significance (J. B. W. Williams, Rabkin, Remien, Gorman, & Ehrhardt, 1991).

Not surprisingly, the most frequently diagnosed clinical syndrome associated with HIV infection is adjustment disorder with features of anxious, depressed, or mixed mood (O'Dowd, Natali, Orr, & McKegney, 1991). O'Dowd et al. (1993) identified two thirds of people with HIV infection as having adjustment disorder. Rundell, Paolucci, Beatty, and Boswell (1988) diagnosed adjustment disorder in 64% of admissions to an Air Force HIV clinic. Chuang, Jason, Pajurkova, and Gill (1992) also found that the most prevalent psychiatric diagnosis in HIV infection is adjustment disorder, and this diagnosis best differentiated HIV seropositive from HIV seronegative individuals. O'Dowd and McKegney (1990) found that 42% of HIV-seropositive injection drug users, most of whom were women of color, were diagnosed with adjustment disorder. However, this rate was only slightly higher than that of a non-HIV-infected medical-patient comparison group. McKegney and O'Dowd (1992) reported that one third of patients with AIDS and other HIV seropositive patients referred for psychiatric evaluations were diagnosed with adjustment disorder, a rate comparable to non-HIV-infected medical patients. Interestingly, a similar situation exists for cancer patients, where 68% of patients with a *DSM-III-R* diagnosis have an adjustment disorder (Derogatis et al., 1983). These findings are influenced by the inclusion of an identified stressor, such as a medical illness, for the diagnosis of adjustment disorder. Depression, anxiety, somatization, and other emotional reactions, although not mutually exclusive, are addressed individually in the following sections.

Depression

Depression can be as or more debilitating than the chronic medical illnesses with which it is often associated (Hays, Wells, Sherbourne, Rogers, & Spitzer, 1995). Depression is common in people with cancer, with similar patterns observed in people with HIV–AIDS (Engel, 1980; S. E. Taylor & Aspinwall, 1990). However, affective disturbances often predate a diagnosis of HIV. For example, Perry, Jacobsberg, Fishman, Frances, et al. (1990) reported that 43% of men and 49% of women at risk for HIV infection who elected to undergo HIV antibody testing had a history of mood disorders, a rate nearly seven times that of age-matched community samples. Similarly, more than one third of injection drug users have depression unrelated to HIV infection (Tross & Hirsch, 1988), one third of HIV seronegative African American gay men report symptoms of depression (Cochran & Mays, 1994), one third of people with HIV infection report a lifetime history of depression (J. B. W. Williams et al., 1991), and HIV-seropositive military-benefit recipients evidence high lifetime rates of depression (M. A. Carey, Jenkins, Brown, Temoshok, & Pace, 1991).

Depression has been reported with great consistency in several studies of HIV-seropositive patients. Although less common than once believed, depression is among the most frequent responses to HIV infection (Rabkin, 1994). HIV-seropositive gay men (e.g., Cochran & Mays, 1994; Mulder et al., 1992), injection drug users (Lipsitz et al., 1994; Rabkin, Johnson, et al., 1997), army recruits (e.g., Ritchie & Radke, 1992), hemophiliacs (e.g., D. Miller & Riccio, 1990), as well as others (e.g., Perry et al., 1993; Perry, Jacobsberg, Fishman, Weiler, et al., 1990), are more likely depressed than non-HIV-infected populations. Dew, Ragni, and Nimorwicz (1990) reported that 42% of HIV-seropositive hemophiliacs met *DSM-III-R* criteria for depression, and Bornstein et al. (1993) found that 29% of asymptomatic gay men exceeded the clinical cutoff on the *Beck Depression Inventory*. Using the *Centers for Epidemiology Studies–Depression* (*CESD*), Kelly, Murphy, Bahr, Koob, et al. (1993) found that their sample of mostly gay men, all of whom were HIV seropositive, far exceeded the clinical cutoff for depression. Also using the *CESD*, Cochran and Mays (1994) found that 32% of asymptomatic and 47% of symptomatic HIV-seropositive gay men met the depression cutoff. Similarly, Cleary, Van Devanter, et al. (1993) found that 31% of HIV-seropositive blood donors exceeded the cutoff for depression on the *CESD* at the time of HIV-test result notification, as well as at follow-up assessments. Katz et al. (1996) also found 37% of HIV-seropositive men without AIDS exceeded the clinical cutoff for depression on the *CESD*.

Studies using clinical and diagnostic interviews to evaluate depression have obtained similar results. Atkinson et al. (1988) reported that 65% of people living with AIDS met diagnostic criteria for recurrent major depression. Also using psychiatric diagnoses, Bornstein et al. (1993) reported that 19% of HIV-seropositive gay and bisexual men had a *DSM-III-R* affective disorder. Similar results have been reported in other studies (e.g., Rabkin, Goetz, et al., 1997). Interpretation of these findings, however, must recognize the pre-HIV histories of depression supported in several studies. Lipsitz et al. (1994), for example, found that 30% of HIV-seropositive injection drug users were diagnosed with a depressive disorder, a rate considerably higher than community samples but not different from HIV-seronegative injectors.

Estimates of affective disorders in HIV-seropositive people, measured by both self-report and interview assessments, may be inflated because of symptom overlap between depression and HIV infection (Kalichman, Sikkema, & Somlai, 1995). To control for this potential confound, Belkin et al. (1992) used a depression screening instrument that was void of behavioral and physical symptoms of depression. Belkin et al. found that 41% of men and 54% of women with HIV infection still showed substantial evidence of depression, relative to 22% of non-HIV-infected primary care medical outpatients screened on the same instrument.

Although depressed mood is associated with HIV infection, some studies have found that relatively few HIV-seropositive people are clinically depressed. For example, Kessler et al. (1988) reported that only 12% of people with HIV infection scored beyond the psychiatric-outpatient mean on the *Hopkins Symptoms Checklist Depression Scale*, with most scores falling between psychiatric outpatients and the general population. Likewise, O'Dowd and McKegney (1990) reported that, although one third of injection drug users with AIDS were depressed, the rate of depression was similar to depression among HIV-seronegative medical patients. A study of gay men found similar rates of depression for HIV-seropositive and HIV-seronegative men; previous history of an affective disorder was the best predictor of depression regardless of HIV serostatus (Perkins et al., 1994). In two large cohorts, approximately one in five HIV-seropositive gay men exceeded the clinical cutoff on the *CESD* (Burrack et al., 1993; Lyketsos, Hoover, et al., 1993). Finally J. B. W. Williams et al. (1991) found that HIV-seropositive gay men scored relatively low on the *Hamilton Rating Scale for Depression*. Williams et al. also found that depression among HIV-seropositive men was not significantly different from depression observed in their HIV-negative counterparts. Therefore, although depression is common to HIV infection, affective disturbances are not universal and do not necessarily reach clinical proportions.

Golden, Gersh, and Robbins (1992) described four interactive dimensions of depression: (a) emotional–affective symptoms (e.g., sadness, crying), (b) cognitive symptoms (e.g., pessimism, negative beliefs), (c) behavioral symptoms (e.g., lethargy, diminished motivation), and (d) vegetative symptoms (e.g., anorexia, sleep disturbances). All four dimensions of depression are observed in depressed HIV-seropositive people, expressed in sadness, demoralization, diminished self-esteem, sense of worthlessness, disturbances in eating and sleeping, psychomotor retardation, and social withdrawal (Treisman, Lyketsos, Fishman, & McHugh, 1993). Some features, however, are particularly prominent in clinically and subclinically depressed people with HIV infection. For example, depressed affect was the most frequently endorsed indicator of depression on the *CESD* in the Chicago Multicenter AIDS cohort (MAC; Ostrow et al., 1986). Bornstein et al. (1993) noted that psychomotor slowing in depression has a significant effect on concentration, attention, and memory and could lead to illusory concerns about early HIV encephalopathy. However, depression has not been reliably associated with neuropsychological test performance decrements in people with HIV infection.

Social disturbances are another common feature in HIV-related depression. It is well recognized that social supports insulate people from depression. HIV-seropositive men with greater social supports, for example, experience less depressive symptomatology (Katz et al., 1996). Because HIV infection has thus far been concentrated in groups that are socially marginalized, individuals with HIV infection may be particularly vulnerable to depression. Social relationships can influence depressed mood in important ways. Men who identify themselves as exclusively homosexual report less depression than do bisexual men (Ostrow, Joseph, et al., 1989), possibly explained by stronger bonds to supportive networks in gay communities and opportunities to establish secure relationships. Social integration may therefore affect the prevalence and course of depression in people with HIV infection (Kiecolt-Glaser et al., 1987).

Hopelessness is another feature of depression particularly relevant to HIV infection. Rabkin, Williams, Neugebauer, Remien, and Goetz (1990) provided the most extensive study of hopelessness in people with HIV–AIDS. Among HIV-seropositive gay men in New York City, Rabkin et al. found that 24% had obtained elevated scores on the *Beck Hopelessness Scale*, classifying them with moderate to severe hopelessness. Rabkin et al. also found that hopelessness was closely related to depression, over and above the number of HIV symptoms. This is an important finding because unlike most measures of depression, including the *Beck Depression Inventory*, hopelessness is primarily a cognitive and affective response, uncontaminated by overlapping physical symptoms. Rabkin, Goetz, et al. (1997) extended these findings to show that hopelessness increases as HIV illness advances. D. Miller and Riccio (1990) reported similar findings in a study of hopelessness among HIV-seropositive hemophiliacs.

Similar to hopelessness, lack of perceived control over the course of HIV infection is related to the onset and course of depression. Recognizing the limitations of anti-HIV treatments, for example, correlates with depression in HIV-seropositive blood donors (Cleary, Van Devanter, et al., 1993). Female blood donors with HIV infection who experience little control over the course of HIV infection are more inclined to report feeling depressed (Cleary, Van Devanter, et al., 1993). Kelly, Murphy, Bahr, Koob, et al. (1993) showed that attributing the progress of HIV–AIDS to external forces significantly predicts *CESD* scores, over and above number of HIV symptoms and length of time since testing HIV seropositive.

In summary, many people living with HIV–AIDS have preexisting histories of depression. The social isolation of AIDS and the fact that

HIV is a chronic life-threatening illness increase vulnerability to depression. Illness and non-illness-related events, particularly declining health and other losses, also complicate depression in HIV–AIDS.

Social Losses, Grief, and Bereavement

A positive HIV-antibody test result can lead to loss of employment, the threat of eviction, denial of health and life insurance, refusal of professional services, and loss of health and dental care. Table 4.1 summarizes the potential sources of social loss associated with HIV infection. It is indeed unfortunate that many people with HIV suffer disruptions to their most intimate relationships. Sexual practices entail protecting sex

Table 4.1
Losses Associated With HIV Infection–AIDS

Loss	Cause of Loss
Employment	Infection status or disability
Family	Fears and stigmas or inability to cope
Friends	Fears and stigmas, inability to cope or to face AIDS-related death
Health care	Inability to obtain insurance benefits
Financial	Health care costs coupled with diminished employment
Social supports	Fears and stigmas or inability to cope
Self-esteem and pride	Self-blame for the epidemic and personal infection
Physical/affectionate contact	Irrational fears of casual transmission
Future goals and aspirations	Facing a chronic life threatening illness
Sexual partners	Fears or inability to cope
Physical functioning	Disease progression
Pets	Potential to carry pathogens
Lifestyle changes	Potential ill effects on health, such as smoking and alcohol use

partners from infection, as well as protecting people with HIV from reinfection and exposure to other sexually transmitted infections. Disclosure of HIV infection to a partner for his or her protection may place people at risk for violent repercussions (Wingood & DiClemente, 1997). Fears of losing a partner at a time when support is most needed may therefore inhibit disclosing serostatus altogether.

The most common source of loss for many HIV seropositive people is the death of partners and friends to AIDS. Complex cognitive, affective, and behavioral reactions occur in response to losing someone (Calabrese, Kling, & Gold, 1987). Thus far, multiple bereavement resulting from AIDS-related deaths have been observed mostly in gay men. In a large Chicago cohort studied relatively early in the epidemic, 45% of gay men reported knowing someone with AIDS, and 35% knew someone who had died of AIDS (Kessler et al., 1988). In a cohort of over 700 gay men who have sex with men in New York City who were asymptomatic for HIV-related illnesses, 27% had lost a sex partner or close friend to AIDS (J. L. Martin, 1988). Among those classified as bereaved, 18% lost two and 15% lost three or more people to AIDS. When J. L. Martin included men who lost any friends to AIDS, 52% of the cohort was considered bereaved. Perry, Fishman, Jacobsberg, and Frances (1992) also found 55% of people with HIV infection in New York City to have suffered the death of someone because of AIDS. Similarly, a study of gay and bisexual men in New York City found that more than half had lost one close friend to AIDS, 11% reported two such losses, and 18% had lost three or more close friends (Neugebauer et al., 1992). Although multiple losses occur frequently in high-AIDS-incidence areas, men who are HIV infected themselves suffer the greatest number of AIDS-related losses; the fact that HIV is spread through social–sexual networks increases this likelihood.

Bereavement is a well known, multidimensional source of stress, and multiple losses have additive effects. J. L. Martin (1988) described a dose response relationship between psychological trauma and the number of bereavements from AIDS a person suffers. Martin observed demoralization, sleep disruptions, affective disturbances, intrusive thoughts, and illicit and prescription drug use that increased proportionally with numbers of AIDS-related deaths. Following the same co-hort studied by J. L. Martin (1988), J. L. Martin and Dean (1992) identified persistent distress among both HIV-seropositive and HIV-seronegative gay men. Men who lost someone to AIDS at any point in this 7-year study showed the greatest signs of trauma, and emotional distress increased in conjunction with the number of losses suffered. Similar results were reported by Neugebauer et al. (1992), finding an increased number of bereavement symptoms, such as preoccupation with and searching for the deceased person, with increased numbers of deaths from AIDS. Bereaved individuals with HIV–AIDS may identify with the deceased in terms of their own mortality (Mulder & Antoni, 1992), and deaths from AIDS exacerbate fears of developing AIDS (Solomon et al., 1991).

Women with HIV infection are likely to suffer additional losses. Women often contend with their own HIV infection while serving as the primary caregiver for their HIV-seropositive partner (although not unique to women with HIV), as well as while caring for their children. Obviously having an HIV-seropositive child further contributes to a sense of impending loss. Caring for her children and concerns about whom will care for them should she become ill are the most significant stressors for a woman with HIV (Hackl et al., 1997).

Two factors appear important in determining responses to AIDS-related losses: the number of losses incurred over a period of time and the HIV serostatus of the bereaved person. Multiple losses to AIDS close in time result in severe emotional disturbances (J. L. Martin, 1988; J. L. Martin & Dean, 1993). Nearly one third of bereaved gay men in New York City experienced two or more losses in the past year, and nearly half of those men had three or more losses in that time (J. L. Martin & Dean, 1993). Such rates of death among young adults have been virtually unknown outside of war (Capitanio, 1994).

Trends in psychological reactions to AIDS-related deaths have changed over the course of the AIDS epidemic. Neugebauer et al. (1992) observed a pattern of decreasing adverse effects of loss over the second decade of AIDS among gay men in New York City. Neugebauer et al. concluded that the expanding scope of the epidemic has led to a gradual normalization and expectation for death at young ages. Social and political mobilization against AIDS in gay communities may also have buffered against emotional distress at later points in the epidemic. J. L. Martin and Dean (1993) observed similar diminishing trends in bereavement intensity in New York City gay communities. Although bereavement was closely tied to distress among gay men in 1985, this association was not observed in 1990. Martin and Dean noted that one's own health and physical functioning seemed to replace AIDS-related loss as the focus of concern among gay and bisexual men.

Suicidal Risk

Given the prevalence of HIV-related depression, the social stigma of being HIV infected, and the isolation experienced by those infected, it would not be surprising if people living with HIV were at increased risk for suicide. People with HIV infection have more frequent thoughts of suicide and more frequent suicide attempts when compared with HIV negative people. However, the risk for completing suicide is only modestly higher for people with HIV–AIDS (Marzuk et al., 1997; Zamperetti et al., 1990). Perry, Jacobsberg, and Fishman (1990) reported that suicidal thoughts, but not attempts, occurred after receiving HIV-test results in more than 15% of individuals who test HIV seropositive. People who are uninfected but at risk for HIV, however, frequently have histories of suicide attempts. For example, Pergami et al. (1993) found that attempted suicide was prevalent in people seeking HIV testing; a history of self-inflicted harm was found for 14% of people who were getting tested and who subsequently tested HIV seropositive and for 22% of those who were to test HIV seronegative. However, after receiving HIV-test results, 21% of seropositives attempted suicide, compared with none of those who tested HIV seronegative. Similarly, Belkin et al. (1992) reported that 17% of HIV-seropositive men and women considered attempting suicide at least once in the previous week. In a study of 2,363 psychiatric consultations in New York Hospital, Alfonso et al. (1994) reported that one in five HIV-seropositive individuals exhibited suicidal behavior compared with 13% of patients with unknown HIV serostatus.

O'Dowd and McKegney (1990) also reported that injection drug users with AIDS had inclinations to attempt suicide. However, O'Dowd and McKegney found a comparable number of non-HIV-infected medical patients had thoughts of suicide. Similar results were reported in a study of over 4,000 military recruits who screened HIV seropositive (Dannenberg, McNeil, Brundage, & Brookmeyer, 1996).

In a prospective study, Perry, Jacobsberg, and Fishman (1990) used the suicide item on the *Beck Depression Inventory* as an index of suicidal tendency. Nearly one third of individuals undergoing HIV-antibody testing reported thoughts of suicide before being tested, with 27% of HIV-seropositive and 17% of HIV-seronegative individuals continuing to consider suicide one week after receiving their test results. Perry et al. found that many HIV-seronegative people continue to have thoughts of suicide two months following test result notification.

Studies have reported that suicides attempted by people with HIV infection occur relatively early in HIV infection, with risk for suicide most elevated for people with early symptoms of infection. Marzuk et al. (1997) showed that 70% of people with HIV in New York City who committed suicide had no HIV-related illnesses at autopsy. In a large study of medical patients referred for psychiatric evaluation, McKegney and O'Dowd (1992) found that 39% of HIV-seropositive people who had not been diagnosed with AIDS had thoughts of suicide, a rate that exceeded both the thoughts of HIV-seronegative people and people living with AIDS. AIDS patients demonstrated similar suicide risk as non-HIV-infected medical patients facing other life-threatening illnesses. A study of male HIV-seropositive asymptomatic army personnel found more than half had considered suicide since their initial diagnosis (Ritchie & Radke, 1992). O'Dowd et al. (1993) showed that having HIV infection and symptoms of illness were as strong predictors of suicidal ideation as was a history of suicide attempts. O'Dowd et al. also found that individuals with AIDS experienced fewer thoughts of suicide than both people with early HIV symptoms and those who were asymptomatic. The onset of HIV symptoms may therefore be an important factor in prompting thoughts of suicide. Individuals diagnosed with AIDS who are not currently ill, either because their diagnosis was based on CD4 cell counts or because an AIDS-defining condition was successfully treated, may also be at increased risk for suicide because of increased energy to commit the act (Frierson & Lippmann, 1988).

Belkin et al. (1992) and Donlou et al. (1985) both reported close associations between contemplating suicide and HIV symptom intensity and chronicity. In both studies, physical symptoms mediated relationships between depression and suicidal tendencies. Along with the physical decline of a progressive illness, the threat of long-term dependency increases risk for suicide (Marzuk et al., 1988). Rabkin, Wilson, and Kimpton (1993) found that people wishing to die, although not necessarily wishing to commit suicide, almost always did so under the threat of serious debilitating illness, particularly when faced with an impending hospital admission. Belkin et al. (1992) also reported that the relationship between physical symptoms of HIV disease and suicidal ideation was mediated by the number of days that a person was bed-bound, with physical symptoms and immobility predicting thoughts of suicide. Other AIDS-related events, such as bereavement and caregiving, can also prompt thoughts of suicide (Rosengard & Folkman, 1997).

Predictors of suicidal tendencies in HIV infection parallel those seen in the general population. Suicide risk is greatest among people who have preexisting or coexisting cognitive and affective disturbances, substance use disorders, and poor social supports (Marzuk et al., 1997; Perry, Jacobsberg, & Fishman, 1990). Consistent with the general population, O'Dowd et al. (1993) reported that an inpatient psychiatric history was significantly associated with suicide risk across stages of HIV infection and that risk was greatest for those with a prior history of attempting suicide. O'Dowd et al. also found that 90% of HIV-seropositive individuals who attempted suicide indicated that their first attempt was unrelated to their HIV infection status. HIV-seropositive African American men admitted for inpatient crisis services are frequently at greater risk for suicide than are their HIV-seronegative counterparts (Wood, Nairn, Kraft, & Kiegel, 1997).

Aside from documenting its prevalence, few studies have investigated the dimensions underlying suicidal risk in HIV infection. An exception is Schneider, Taylor, Hammen, Kemeny, and Dudley (1991), who investigated predictors of suicidal ideations among 100 HIV-seropositive and 112 HIV-seronegative men in the Los Angeles MACS cohort. Notification of positive HIV-test results, onset of HIV symptoms, number of close friends diagnosed with HIV, knowing someone who died from AIDS, and perceived risk of developing AIDS significantly predicted intentions to attempt suicide. Not having a close friend or confidant, and feelings of loneliness, also predicted suicidal ideations. In contrast, suicide risk for HIV-seronegative men was predicted, as expected, only by depression and loneliness. Path analyses showed that AIDS-related events and perceived risks of developing AIDS were significantly stronger predictors of suicide intent among HIV-seropositive men than for HIV-seronegative men. Further analyses showed that AIDS-related events specifically predicted suicidal ideations independent of dysphoria.

Although suicide risk in HIV infection is related to pessimism, depression, hopelessness, and grief, suicide risk may also emerge from decisions to "rationally" end one's life to avoid protracted pain, dependence, and economic decline (Frierson & Lippmann, 1988; Zich & Temoshok, 1990). The terminally ill in general may desire to die as a result of their illness (Chochinov et al., 1995). Planning to avoid suffering by hastening death is common among the terminally ill and older people, who often seek information about the lethality of suicide methods (Humphry, 1991; McIntosh, Santos, Hubbard, & Overholser, 1994). Rabkin, Remien, et al. (1993) found one in four long-term survivors with AIDS made arrangements to end their lives should their condition advance to where their quality of life would deteriorate. Furthermore, with advancing disease people may refuse treatment and seek control over the course of their life and death. Progressive illness may therefore inhibit accepting medical interventions and life-sustaining supports (Fogel & Mor, 1993). Caregivers may also be asked to help hasten death. One study found that 12% of caregivers of gay men who died of AIDS in San Francisco acknowledged increasing medication doses to hasten death for the person they were caring for (Folkman, Chesney, Cooke, Boccellari, & Collette, 1994).

Anxiety

A condition such as HIV–AIDS is expectedly associated with anxiety. Nearly half of individuals who decline to receive their HIV antibody test results indicate that they would rather not know their HIV serostatus in fear of being unable to cope with the result (Lyter, Valdiserri, Kingsley, Amoroso, & Rinaldo, 1987). Among HIV seropositive gay men, Kessler et al. (1988) reported that 12% of their cohort showed obsessive–compulsive symptoms. Dew et al. (1990) found 45% of HIV-infected hemophiliacs had greater anxiety than an HIV-seronegative comparison group. Similarly, Pace et al. (1990) reported that 23% of HIV-seropositive Air Force personnel had generalized anxiety disorder and that one in five had a simple phobia. A clinic chart review of depressed patients with HIV infection showed significantly more use of antianxiety medications than a non-HIV-infected but depressed comparison group matched on sociodemographic characteristics, illustrating comorbidity of depression and anxiety in HIV infection (Hintz et al., 1990).

HIV anxiety is associated with several HIV-related events including concerns about becoming physically disabled, rejected, and isolated (Maj, 1990; Snyder et al., 1992). Because HIV is transmissible, people with HIV may feel pressure to protect others from infection while simultaneously protecting themselves from rejection and isolation. Loss of friends to AIDS may serve as a salient reminder that HIV infection leads to early death, further heightening anxiety (J. L. Martin, 1988; J. L. Martin & Dean, 1993a). Environmental cues such as AIDS-related newspaper articles, television news stories, public service announcements, and comments by friends can all provoke anxiety.

The prospect of dying is, of course, a major source of anxiety (Wolcott, Namir, Fawzy, Gottlieb, & Mitsuyasu, 1986). Catania, Turner, et al. (1992) found that 85% of HIV-seropositive gay men reported concerns about death, relative to 64% of HIV-seronegative gay men. Death anxiety is greatest when HIV symptoms develop and increases with time (Catania, Turner, et al., 1992; Kurdek & Siesky, 1990). Impeding physical decline and becoming dependent on others are closely associated with the dying process, and these concerns can supersede fears of death itself.

Somatization and Hypochondriasis

Somatization illustrates how HIV infection can become interwoven with symptoms of emotional distress. *Somatization* is the tendency to amplify somatic symptoms of emotional distress and attribute them to physical illness in the absence of corroborating organic pathology (Bakal, 1992; Lipowski, 1988). Body vigilance and symptom expectancies can produce vague and diffuse physical complaints. In HIV-related somatization, minor physical discomforts often associated with depression and anxiety can heighten illness concerns. Misperceptions of innocuous bodily sensations may exacerbate anxiety, intensifying stress responses that are open to further misinterpretation (Warwick, 1989). Figure 4.5 presents a model of the relationship between body vigilance and anxiety adapted from Schmidt, Lerew, and Trakowski (1997). As shown in the figure, sensations stem from fear arousal feedback and increase fear arousal.

Receiving a positive HIV test result can lead to preoccupations with

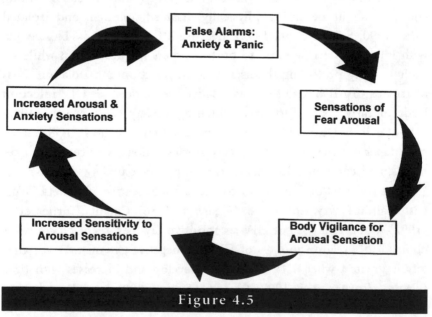

False Alarms: Anxiety & Panic

Increased Arousal & Anxiety Sensations

Sensations of Fear Arousal

Increased Sensitivity to Arousal Sensations

Body Vigilance for Arousal Sensation

Figure 4.5

Model of body vigilance and anxiety.

physical health. Repeated body checking and palpating for swellings, discolorations, blemishes, and other bodily changes that are indicative of HIV-related illnesses can take on an obsessive quality, becoming maladaptive and disabling (Kessler et al., 1988). Preoccupations with physical functioning and compulsive symptom checking may develop from premorbid histories of obsessive–compulsive behaviors among both HIV seropositive (D. Miller, 1990) and non-HIV-infected medical patients (Burns & Howell, 1969). AIDS-related events, such as declines in immunologic markers, increased viral load, testing anniversaries, or illnesses among friends can serve as external cues for disease progression and contribute to somatization. J. L. Martin and Dean (1993) found that AIDS-related bereavement increased physical preoccupations and perceptions of developing AIDS. This finding is consistent with descriptions of somatic preoccupations in non-HIV-infected populations, where a death can increase a sense of vulnerability to that illness (Barsky, Wyshak, & Klerman, 1990).

HIV-related somatization is also facilitated by non-HIV-related illnesses, such as a cold or the flu. Symptoms of relatively innocuous illnesses can lead to perceptions of progressing to AIDS. Early symptoms of HIV infection, such as persistent fever or diarrhea, can be exacerbated by psychosomatic reactions. However, physical signs of HIV disease appear less important in somatization than attribution processes. Ostrow, Monjan, et al. (1989) found that gay men with HIV infection who reported swollen lymph nodes experienced significant emotional distress, regardless of whether enlarged lymph nodes were actually detected upon physical examination. Kessler et al. (1988) demonstrated that physical illness mattered less in HIV-related somatization than perceptions that HIV disease was progressing. Perry, Ryan, Ashman, and Jacobsberg (1992) found that, although markers of immune system functioning are not related to concurrent emotional distress, awareness of one's CD4 cell counts and the experience of intrusive thoughts of physical functioning did predict emotional distress. In addition, people notified of declines in their immune system become more preoccupied with physical illness compared with people with stable immune systems. The use of CD4 counts and measures of viral load as benchmarks for immune system status may also become a means for self-monitoring disease progression. When CD4 cells decline or viral load increases, individuals typically expect illness symptoms to quickly follow, with such expectations increasing somatic anxiety.

HIV-related somatization appears similar to the condition *transient hypochondriasis* (Barsky et al., 1990), a subclinical form of hypochondriasis characterized by multiple and diffuse somatic complaints attributed to undetected medical illness. Several aspects of transient hypochondriasis suggest that it may occur in HIV infection. Transient hypochondriasis tends to develop in the context of life-threatening and terminal conditions and is related to perceptions of treatments as ineffective (Barsky, Cleary, Sarnie, & Klerman, 1993; Barsky et al., 1990). Distortions of physical symptoms tend to focus on a specific ailment like HIV infection (Jenike & Pato, 1986). Finally, people most susceptible to transient hypochondriasis tend to have fewer coping resources compared with individuals who are free of somatic symptoms (Barsky et al., 1990).

Somatization and physical preoccupation are not universal to HIV infection. Kessler et al. (1988) found that HIV-seropositive gay men often underdetected recognizable symptoms of HIV-related illnesses, where only 9% to 14% of men who had medically diagnosed lymphadenopathy detected enlarged nodes themselves. Similar underdetection occurred for fever and weight loss. Thus, not all patients with HIV infection become preoccupied with physical functioning and symptom checking. Many probably do not recognize actual illness symptoms because they lack awareness of their meaning or are unaware of proper methods of self-detection.

Anger and Guilt

Anger is a common emotional reaction to a life-threatening illness. Guilt, on the other hand, typically accompanies diagnoses of sexually transmitted infections. Anger and guilt are therefore probably common responses to HIV infection. However, surprisingly few studies have assessed anger and guilt in HIV–AIDS. In one of the few studies that assessed anger, McCusker et al. (1988) found that HIV-seropositive gay men experienced greater anger than HIV-seronegative men did.

Guilt is a common reaction to sexually transmitted infections, as is the case for HIV–AIDS (Christ & Wiener, 1985; Dilley, Ochitill, et al., 1985). Self-blame, shame, and self-devaluation are among the first emotional responses to an HIV-positive test result (Chuang et al., 1992). These emotions often stem from beliefs about having engaged in behaviors that resulted in becoming infected, beliefs that HIV infection is a form of moral retribution or punishment, and beliefs about the social disapproval of others (Catalan, 1988; D. Miller & Riccio, 1990; Nichols, 1985). Guilty feelings also arise in response to surviving when lovers and friends have died of AIDS. Survivor guilt was common among Nazi holocaust survivors and occurs in AIDS-devastated communities for similar reasons. Guilt may arise when one is successfully treated for HIV–AIDS because many others fail. HIV-related guilt may become internalized homophobia among men who contracted HIV through same-sex practices. Guilt is also facilitated by the social stigmas of sexual and drug-use behaviors. Finally, guilt may arise from thoughts of having possibly infected others before or after testing HIV positive.

QUALITY OF LIFE

Emotional well being is but one dimension of quality of life. Health-related quality of life is the bridge between life events and health status (Vanhems, Toma, & Pineault, 1996). Most frameworks of health-related quality of life include sensory functioning, physical mobility, emotional well being, cognitive functioning, self-care and independence, and degrees of pain and discomfort. Perceptions of health, social functioning, and energy level in their definitions of quality of life have also been included in definitions of health-related quality of life (R. D. Hays, Cunningham, Ettl, Beck, & Shapiro, 1995). Although HIV infection has unique features that influence quality of life, there are no domains of quality of life specific to people living with HIV–AIDS (Vanhems et al., 1996).

Given the range of devastation that occurs as HIV progresses, quality of life would be expected to decline over the course of HIV infection.

However, there is little evidence available to support this presupposition. In fact, studies of long-term survivors with AIDS support the opposite view; many people with late stage HIV infection maintain high levels of quality of life. Quality of life in the context of a chronic illness, however, is a dynamic process that requires periodic redefining. The relative importance of various aspects of quality of life shifts as functioning is limited and losses are suffered. With greater access to more effective treatments, quality of life will improve even after periods of significant illness. In some studies, activity levels and employment status at later stages of disease do not differ from those at earlier stages (Leigh, Lubeck, Farnham, & Fries, 1995). Adaptation to changes in quality of life, both negative and positive, are among the most significant challenges facing people living with HIV–AIDS.

EMOTIONAL DISTRESS AND HEALTH

Psychoneuroimmunology, the study of central nervous system and immune system interactions, has extensively investigated the mechanisms underlying psychological influences on immune diseases. There is a substantial body of evidence that shows both acute and chronic stressful life events affect several branches of the immune system (for reviews, see S. Cohen & Williamson, 1991; Herbert & Cohen, 1993; O'Leary, 1990). Negative life events and lack of social supports also increase the likelihood of becoming ill (Sarason, Sarason, Potter, & Antoni, 1985). The persistent stress of caring for a person with a chronic illness, for example, suppresses immune responses, including declines in the number of T-helper lymphocytes and natural killer cell responses (Esterling, Kiecolt-Glaser, Bodnar, & Glaser, 1994; Kiecolt-Glaser et al., 1987). Chronic stress associated with living through an environmental catastrophe also adversely affects immune functioning (Schaeffer & Baum, 1984). Minor and acute life stressors can have important effects on the immune system in healthy and resourceful populations, such as the observed effects of exams on the immune functioning of medical students (Kiecolt-Glaser et al., 1984). Minor stressful life events can accumulate over time and act as chronic stressors, with similar effects on the immune system. The effects of stress on the immune system have therefore been widely observed, but it has not been determined if the nature and magnitude of such changes alter susceptibility to disease (S. Cohen & Williamson, 1991).

Several studies have reported links between depression, immune functioning, and disease, but these findings are not conclusive (Schleifer, Keller, Bond, Cohen, & Stein, 1989; Schleifer, Keller, Siris, Davis, & Stein, 1985; Stein, Miller, & Trestman, 1991; Zonderman, Costa, & McCrae, 1989). Depression can alter several branches of immunity (Kiecolt-Glaser & Glaser, 1988a). Suppressed immune activity results from bereavement following the death of a spouse, independent of the stress effects of caregiving (Bartrop, Luckhurst, Lazarus, Kiloh, & Penny, 1977; Schleifer, Keller, Camerino, Thorton, & Stein, 1983). Similar changes occur in people with poor marital satisfaction and those who experience marital separation (Kiecolt-Glaser, Fisher, et al., 1987; Kiecolt-Glaser et al., 1988).

The immune system is affected by stress through complex interactions between central nervous and endocrine systems. Laboratory experiments show that changes in the immune functions occur within 15 minutes following exposure to a mild stressor and that changes can persist over extended times (Zakowski, McAllister, Deal, & Baum, 1992). Perceptions of threat activate the sympathetic branch of the autonomic nervous system to invoke a "flight or fight" response. Hormones released during stress can also mediate central nervous system and immune system activities, for example, cortisol released under stress, during depression, and following periods of social deprivation. Cortisol suppresses immune responses, particularly with regard to reductions in T-helper lymphocytes (Kemeny, 1991; O'Leary, 1990). Stressful life events are predictive of upper-respiratory illnesses and a number of bacterial infections (S. Cohen & Williamson, 1991; R. Glaser, Kiecolt-Glaser, Speicher, & Holliday, 1985; Kemeny, 1991; Kemeny, Cohen, Zegans, & Conant, 1989). Evidence therefore shows that stress can modulate immune processes involved in controlling infections. Because these processes are directly related to cell-mediated immunity and can activate latent viruses, it is reasonable to propose stress as a cofactor in the progression of HIV infection.

There are several potential mechanisms by which stress can theoretically complicate the course of HIV infection. First, stressful events,
as they affect the central nervous and endocrine systems, may directly
affect branches of the immune system of relevance to HIV infection.
Cortisol is of particular importance because it affects the blood concentration and functions of T-helper lymphocytes (Fauci & Dale, 1975).
A second potential role that stress may play in HIV progression involves
the activation of HIV in vitro. For example, Markham, Salahuddin,
Veren, Orndorff, and Gallo (1986) found that corticosteroids and other
stress-related hormones enhance the expression of HIV. Thus, people
with impaired immune defenses may be more vulnerable to the immune-suppressing effects of stress (Kiecolt-Glaser & Glaser, 1988b).

Despite the evidence that stress has immunologic effects, the likelihood that stress-related reactions interact with the expression of infectious disease, and the logical formulation of hypotheses that stress reactions interact with HIV disease, research findings on these relations
have been mixed. For example, a study of asymptomatic men with HIV
infection did not find bereavement or clinical depression to predict any
of several markers of immune functioning significantly (Kemeny et al.,
1994). This study did report, however, that for men who were not bereaved, depressed mood, although not clinical depression, was correlated
with immune markers relevant to HIV disease. The authors acknowledged that these relationships may have been mediated by awareness of
physical decline that may accompany both immunosuppression and depressed mood. In another study, researchers failed to identify relationships between emotional distress and immune functions in HIV infection, although an active coping style did correlate with some immune
markers (Goodkin et al., 1992). Thus, some studies have suggested relationships among psychological factors and immune functions in HIV
infection, but there has not been a consistent pattern of results.

Research has typically failed to identify any stress–immune system
relationships of clinical relevance in HIV infection. In one study, stress-
induced activation of the sympathetic nervous system did not result in
loss of T-helper lymphocytes beyond that already seen in the early
phases of HIV infection (Gorman et al., 1991). A follow-up study of

this sample also failed to identify relationships among distress, levels of cortisol, and immune functioning (Kertzner et al., 1993). In addition, widely accepted effects of depression on immune system functioning are not observed among HIV-infected individuals (Rabkin et al., 1991; Saahs et al., 1994). Stressful life events do not predict the onset of HIV-related symptoms in gay men (Kessler et al., 1991). Cross-sectional analyses by J. B. W. Williams et al. (1991) failed to find relationships between distress and markers of immune functioning in HIV-seropositive gay men. In yet another prospective study of people with HIV infection not diagnosed with AIDS, Perry, Ryan, Ashman, and Jacobsberg (1992) found that emotional distress was not associated with immune markers, in both concurrent and prospective analyses. Thus, several immune system responses to stress seen in HIV-seronegative populations have not been observed in similar studies of HIV-seropositive individuals.

The most compelling evidence against effects of emotional distress on HIV disease progression comes from two longitudinal studies, the MACS (Lyketsos, Hoover, et al., 1993), and the San Francisco Men's Health Study (Burrack et al., 1993). Both studies reported several years of prospective data on large samples of gay and bisexual men. In both studies, cohort members were assessed using the CESD at study entry, before the HIV-antibody test was available. Blood samples were stored and later evaluated after the HIV test was developed. Baseline depression, which could not have been affected by knowledge of HIV status, although potentially affected by the onset of HIV symptoms, were used to predict declines in T-helper lymphocyte counts, the onset of AIDS, and death. For both studies, multivariate statistical techniques and survival analyses failed to demonstrate depression as a significant predicator of AIDS or death. Although Burrack et al. found a statistically significant relationship between baseline depression and T-helper cell counts, the degree of association was small and of questionable clinical significance (Perry & Fishman, 1993). Data from these two studies therefore suggest that effects of negative emotions on the clinical status of HIV infection may be negligible.

There are, however, studies that suggest clinically relevant effects of stress and adjustment on immune functioning in people living with

HIV–AIDS. Progression of HIV disease, for example, may be accelerated when stressful life events occur at an earlier point in infection. Evans et al. (1997) observed a fourfold increase in early disease progression in HIV-seropositive men who experienced severe life stress. HIV-positive men who experience the stress of homophobia and conceal their sexual identity may also suffer ill health effects, including accelerated rates of decline in immune functions (Cole, Kemeny, Taylor, & Visscher, 1996; Cole, Kemeny, Taylor, Visscher, & Fahey, 1996). Negative effects of stress, therefore, may have bearing on clinically relevant health outcomes in some people living with HIV–AIDS.

Coping resources may moderate stress–immune associations in people living with HIV. Benight et al. (1997) found that self-efficacy for effective coping was related to cortisol levels for HIV-seropositive men following Hurricane Andrew in Miami, an association not observed in HIV-negative men. No effects, however, were reported for direct immune functioning. Cognitive attributions also may play a role in immunity. A prospective study reported that HIV-seropositive men who attribute negative events to internal characterological causes show more rapid declines in CD4 cell counts (Segerstrom, Taylor, Kemeny, Reed, & Visscher, 1996), losing on average 125 CD4 cells over 18 months compared to 75 lost for men with less internal attributions, a sizeable difference but with unclear clinical meaning. Finally, HIV-seropositive men participating in a cognitive–behavioral skills management intervention showed reductions in herpes simplex virus-2 antibody not seen in control group participants, suggesting a positive effect on the immune system (Lutgendorf et al., 1997). However, measures of more direct relevance, such as CD4 cell counts, did not differ between conditions.

The limited associations between emotional reactions to stress and immune system responses among people with HIV infection are in some ways not surprising given the pervasive damage that HIV causes to the immune system. That is, immune responses in the context of HIV infection are likely different from normal immune responses (Coates, McKusick, Kuno, & Stites, 1989; Ironson et al., 1990; Mulder & Antoni, 1992). Even if stress does affect immune functioning in HIV-seropositive individuals, the stress–immune relations will likely differ at various phases of HIV disease, making any such relationships far more complex than they are in typical cases. In summary, although proposed relationships between stress and HIV-disease progression are based on studies of stress—immune interactions in the psychoneuroimmunology literature, the relatively small number of studies, their methodological limitations, underrepresentation of women and ethnic minorities, and lack of positive findings precludes conclusions of stress—immune relationships in HIV infection. Thus, although stress seriously affects the quality of life for people living with HIV infection, it is not clear whether stress influences HIV-disease progression.

CONCLUSION

Living with HIV—AIDS has been described as an emotional roller coaster, with rapid changes in feelings coinciding with changes in health and the social environment. The experience of living with HIV therefore differs for each individual. For people whose mental health diminishes with HIV progression, overlapping HIV disease and psychological symptoms complicate both medical and psychological clinical assessments. The interrelationships between HIV-related illnesses, depression, anxiety, and somatization are difficult to sort through. People can mislabel HIV symptoms as depression or other mental states, potentially delaying medical attention to declining health. Conversely, symptoms of depression or anxiety are easily misinterpreted as HIV-related symptoms, delaying adequate mental-health services. Patient education, both in medical and nonmedical service delivery settings, must inform people with HIV about overlapping symptoms. The ability to recognize the differences between psychogenic and HIV-related symptoms will enhance a sense of internal control and likely improve quality of care. Similarly, symptoms of HIV-related central nervous system disease are confused for other conditions, further complicating accurate diagnoses and treatment. The nature of HIV's involvement in the nervous system is the topic of chapter 5.

5

Neuropsychological Sequelae

The human immune system is the principal site of HIV infection, but numerous other organ systems are vulnerable to HIV. Early in the epidemic, HIV was thought to invade the central nervous system only at the latest stages of infection, and there were theories that brain damage observed in people with AIDS was actually caused by cytomegalovirus (Sharer, 1992). However, we now know that HIV itself crosses the blood–brain barrier to infect CD4 cells in the brain (Levy, Shimabukuro, Hollander, Mills, & Kaminsky, 1985; Shaw et al., 1985). A diagnosis of *AIDS dementia complex*, introduced in 1987, serves to describe the clinical constellation of neuropsychological symptoms of AIDS. However, most people develop more generalized HIV infection of the central nervous system, with 30% to 60% of all AIDS patients developing symptoms of central or peripheral nervous system disease (Collier et al., 1992). AIDS can also involve opportunistic infections and malignancies of the nervous system, which include toxoplasmosis, Cryptococcal meningitis, progressive multifocal leukoencephalopathy (PML), and non-Hodgkin's lymphomas.

Distinguished from opportunistic illnesses, AIDS dementia complex is defined by cognitive and behavioral deterioration in the absence of a neurological opportunistic illness (Aronow, Brew, & Price, 1988; Egan, 1992). AIDS dementia complex is therefore self-evident: *AIDS* reflects a complication of HIV infection; *dementia* denotes acquired and persistent declines in cognitive functioning observed over the course of late-stage HIV infection; and *complex* indicates the triad of cognitive, motor, and behavior disturbances it involves (see Table 5.1). Like other dementias, such as Alzheimer's and Huntington's diseases, AIDS dementia complex causes persistent impairment in multiple spheres of mental activity, including, but not limited to, motor control, attention, concentration, language, memory, visual–spatial skills, emotion, reasoning, and cognitive flexibility. Similar to organic mental disorders in general, the essential feature of AIDS dementia complex is a loss of intellectual abilities of sufficient severity to interfere with social or occupational functioning (American Psychiatric Association, 1987). Although any person with AIDS can develop dementia, children are more susceptible than adults (Egan, 1992). Children with AIDS dementia demonstrate significant developmental delays, motor disturbances, multiple sensory and memory deficits, and brain structure abnormalities (Boivin et al., 1995; Janssen et al., 1991). The threat of losing personal control and independence makes neurological clinical symptoms among the most frightening consequences of HIV–AIDS.

Table 5.1
Clinical Manifestations of HIV-Related Dementia

Domain	Early Manifestations	Late Manifestations
Cognitive	Reduced attention and concentration, increased forgetfulness	Generalized dementia
Motoric	General slowing, clumsiness, disrupted walking	Paraplegia
Behavioral	Apathy, agitation	Mutism

DIAGNOSIS AND CLASSIFICATION

Diagnostic and classification schemes for HIV central nervous system disease have undergone many revisions. Because AIDS dementia complex (ADC) has a specific and identifiable etiological agent, the *Diagnostic and Statistical Manual* criteria for organic mental disorder provides an adequate diagnosis. However, only considering the symptoms of dementia provides an incomplete description of the neurocognitive effects of HIV infection. First, although ADC describes a loss of cognitive and motor functioning not attributable to opportunistic infections, malignancies, or systemic HIV disease, dementia does not accurately describe HIV-related deficits that can be outside of the cognitive, motor, and behavioral domains (Vitkovic & Koslow, 1994). Second, HIV infects the brain early in the course of HIV infection, inconsistent with the notion that central nervous system involvement is only associated with AIDS. Finally, earlier and less severe neurological symptoms of HIV infection clearly cause cognitive decline but do not approach the level of impairment seen in dementia (See Table 5.2).

Several diagnostic labels have been proposed to replace ADC, including *HIV-associated neurobehavioral deficit* (Bornstein et al., 1992), and *HIV-related* or *HIV-induced organic mental disorder* (Markowitz & Perry, 1992; Perry & Marotta, 1987). The Working Group of the American Academy of Neurology AIDS Task Force introduced one of the more widely used nomenclatures (Janssen et al., 1991). This system distinguishes two subclasses of HIV-related disorders, *HIV Associated Minor Cognitive/Motor Disorder* and *HIV Associated Dementia Complex*. HIV Associated Minor Cognitive/Motor Disorder includes mild functional impairment, such as minimal disruption of social relationships, occupation, or daily living. Severe neuropsychological impairment is diagnosed as HIV Associated Dementia Complex, denoting progressive HIV encephalopathy. The major distinction between the minor and severe subclasses is their degree of functional impairment. The diagnostic classification system, therefore, reserves the term *dementia* for cases with cognitive impairment consistent with such a diagnosis (Worley & Price, 1992). Although HIV Associated Dementia Complex constitutes an AIDS case-defining condition, manifestations of HIV Asso-

Table 5.2	
Clinical Staging of AIDS Dementia Complex	
Stage	Symptoms and Characteristics
0 (normal)	Normal mental and motor function.
0.5 (subclinical)	Either minimal or equivocal symptoms or motor dysfunction characteristic of HIV-related dementia, or mild signs but without impairment of work or capacity to perform activities of daily living; walking and strength are normal.
1 (mild)	Unequivocal symptoms, neuropsychological test performance, or functional, intellectual, or motor impairment characteristic of HIV-related dementia but able to perform all but the most demanding work or daily living tasks; can walk without assistance.
2 (moderate)	Cannot work or maintain demanding aspects of daily life, but able to perform basic activities of self-care; may require assistance in walking.
3 (severe)	Major intellectual incapacity or motor disability, including carrying on conversations, performing daily living tasks; requires walker or personal support in walking; usually motor slowing and clumsiness of arms.
4 (end stage)	Nearly vegetative; intellectual and social comprehension and responses are at very low levels; nearly or absolutely mute; paraplegic with incontinence.

ciated Minor Cognitive/Motor Disorder are insufficient for an AIDS diagnosis.

HIV-Associated Dementia Complex is composed of clinical symptoms that are consistent with disturbances of both subcortical and frontal lobe functioning, including cognitive slowing, memory impairment, and behavioral disinhibition (Egan, 1992; R. W. Price & Sidtis, 1992). HIV predominantly affects subcortical brain structures, with attention deficits and cognitive slowing being the most salient features of HIV-related impairment (Krikorian & Worbel, 1991; E. M. Martin, Sorensen, Edelstein, & Robertson, 1992; Perdices & Cooper, 1990; Sharer, 1992), and dysfunction of the cerebral cortex, such as language, being the least common (Ho, Bredesen, Vinters, & Daar, 1989). Damage to the basal ganglia results in involuntary movements, such as tremors and reduced motor speed, without paralysis.

HIV ENCEPHALOPATHY

HIV can cause structural damage to the brain, but clinical signs of higher-order cortical dysfunction, such as verbal responsiveness, aphasia, and behavioral disinhibition, rarely occur. HIV-related encephalopathy poses nonspecific disturbances that include clouding of consciousness, dysfunction in short-term memory, and psychomotor slowing (Ostrow, 1990). Other neuropsychological conditions of HIV include peripheral neuropathy, causing both sensory numbness and pain in up to 35% of people with AIDS, and myopathy, a slow and progressive weakness of the arms and legs (Koppel, 1992). Although neurological symptoms of HIV overlap with other AIDS-related conditions, particularly in the later stages of HIV disease, HIV Associated Minor Cognitive/Motor Disorder and HIV Associated Dementia Complex are independent manifestations of HIV infection.

HIV-RELATED DISEASE OF THE NERVOUS SYSTEM

HIV was isolated from the brains of people with AIDS early in the epidemic (e.g., Ho et al., 1989; Shaw et al., 1985). Autopsies of AIDS patients consistently found that 70% to 90% showed significant central nervous system disease (Anders, Guerra, Tomiyasu, Verity, & Vinters, 1986; Bornstein, 1993; Koppel, 1992), with structures most affected by HIV being those involved in the transfer of information across brain regions (e.g., central white matter, the thalamus, brain stem, and basal ganglia).

In addition to postmortem studies, imaging techniques have clearly demarcated structural brain damage. Both computed tomography (CT) and magnetic resonance imaging (MRI) reveal a substantial number of AIDS patients with cerebral cortical atrophy (widening of cortical sulci), scattered brain lesions, and ventricular dilation (Markowitz & Perry, 1992). Electroencephalography (EEG) also shows abnormalities in both slowed Alpha rhythms, associated with states of relaxed wakefulness, and diffuse Theta waves, normally associated with sleep in adults (Kandel, Schwartz, & Jessell, 1991; Koppel, 1992). However, structural damage and electrical disturbances in AIDS are not directly linked to functional impairment; some people show clinical signs of dementia without apparent HIV encephalitis, whereas others have gross abnormalities on CT and MRI scans but do not experience functional limitations (Sharer, 1992).

HIV usually enters the central nervous system shortly after viral transmission. HIV antigens are found in the cerebrospinal fluid soon after infection, and HIV is detected in the cerebrospinal fluid of asymptomatic persons within 6 to 24 months following HIV seroconversion (Bornstein, 1993; McArthur et al., 1988; Resnick et al., 1985). HIV infection of the central nervous system principally occurs in monocyte-derived cells, including macrophages and microglia, cells that share the same origin as T-helper lymphocytes and carry out immune functions in the brain (Giulian, Vaca, & Noonan, 1990; Sharer, 1992; Worley & Price, 1992). HIV does not, however, directly infect neurons. HIV infection of macrophages in the brain causes both the loss of neurons and damage to cell dendrites, effectively disabling neurons (Sharer, 1992). Table 5.3 summarizes the areas of the brain most commonly affected by HIV and their associated symptoms.

HIV-related neurological damage can be caused by multiple factors. However, toxins, either created by viral components of HIV or released from HIV-infected neighboring cells cause most of the damage observed in neurons. Neurotoxic substances associated with HIV include the viral envelope glucoprotein *gp120*, the cause of imbalances in the neuronal intracellular chemistry (Bornstein, 1993; Sharer, 1992). In addition, uninfected macrophages respond to HIV envelope proteins by releasing cytokines, which accumulate and interfere with interneuron

Table 5.3
Areas of the Brain Most Commonly Affected by HIV

Structures	Symptoms
Frontal lobes	Apathy, depression, trouble concentrating, loss of organizational skills
Limbic system and temporal lobe	Memory loss and language impairment
Basal ganglia	Impaired eye movements, involuntary movements, tremor
Brain stem	Disturbed gait, eye-movement dysfunctions, visual disturbances
Demyelination	Delayed information processing, slowed responses, impaired fine motor skills, incontinence

communication. Nervous tissues infected by HIV, particularly macrophages and microglia, release additional neurotoxins that compromise neuron metabolic activities. HIV infection can also stimulate macrophage responses, leading to an additional release of toxic substances (Lipton & Gendelman, 1995). Diffuse encephalopathies caused by metabolic and toxic disturbances have been confirmed by MRI scans of AIDS patients (Bottomley, Hardy, Cousins, Armstrong, & Wagle, 1990).

Concurrent with primary HIV infection of the brain, damage results from opportunistic infections and malignancies within and outside of the nervous system. For example, pneumonia can cause hypoxia, reducing oxygen flow to the brain (R. W. Price & Brew, 1991; Worley & Price, 1992). Reduced cerebral blood flow early in HIV infection can also cause encephalopathy (Schielke et al., 1990). Co-infection with other viruses, including HTLV-I, HTLV-II, and cytomegalovirus, serve as additional sources of neurological damage (I. Grant & Heaton, 1990). Finally, neurological symptoms may stem from iatrogenic factors, such as the direct effects and side effects of treatments for HIV infection and associated ailments. For example, most antiretroviral medications, including AZT, ddC, and ddI, can cause neuropathy and in extreme cases even seizures (Koppel, 1992). Like other aspects of HIV disease, multiple sources of damage can become superimposed upon each other. Multiple etiologies and interrelated symptoms cause a complex array of neuropsychological impairments, as well as a variety of neuropsychological disturbances across the HIV disease spectrum. Before reviewing specific neuropsychological deficits related to HIV Associated Minor Cognitive/ Motor Disorder and ADC, some conditions to consider for possible differential diagnosis are presented in the next section.

DIFFERENTIATING NEUROPATHOLOGY FROM OTHER CONDITIONS

Several conditions that compromise cognitive abilities can be confused for HIV-related neuropsychological dysfunction. For example, depression potentially confounds neuropsychological testing by slowing or decreasing motivation and cognitive processing speed, attention, concentration, and motor functioning (Hinkin et al., 1992; van Gorp, Satz, Hinkin, Evans, & Miller, 1989). In contrast with earlier findings, however, there is substantial evidence that depression does not seriously threaten the interpretation of neuropsychological tests of most people with HIV infection (Markowitz & Perry, 1992). Many studies fail to identify meaningful associations between measures of depression and functional impairment (I. Grant et al., 1993), performance on standardized neuropsychological batteries (Hinkin et al., 1992), screening measures of cognitive functioning and attention (Belkin, Fleishman, Stein, Piette, & Mor, 1992), and tests of memory (Egan, Chiswick, Brettle, & Goodwin, 1993). For example, Goggin et al. (1996) compared depressed HIV-seropositive men to a carefully matched nondepressed control group. Results showed that although depressed persons demonstrated poorer performance on tests of retentive memory, attention, and learning, both groups performed within the normal range. Nevertheless, relationships between depression and neuropsychological testing may be attenuated by the limited neuropsychological impairment observed during asymptomatic HIV infection and the severe impairment of later phases of ADC. Multiple other factors can also create problems interpreting neuropsychological symptoms. Concomitant opportunistic illnesses, past and current prescription and nonprescription drug use, sleep deprivation, and poor nutrition potentially impede neuropsychological testing. In addition, education and socioeconomic status may influence neuropsychological test performance, particularly in studies of gay men with higher education as well as injection drug users, whose education and socioeconomic status are typically low (Krikorian & Worbel, 1991; Selnes & Miller, 1992).

Antiretroviral medications can also disrupt neuropsychological performance through fatigue and reduced concentration (Koppel, 1992; Markowitz & Perry, 1992). On the other hand, AZT, particularly at higher doses, may reduce cognitive symptoms of HIV associated dementia complex and therefore improve neuropsychological test performance (Bornstein, 1993; Catalan & Burgess, 1991; Koppel, 1992; Schmitt et al., 1988; Worley & Price, 1992). In either case, neurological functioning of people taking AZT and perhaps other reverse transcriptase inhibitors could be influenced by effects and side effects of these drugs (Clifford, Jacoby, Miller, Seyfried, & Glicksman, 1990). Protease inhibitors, on the other hand, do not cross the blood–brain barrier and therefore offer no effects on HIV in the brain (Rabkin & Ferrando, 1997).

Another critical factor that can influence how neuropsychological tests are interpreted are the expectations for people with HIV to experience neurological deficits. From the perspective of the HIV-infected person, loss of cognitive abilities causes great anxiety and can prompt overinterpreting what may be normal lapses in memory or subtle neuropsychological disruptions related to medications, stress, or any number of factors. Similar expectations held by family, friends, and health care providers may subtly influence behavior. The expectation that HIV infection inevitably leads to cognitive decline should be addressed directly within the context of other forms of misinformation and inaccurate beliefs about HIV disease processes.

Acute Infection	Asymptomatic Infection	Early Symptoms	Late-Stage AIDS
Absence of HIV-Related Neurocognitive Deficits		Possible Mild Neurocognitive Deficits Mental and Motor Slowing Memory Lapses	Possible Significant Neurocognitive Deficits Opportunistic Illnesses AIDS Dementia

Figure 5.1

Manifestations of nervous system disease over the course of HIV infection.

NEUROPSYCHOLOGICAL MANIFESTATIONS

HIV enters the central nervous system shortly after infection and many individuals with AIDS suffer cognitive decline. Neuropsychological decrements have been described at early, asymptomatic, and later phases of HIV disease. Figure 5.1 shows the typical time line of neurological disorders in relation to the course of HIV disease, with most central nervous system manifestations occurring at later stages of AIDS. Unfortunately, most studies of HIV-related neuropsychological sequelae have relied on cross-sectional research designs, and few longitudinal studies have provided information on the progression of neuropsychological impairment.

EARLY HIV INFECTION

Although most people do not experience cognitive or motor symptoms early in the course of HIV infection, a small number of newly infected persons show signs of neurological impairment. Acute meningitis and meningoencephalitis occur soon after HIV crosses the blood–brain barrier (Bornstein et al., 1992; Markowitz & Perry, 1992). Early neurological symptoms, when present, usually overlap with other acute symptoms of HIV infection, including fatigue, headache, sensitivity to light (photophobia), pain around the eyes and facial areas, and leg weakness (Tindall, Imrie, Donovan, Penny, & Cooper, 1992; Worley & Price, 1992).

The prevalence of early neurological symptoms differs across age groups. Infants and young children demonstrate early neuro-deficits more often than adolescents and adults, with progressive encephalopathy in infants beginning as early as 2 months of age. Young children with HIV infection usually fail to reach developmental milestones, such as sitting up and walking, and milestones achieved are often lost (Ho et al., 1989; Janssen et al., 1991). Children with HIV infection otherwise show the same features of neuropsychological deficits observed in adults. The course of central nervous system involvement varies in children and, as in adults, can be either progressive or stable (Worley & Price, 1992).

ASYMPTOMATIC HIV INFECTION

There is considerable controversy concerning possible central nervous system dysfunction before the onset of significant immune suppression and opportunistic illnesses. Several studies with small samples and extensive testing batteries have found HIV-related neuropsychological impairment prior to other HIV-related illness. Early neurological symptoms would suggest that HIV can cause insidious damage to the central nervous system prior to symptomatic HIV disease (Markowitz & Perry, 1992). Using a one-standard-deviation difference from a control group mean as a criterion for neuropsychological impairment, Bornstein et al. (1992) classified 26% of HIV-seropositive men as neurocognitively impaired, relative to 15% of HIV-seronegative men. Bornstein et al. showed that degrees of neurocognitive impairment for the HIV-seropositive sample were twice the magnitude of those observed among HIV-seronegative individuals. The study also found that neuropsychological impairment was not accounted for by clinical depression and that neuropsychological test performance agreed with self-reported ratings of functional limitations. In another study, Saykin et al. (1989) found that asymptomatic HIV-seropositive individuals were more neuropsychologically impaired than a control group, but HIV-seropositive people on average performed within normal limits. Thus, studies that do find neuropsychological deficits in asymptomatic HIV infection suggest that only a subgroup, and probably a small group at that, evidences such decline.

The Multicenter AIDS Cohort (MAC) provided neuropsychological data from a large sample: 727 HIV-seropositive asymptomatic gay men, 84 men with symptoms of HIV disease, and 769 HIV-seronegative men (E. N. Miller et al., 1990). An extensive neuropsychological battery, including the Trial Making Test, Digit Span, a verbal fluency test, Grooved Pegboard Test, Symbol Digit Modalities Test, and the Rey Auditory Verbal Learning Test, showed no significant differences between HIV-seropositive asymptomatic and HIV-seronegative men. Using a two-standard-deviation difference from the HIV-seronegative group mean as a criterion for impairment, Miller et al. classified 6% of HIV seropositive men as impaired relative to 4% of HIV-seronegative men. When the criterion for impairment was relaxed to one standard deviation, Miller et al. classified 37% of HIV-seropositive and 34% of HIV-seronegative men as cognitively impaired. Miller et al. also failed to find relationships between immunology markers and neuropsychological functioning. Subdividing men on the basis of duration of HIV infection also did not show any associations with impairment. These findings argue against neuropsychological impairment in asymptomatic individuals and suggest that when deficits do occur they are usually modest. The degree to which these results are generalizable to women, however, is not known.

Additional research has failed to find neuropsychological impairment in otherwise asymptomatic HIV-seropositive people. Selnes et al. (1990), also from the MACS, administered a battery of neuropsychological tests to HIV-seropositive and HIV-seronegative men over a period of one and a half years. The study did not find significant differences between the two groups in neuropsychological changes over time. Furthermore, HIV-seropositive men did not decline in neuropsychological functioning over time. Consistent with these findings, Egan, Brettle, and Goodwin (1992) and Bono et al. (1996) found no evidence for significant cognitive impairment prior to the onset of other HIV-related symptoms in HIV-seropositive injection drug users. Other studies using more extensive neuropsychological batteries (e.g., E. M. Martin et al., 1993) and experimental memory tasks (e.g., Clifford et al., 1990) have failed to distinguish asymptomatic HIV-seropositive from HIV-seronegative individuals. In addition, studies that have identified central nervous system electrophysiological and structural changes in HIV-seropositive individuals, such as EEG abnormalities and cerebral atrophy, have not consistently related such abnormalities to clinical symptoms.

In their comprehensive review of 36 cross-sectional and 9 prospective studies of neuropsychological effects of HIV infection, Newman, Lunn, and Harrison (1995) found little evidence for neuropsychological dysfunction in asymptomatic HIV infection. Almost half of cross-sectional studies and two thirds of longitudinal studies failed to show any significant decrements in neuropsychological performance in asymptomatic persons. In addition, most differences were reported in studies with small samples that administered multiple test batteries. Newman et al. concluded, therefore, that there is insufficient evidence to suggest any increased prevalence of neuropsychological deficits in asymptomatic HIV-infected people.

Research conducted thus far does not indicate that HIV associated dementia is a progressive disorder that has an early onset and evolves during asymptomatic periods (Bornstein et al., 1992; Catalan & Thornton, 1993). We also do not know whether minor and severe forms of impairment are the same disease entity expressed to different degrees or whether people with minor forms of cognitive decline inevitably progress in severity. An absence of detectable cognitive decline over asymptomatic HIV infection further suggests that HIV-related neuropsychological impairment follows immune suppression and usually coincides with opportunistic illnesses, although not necessarily opportunistic illnesses afflicting the central nervous system. When the immune system is relatively healthy, viral expression of HIV remains generally suppressed in the central nervous system. Therefore, a competent immune system may delay the onset of HIV-related cognitive symptoms, encephalitis, and opportunistic illness (Sharer, 1992). In summary, although some people may experience acute episodes of meningitis near the time of seroconversion, asymptomatic phases of HIV infection are rarely associated with impaired occupational, social, or daily functioning. However, these conclusions remain tentative because some studies, mostly with small sample sizes using extensive test batteries, have identified a small subgroup of asymptomatic HIV-seropositive individuals with cognitive deficits. In contrast, there is general agreement that neuropsychological deficits are common to the late phases of HIV disease.

LATE HIV INFECTION AND AIDS

Neurological dysfunction associated with HIV infection is most likely to occur at times of severe immune suppression (Mapou & Law, 1994). Cognitive deficits appear in 40% to 50% of people with symptoms of HIV infection and 33% to 87% of people with AIDS (I. Grant et al., 1993; R. W. Price & Brew, 1991). As many as 15% of AIDS cases demonstrate abnormal brain structures on CT and MRI scans (Ostrow, 1990). Studies of the clinical symptomatology of HIV-associated neurological impairment suggest that one third of individuals eventually develop severe cognitive impairment, one third show mild disturbances, and one third experience few or no neurocognitive symptoms (Bornstein, 1993). Even when neurological problems do occur, only a minority of people progresses to full-blown dementia (Egan et al., 1992). Thus, although many individuals with later HIV infection do not demonstrate serious cognitive decline, a sizable number of people with AIDS do experience some degree of neurological impairment.

A broad range of neurocognitive disturbances occur in later-stage HIV infection. The earliest signs include diffuse and nonspecific symptoms such as lethargy; social withdrawal; psychomotor slowing; attention, concentration, and retrieval deficits; derailed train of thought; increased difficulty with complex tasks; forgetfulness; clumsiness; and complaints of sluggish thought processes (R. W. Price & Brew, 1991; Sharer, 1992; Worley & Price, 1992). These symptoms reflect HIV Associated Minor Cognitive/Motor Disorder. Severe cognitive disturbances, such as those in dementia, occur late in HIV infection and include disruptions to social, occupational, and daily routines; confusion; disorientation; motor losses; and eventual degeneration into a vegetative state.

Many HIV-related cognitive symptoms correspond to damaged subcortical brain structures (Koppel, 1992). Most commonly, deficits occur in information-processing speed and efficiency; memory and learning; and motor abilities. Cognitive slowing is, however, the most widely observed feature of HIV-associated neurocognitive impairment (Derix, de Gans, Stam, & Portegies, 1990; I. Grant et al., 1993). Reaction-time tasks provide a valuable index of cognitive-processing speed because they are sensitive to cognitive dysfunction without ceiling effects. Simple reaction-time tasks, in which a key is pressed as quickly as possible in response to a stimulus, consistently show that people with HIV infection have slower response times than do HIV-seronegative individuals (e.g., E. M. Martin, Sorensen, Edelstein, & Robertson, 1992). Choice reaction-time tasks, in which a key is pressed as quickly as possible with one hand in response to a target stimulus and another key is pressed with the other hand in response to a different stimulus, have also demonstrated cognitive slowing in HIV infection. E. M. Martin, Sorensen, Edelstein, et al. (1992) found that both asymptomatic and symptomatic HIV-seropositive gay men have slower decision-making speed in choice reaction time relative to their HIV-seronegative counterparts. Similar effects occur for choice reaction-time tasks with injection drug users (Egan et al., 1993). In a study of hemophiliacs with known dates of HIV seroconversion, duration of time since contracting HIV infection correlated with declines in decision speed as indexed by choice reaction time (Kokkevi et al., 1991). It should be noted, however, that most reaction-time differences occur in comparing symptomatic HIV-seropositive and HIV-seronegative groups rather than in observing declines in the performance of HIV-seropositive individuals.

Attention and concentration deficits are also found in relation to HIV infection. E. M. Martin, Sorensen, Robertson, Edelstein, and Chirurgi (1992) found that HIV-seropositive men performed less accurately on a subtle visual attention task relative to HIV-seronegative men. Another study using the same sample reported by E. M. Martin, Sorensen, Robertson, Edelstein, et al. (1992) showed further evidence for disrupted attention using the Stroop color–word naming task (E. M. Martin, Robertson, Edelstein, et al., 1992). HIV-seropositive men had more difficulty than HIV-seronegative men with controlled cognitive functions on a Stroop task that requires effortful, voluntary actions and places greater demands on attention. Additional evidence from divergent neuropsychological measures has suggested that cognitive and perceptual information-processing disturbances occur at later rather than earlier stages of HIV infection.

HIV-infected people perform less accurately than HIV-seronegative people on tests of long-term and short-term memory and on verbal learning tasks (Egan et al., 1993; Krikorian & Worbel, 1991). In one study using a neuropsychological battery, HIV-seropositive men differed in short-term and long-term verbal memory when compared to other medical patients matched for education and socioeconomic status (McKegney et al., 1990).

Motor deficits are also common to HIV infection. E. N. Miller et al. (1990) found that symptomatic men in the MACS cohort showed the greatest degree of neurocognitive deficits on measures of manual dexterity and psychomotor speed, including the Grooved Pegboard Test, Symbol Digit Modalities, and the Trail Making Test. HIV-seropositive injection drug users also experience difficulty with the Finger Tapping Test, an index of fine motor speed (McKegney et al., 1990). Motor slowing, leg weakness, and loss of mobility can occur without any other cognitive or intellectual dysfunction (Worley & Price, 1992). In summary, information-processing speed, attention processes, learning, memory, and motor abilities are affected by HIV infection. Such deficits are most apparent when measured by sensitive cognitive tasks at later infection stages.

The risk for neuropsychological impairment increases as HIV disease progresses. Of people with AIDS, 25% develop clinically significant impairment within 9 months of their first AIDS-defining condition, and another 25% show impaired functioning within 1 year of diagnosis (Markowitz & Perry, 1992). Rather than starting slowly and gradually progressing during asymptomatic phases, HIV-associated neurological deficits seem to follow the onset of other manifestations of HIV infection, and the progression is usually rapid (I. Grant & Heaton, 1990; Selnes et al., 1990). Although both longer duration of infection and accelerated rates of CD4 cell declines are associated with cognitive impairment, immune suppression does not reliably predict developing neurocognitive deficits. Immune and neurological declines are therefore correlated but not causally linked. Because cognitive deficits correlate with immune suppression, it is likely that cognitive impairment will occur with illnesses. Later HIV infection therefore involves simultaneous vulnerability to HIV-related symptoms, HIV-related neurological disorders, and opportunistic infections and malignancies that have distinctive neurocognitive consequences.

OPPORTUNISTIC ILLNESSES OF THE CENTRAL NERVOUS SYSTEM

Advancing declines in the immune system lead to an increased susceptibility to infections and malignancies, including those of the nervous system (see Table 5.4). AIDS-related central nervous system conditions are typically diagnosed using CT and MRI scanning, as well as through

Table 5.4

AIDS-Related Diseases of the Central Nervous System

Manifestation	Causal Agent
Opportunistic viral infections	Cytomegalovirus
	Herpes Simplex I & II
	Herpes Zoster
	Papovavirus (PML)
Fungal and protozoan infections	Toxoplasmosis
	Cryptococcus
	Candida
	Mycobacterium
Malignancies	Primary lymphoma
	Metastatic lymphoma
	Metastatic Kaposi's sarcoma
Cerebrovascular	Hemorrhage
	Infarction

attempts to medically treat neurological symptoms. Among the least frequent initial AIDS diagnoses, opportunistic illnesses of the nervous system develop during the later stages of AIDS.

Cytomegalovirus (CMV)

This infection is highly prevalent, with 95% of HIV-seropositive gay men carrying antibodies for cytomegalovirus (Markowitz & Perry, 1992). Although an infrequent manifestation, cytomegalovirus can cause meningoencephalitis, resulting in clouding of consciousness and a variety of other cognitive problems (Worley & Price, 1992). More commonly, cytomegalovirus infects the retinas (CMV retinitis), threatening partial and complete blindness. Cytomegalovirus can also cause demyelination of brain white matter and a subacute encephalitis (Koppel, 1992).

Progressive Multifocal Leukoencephalopathy (PML)

This demyelinating disease is caused by activation of a latent papovavirus infection. Progressive deterioration of white matter occurs because the papovavirus attacks oligodendrocytes, resulting in loss of nerve fiber insulation. Changes in mental status, memory loss, motor weaknesses, loss of vision and other sensory problems, as well as decreased mobility are common consequences of PML (Koppel, 1992; Krupp, Belman, & Schneidman, 1992). Symptoms of PML develop gradually and can be fatal.

Toxoplasmosis

The protozoan *Toxoplasma gondii* principally infects the central nervous system as a generalized encephalopathy as well as causes brain lesions (Koppel, 1992; Mariuz & Luft, 1992). Toxoplasmosis is the most common central nervous system infection in adults with AIDS (Koppel, 1992). The symptoms of toxoplasmosis encephalopathy include headache, fever, confusion, lethargy, changes in personality, and delirium. Focal neurologic damage resulting from brain lesions can cause seizures and specific cognitive deficits depending on location of the lesion (Levy,

Kaminsky, & Bredesen, 1988). In general, cerebral toxoplasmosis progresses rapidly and seriously threatens permanent brain damage. However, once diagnosed, several treatments can clear toxoplasmosis and provide relatively fast symptom relief.

Cryptococcal Meningitis

Caused by the fungus cryptococcus, an encapsulated yeast, Cryptococcal meningitis is the most common central nervous system fungal infection in late HIV infection, affecting up to one in four people with AIDS (Koppel, 1992; Masci, Poon, Wormser, & Bottone, 1992). The symptoms of Cryptococcal meningitis are similar to those of other meningitides, including neck stiffness, headache, photophobia, lethargy, declines in mental functioning, confusion, nausea, and vomiting. Symptoms can range from mild to severe and can result in encephalitis, possibly mimicking signs of depression (Markowitz & Perry, 1992).

Lymphoma

Central nervous system lymphomas are experienced by 5% of people with AIDS (Worley & Price, 1992). Although the brain is rarely the site of primary lymphoma, people with AIDS are nearly 100 times more likely to develop primary central nervous system lymphoma than are the general population (Koppel, 1992). In addition, B-cell lymphomas that originate as systemic disease can spread secondarily, resulting in metastatic lymphoma to the central nervous system, causing single or multiple lesions. Symptoms include headache, lethargy, and damage to cranial nerves, as well as damage to specific sites of tumor growth.

Other Nervous System Complications

Several additional HIV-related conditions can spread to the central and peripheral nervous systems, although such occurrences are relatively rare. Herpes simplex viruses I and II can cause encephalitis and meningitis, with acute symptoms of headache, fever, seizures, and abrupt behavioral disturbances (Koppel, 1992). In addition to its characteristic painful outbreaks of blisters, herpes zoster virus can also cause encephalitis (Koppel, 1992). Candidiasis, a common fungal infection in HIV, can cause brain abscesses in people with AIDS (Koppel, 1992). Coccidioidomycosis and histoplasmosis, also fungi, can cause chronic meningitis. Mycobacterium infection can cause meningitis and brain abscesses (Aronow et al., 1988). Neurosyphilis may develop or recur with suppressed immunity and is more difficult to treat than primary syphilis. Kaposi's sarcoma may also spread to the central nervous system. In addition to infections and malignancies, people with AIDS can suffer strokes as a result of cerebral vascular changes and changes in blood flow, as well as cerebral hemorrhage from HIV-related disruptions to blood clotting factors.

NEUROPSYCHOLOGICAL ASSESSMENT

Neuropsychological testing in HIV infection is most useful in evaluating subjective reports of decline in cognitive functions, including but not limited to attention, concentration, abstraction, reasoning, visual-perceptual skills, problem solving, mental and motor processing speed, and language. Neuropsychological evaluations inform clinicians of cognitive deficits and can disconfirm mistaken beliefs about declining cognitive abilities (Greenwood, 1991). Factors such as expectancies, anxiety, depression, and illness can contribute to the presence or absence of early neuropsychological symptoms. Because most cognitive changes in HIV infection are subtle, clinical mental status exams lack adequate sensitivity for reliable assessment (I. Grant & Heaton, 1990). Screening tests specific for detecting HIV associated cognitive impairment have also been developed. For example, a five item test of memory, attention, psychomotor speed, and manual construction showed 80% sensitivity and 91% specificity for detecting HIV-related dementia (Power, Selnes, Grim, & McArthur, 1995). However, screening positive for neuropsychological deficits requires confirmation with a complete assessment battery. Therefore, comprehensive neuropsychological evaluations that assess multiple mental faculties, although time consuming, labor intensive, and expensive, remain the most effective method for evaluating cognitive capacities.

There are several comprehensive neuropsychological assessment batteries that provide optimal sensitivity to neurocognitive deficits associated with HIV infection. For example, Janssen et al. (1991) suggested assessing attention and concentration (Trail Making Test A; Continuous Performance Test), information processing speed (Trail Making Test A and B; Digit Symbol Modalities; choice reaction-time task), motor functioning (Finger Tapping Test; Grooved Pegboard Test; Thumb–Finger Sequential Test), abstract reasoning (Wisconsin Card Sorting Test; Halstead Category Test), visual–spatial skills (Weschler Adult Intelligence Scale-Revised, Block Design Subtest), concentration (Serial Sevens; Digit Span), memory and learning (Rey Auditory Verbal Learning Test; California Verbal Learning Test; Weschler Memory Scale; Verbal Reproduction; Logical Prose Test), and speech-language abilities (Verbal Fluency Test; Vocabulary; Boston Naming Test). Although Janssen et al. recommended these areas of assessment and suggested specific tests, they did not propose a standardized evaluation battery.

To address the need for a standardized battery for use with HIV infection, a workshop sponsored by the National Institute of Mental Health assembled a 7- to 9-hour battery for assessing HIV-related cognitive impairment (N. Butters et al., 1990). Tests were compiled with the intention of maximizing sensitivity to cognitive functions most affected by HIV infection. Both widely used standardized clinical tests and tasks drawn from experimental cognitive psychology broadened the battery's complexity and increased its sensitivity. The battery included 10 cognitive domains assessed by 26 tests (see Table 5.5). Administration of the full battery was meant to cast a broad net across a wide range of cognitive and motor functions.

Unfortunately, administration of the battery recommended by N. Butters et al. (1990) poses several limitations, including the use of experimental cognitive-psychology tasks often unavailable in clinical settings. Furthermore, experimental psychology procedures do not provide normative information and cannot define clinical diagnostic criteria. The battery is also long and taxing for both the test taker and administrator. For these reasons, N. Butters et al. abbreviated the battery to require only 1 to 2 hours for administration.

Table 5.5

Neuropsychological Test Battery Recommended by an NIMH Sponsored Workshop

Cognitive Function	Assessment Instrument
Premorbid intelligence	*WAIS-R Vocabulary
	National Adult Reading Test
Attention	WMS-R Digit Span
	*WMS-R Visual Span
Processing speed	Sternberg Search Task
	Simple and Choice Reaction Time
	*Paced Auditory Serial Addition test
Memory	*California Verbal Learning Test
	Working Memory Test
	Modified Visual Reproduction Test
Abstraction	Category Test
	Trails Making Test A and B
Language	Boston Naming Test
	Letter and Category Fluency Test
Visual spatial ability	Embedded Figures Test
	Money's Standardized Road-Map Test of Direction Sense
	Digit Symbol Substitution
Construction ability	Block Design Test
	Tactile Performance Test
Motor abilities	Grooved Pegboard
	Finger Tapping Test
	Grip Strength
Psychological distress	Diagnostic Interview Schedule
	*Hamilton Depression Rating Scale
	*State-Trait Anxiety Inventory
	Mini-Mental Status Examination

NOTE: Data from Butters et al., 1991. *Tests included in the abbreviation battery recommended by Butters et al. (1991). WMS-R = Weschler Memory Scale–Revised; WAIS-R = Weschler Adult Intelligence Scale–Revised

Clinical findings from a neuropsychological battery usually lack sufficient specificity to diagnose HIV-related neuropsychological impairment (Janssen et al., 1991; Markowitz & Perry, 1992). Neuropsychological testing is most limited early in the course of HIV-related central nervous system disease. When present, early symptoms are usually subclinical and cannot be reliably detected by standard instruments (Martin, Sorensen, Robertson, et al., 1992). In addition, although neuropsychological assessments can indicate focal lesions, underlying disease processes cannot be determined by testing alone. The interpretation of neuropsychological tests should therefore occur in conjunction with neuroimaging and neurological exams as well as in consultation with infectious disease specialists.

Differential diagnosis of cognitive deficits and affective disorders can pose another obstacle to neuropsychological assessment, particularly in earlier phases of HIV infection. Even when symptoms of depression and anxiety are somewhat distinct from those of mild neurocognitive impairment, emotional distress can disrupt neuropsychological test performance. Neurological conditions are often accompanied by a sense of indifference, apathy, social withdrawal, emotional blunting, and lethargy (Navia, Jordan, & Price, 1986). Reduced motivation, attention, and concentration can impede neuropsychological test performance, so most batteries include evaluations of associated mental health problems.

FUNCTIONAL DEFICITS

The deficits that may result from neurological complications of HIV infection range from complete absence of impairment to severe disability. People with central nervous system HIV infection, determined either through examinations of cerebral spinal fluid or radiological imaging, are often completely unaffected by cognitive impairment. In HIV Associated Minor Cognitive/Motor Disorder, most complex daily living skills are minimally disrupted. Asymptomatic HIV infection also rarely involves cognitive and motor dysfunction (Selnes et al., 1990). Early symptoms of HIV infection may include slowed information-processing speed and deficits in verbal memory, but neither of these domains are affected to such a degree where daily routines are impaired (Sinforiani et al., 1991). Apathy, mental sluggishness, social withdrawal, and avoiding complex tasks may occur, posing problems in differential diagnosis of clinical depression (Markowitz & Perry, 1992). Although decrements in cognitive abilities can mark progressive neurological decline, mild forms of impairment do not indicate the onset of ADC.

Among the far-reaching complications of neurocognitive deficits are their effects on coping capacity. Even the most minor cognitive impediments can compromise problem solving abilities and decision making. In a study of asymptomatic HIV infected men, Manly et al. (1997) examined the use of coping strategies to manage daily stressors and found that persons who were experiencing impaired attention, slowed information-processing speed, and deficits in verbal skills were more likely to use confrontive behaviors as coping strategies. These differences occurred regardless of whether medical symptoms were present. Thus, neuropsychological deficits in early HIV infection can tax coping resources, reducing the capacity to manage stressful situations and leading to more impulsive coping behaviors.

Dementia and most opportunistic infections and malignancies of the central nervous system pose serious threats to functional capacities in the later phases of HIV infection. Impairment can be progressive and affect multiple cognitive and motor abilities. Cognitive and motor disorders related to HIV infection often co-occur with systemic manifestations of HIV as well as opportunistic illnesses outside of the nervous system. True for many dementias, concerns may eventually arise about home safety, wandering, confusion, and severe memory loss. Cognitive impairments also limit coping and adaptation, further complicating efforts to adjust psychologically to HIV infection and AIDS.

CONCLUSION

The prospect of losing mental and sensory abilities is one of the most frightening aspects of HIV infection. Individuals with HIV infection are usually aware of the potential for neuropsychological impairment and may have known others who have experienced cognitive decline. People who expect to lose their mental faculties can become hypervigilant and monitor their day-to-day activities and their performance of even simple tasks. Normal forgetfulness and poor concentration can result from stress, yet when a person with HIV is forgetful, it may be attributed to HIV infection and misinterpreted as the beginnings of dementia.

People living with HIV–AIDS, their families, and others in their support networks usually benefit from education and counseling about the realities of HIV disease. Learning that significant loss of mental abilities rarely occurs before people become quite ill and understanding that many people with HIV infection do not ever experience such difficulties can help alleviate undue anxiety. Individuals should also be informed of how depression, anxiety, and medication side effects can mimic neurological symptoms. HIV-seropositive individuals should be informed of the distinctions between HIV-related encephalopathy and opportunistic illnesses of the central nervous system, as well as the treatment options available for each.

Perhaps as much as any other dimension of HIV disease, central nervous system disease demands the integration of services from a multidisciplinary intervention team. Neurologists, infectious disease specialists, and radiologists can definitively diagnose HIV-related nervous system conditions. Functional evaluations offered by neuropsychological assessments can help to determine degrees of impairment. Behavioral interventions may help ameliorate functional impairments, including altering environmental obstacles to facilitate occupational and daily functioning and using learning and memory aides. Functioning can improve through interventions already widely used by neuropsychologists and rehabilitation specialists who treat cognitive deficits, regardless of their origin.

6

Social Sequelae

All epidemics have far-reaching social repercussions. An invisible microbe that causes illness and death understandably brings irrational fears and widespread panic. History shows that epidemics ultimately caused the persecution of people who became associated with the disease. For example, the 14th-century plague was viewed as divine punishment for sinful behavior; the uninfected often became so terrified they blamed the epidemic on already socially marginalized groups (Kishlansky, Geary, & O'Brien, 1991). Villages in Germany where plague ran rampant sought out Jews as scapegoats, putting many innocent people to death. Similarly, the cholera epidemic of the 1930s was viewed as a moral punishment for unclean and sinful behavior. Not until the early to middle 1900s did fear and prejudice against people with cancer begin to give way to care and compassion, although many discriminatory practices against cancer patients still exist (Stahly, 1988).

The social sanctions suffered by people afflicted with disease fit well under the broader rubric of *social stigmatization*. *Stigma* refers to a visible mark, such as a brand or tattoo, used to disgrace, shame, condemn, or ostracize (Herek, 1990). Stigmas are therefore socially ascribed to discredit those who bear a mark of social disapproval (Goffman,

1963). Discrediting results when a stigma is openly known and visible to others and stigmatization exists to the extent that a person loses social stature and becomes socially isolated.

The social construction of HIV–AIDS in the United States has made it among the most stigmatizing medical conditions in modern history. AIDS is viewed as much more than a transmissible and lethal disease. HIV-related stigmatization constitutes an epidemic in itself—an epidemic of fear, prejudice, and discrimination. Although contributing factors may differ, AIDS stigmatization occurs across societies (Woo, 1992). In the United States, AIDS stigmatization is fueled by misinformation about risks of HIV transmission, as well as by prejudicial attitudes against groups most affected by the epidemic, the sexual and drug-using behaviors that transmit HIV, and fears more generally associated with sickness and death (Herek & Glunt, 1988).

Herek (1990) identified six general dimensions of social stigmas relevant to AIDS: (a) *concealability*, the extent to which a condition is hidden or apparent to others; (b) *disruptiveness*, the degree to which it interferes with social interactions and relationships; (c) *aesthetics*, how others react to the condition with dislike or disgust; (d) *origin*, the responsibility attributed for causing or maintaining the stigmatized condition; (e) *course*, the degree to which the condition is alterable or progressively degenerative; and (f) *peril*, whether the condition will physically, socially, or morally contaminate others. Using these dimensions, Herek illustrated the stigmatization of HIV–AIDS as follows: although cancelable early in its course, later stages of HIV infection and AIDS are rarely hidden from others; HIV infection interferes with social relationships; the disease physically disables and disfigures and is therefore aesthetically repellent; its origin is often, although not always, blamed on behaviors and choices; the course of HIV infection is degenerative and not alterable; and HIV is a high-peril condition in that it poses risks to others. Thus, HIV infection falls on the negative end of all six stigmatization dimensions (see Table 6.1)

Whether related to medical illness or other culturally constructed conditions, social stigmas serve instrumental functions (Pryor, Reeder, Vinacco, & Kott, 1989). Stigmas create social distance to allow a sense

Table 6.1	
Characteristics of AIDS Along Six Dimensions of Social Stigmatization	
Stigma Dimension	Characteristic of HIV–AIDS
Concealability	Apparent at the later stages of disease
Disruption	Disabling and degenerative
Aesthetics	Body disfigurement in later stages
Origin	Blame for contracting and spreading HIV
Course	Progressive and irreversible
Peril	Poses actual and fictive risks to others

of personal security (Kegeles, Coates, Christopher, & Lazarus, 1989; Mondragon, Kirkman-Liff, & Schneller, 1991). Moralistic judgments that hold people responsible for contracting HIV infection serve the purpose of distinguishing between "people like them" and "those like us" (McDonell, 1993). However, stigmas play out in subtle and unexpected ways. For example, what at first may appear as supportive, treating individuals as "special" or with "holiness," becomes patronizing and results in a form of paradoxical stigmatization (Herek, 1990).

People suffer countless social repercussions related to HIV and AIDS. Family, friends, employers, coworkers, and health-care providers can all contribute to social prejudice, discrimination, and isolation. Many people conceal their HIV status from others, often at the cost of their personal welfare. Here I review the attitudes and fears that contribute to stigmatization toward people with HIV–AIDS. Attention is focused on how social stigmas are expressed among human service professionals. The chapter concludes with a discussion of education as a means of combating HIV-related stigmas.

SOURCES OF HIV-RELATED STIGMATIZATION

Prejudice against people with HIV infection primarily stems from three distinct, although not mutually exclusive, sources (Crandall, 1991; V.

211

Price & Hsu, 1992; Taerk, Gallop, Lancee, Coates, & Fanning, 1993). First, social stigmas result from realistic and unrealistic fears of contracting HIV. Although fears can stem from a lack of knowledge about HIV and its transmission, misinformation alone does not completely account for avoiding people with AIDS. Second, the groups most affected by HIV–AIDS are often marginalized prior to ever contracting HIV. Social prejudices that extend beyond HIV itself can therefore serve as a foundation for AIDS stigmatization. Third, the course of HIV–AIDS stirs cultural fears about death and dying and tendencies to avoid the terminally ill. These sources of stigmatization are discussed in the following sections.

Fear of HIV Infection

Fears of contracting HIV are a major contributing factor to HIV-related stigmas. AIDS fears, for the most part, are grounded in misinformation and misperceptions. Many negative attitudes toward HIV–AIDS surfaced early in the epidemic when little was known about AIDS and its cause. Attitudes toward people with HIV infection have not, however, much improved despite new information and understanding of AIDS.

Studies continue to show that the public lacks accurate information about HIV infection and AIDS. For example, the National Health Survey found that, although the majority of people in the United States were aware of the basic facts of how HIV is transmitted, a sizable number continued to hold misperceptions of AIDS that are associated with AIDS stigma (Sweat & Levin, 1995). The link between misinformation about AIDS and attitudes toward people living with HIV–AIDS has been investigated in telephone surveys. For example, Herek and Capitanio (1993) conducted a random phone survey of men and women across the United States and found a high degree of misinformation about HIV–AIDS, and inaccurate information was associated with negative attitudes toward HIV-infected individuals. Nearly half of the respondents believed that HIV infection could result from casual activities such as drinking from the same glass as a person with HIV, using the same toilet seat, being near a person with HIV–AIDS when he or she coughs or sneezes, and being bitten by insects.

Another random-digital-dial survey in 44 states and the District of Columbia showed that 16% of those called believed that insects could transmit HIV (Centers for Disease Control and Prevention [CDC], 1991b). In yet another random-digit-dial phone survey, Mondragon et al. (1991) found associations between misperceptions of HIV transmission from low-risk activities and hostile feelings toward people with AIDS. Similarly, Kegeles, Coates, Christopher, et al. (1989) found that one third of survey respondents believed that they could contract HIV from a physician who carries the virus. Similar fears of casual HIV transmission, including sharing kitchen utensils and bathroom facilities, were a major source of anxiety for caregivers of people with AIDS earlier in the epidemic (Frierson, Lippmann, & Johnson, 1987). People may therefore fear contracting HIV through casual social contacts despite the fact that no cases of HIV transmission have occurred through such modes. Misperceptions of HIV transmission potentially lead to hostile reactions and avoidance of people with HIV–AIDS.

Factors other than misinformation, however, contribute to fears of contracting HIV through casual contacts. Concern about even the most remote possibilities of contracting HIV stem from its high mortality rate. Of course, a great deal of concern is exerted over contacts with very low probabilities of HIV transmission while people continue to freely engage in sexual behaviors that carry real risks for HIV transmission (Gelman, 1993). People are well known to inaccurately judge risks, particularly in estimating the risks of low-probability events (Slovic, Fischhoff, & Lichtenstein, 1982). Frequencies and salience of media images depicting a particular route of transmission are a major source of risk misperceptions. For example, media coverage of six cases of HIV transmission that apparently occurred in one dental practice contributed to near hysteria over contracting HIV from dentists, which in turn brought guidelines from the CDC and the American Dental Association. Policy initiatives to mandate HIV-antibody testing for dentists and to limit the practices of dentists with HIV infection resulted from this one unusual case. Similarly, news reports of a case where HIV was apparently transmitted by kissing a person with bloody gums and open sores, caused considerable public hysteria (CDC, 1997).

Fears of contracting AIDS ultimately leads to the isolation of people with HIV infection. Herek and Capitanio (1993) found that 12% of individuals surveyed would intentionally avoid a close friend if they learned that he or she were HIV positive, 16% would prohibit HIV-infected children from attending schools, 20% would avoid an infected coworker, and 50% would avoid a neighborhood grocer if they knew he or she was HIV positive. Isolating individuals with HIV in prisons and hospitals is a common practice that originated with policies that were put into place before the cause of AIDS was even known. Quarantining people with HIV–AIDS is periodically considered as an option to contain the epidemic. For example, isolating hospital patients with HIV infection is a practice supported by many uninfected patients. A survey of hospitalized patients found that 55% would object to sharing a room with an HIV-infected person because of unfounded fears of contracting HIV (Seltzer, Schulman, Brennan, & Lynn, 1993).

Public misperceptions about HIV transmission may translate to other health policies that reflect prejudicial attitudes. Fears of HIV transmission have justified prohibiting people with HIV infection from entering the United States despite widely held views by public-health experts that such policies only serve discriminatory functions. Fears of contracting HIV infection can also form the basis for discriminatory practices in the workplace. At their worst, fears of AIDS have led to recommendations to persecute people with HIV–AIDS. Kegeles, Coates, Christopher, et al. (1989) found that 29% of survey respondents favored tattooing or otherwise visibly marking individuals who are HIV seropositive. The study also found that 21% to 40% of respondents supported isolating people with AIDS from neighborhoods and public places. Some have even called for quarantines of people with HIV infection, even though such actions may have a public health backlash and result in increased HIV transmission (D. A. Smith & Smith, 1989). Although nowhere in the United States has there been a serious policy to isolate individuals with HIV infection, several states have enacted legislation to restrict the liberties of people with HIV who are known to engage in high-risk behaviors (Gostin, 1989). For example, restrictive measures have been taken against people with HIV infection in Colorado who exposed others to the virus through negligent, reckless, or criminal behavior (Woodhouse, Muth, Potterat, & Riffe, 1993). Related policies include mandated reporting of HIV infection to public health authorities, a practice that will likely keep people from seeking HIV-antibody testing (Kegeles, Coates, Lo, & Catania, 1989); laws requiring disclosure of HIV status to sex partners; and aggressive partner notification programs.

Labeling Risk Groups

HIV-related social stigmas are superimposed upon attitudes that existed long before AIDS. Prejudice and fears are directed toward behaviors viewed as deviant, such as homosexuality and drug abuse. Public perceptions of AIDS combine with sociocultural perceptions of subgroups most visibly affected by the epidemic (Herek & Glunt, 1988). Discrimination against people with HIV infection has therefore grown out of prejudice against gay and bisexual men, the sexually promiscuous, and injection drug users (Kegeles, Coates, Christopher, et al., 1989; Treiber, Shawn, & Malcolm, 1987).

At first, AIDS was referred to as *Gay-Related Immune Deficiency* (GRID), and the *Gay Plague*. Media images of gay activists protesting political silence about the new disease, coupled with the first widely recognized celebrities afflicted with HIV being gay men, served to strengthen perceptions of AIDS as a gay disease (Triplet, 1992). Antigay hostility, homophobia, prejudice, and intolerance became closely associated with AIDS. Shortly later in the U.S. epidemic, injection drug use also became associated with HIV–AIDS.

It is unfortunate that the behaviors that afford efficient transmission of HIV are also socially condemned, fostering perceptions of personal responsibility for contracting the virus. The greatest degree of blame for the epidemic is attributed to individuals who are believed to have knowingly taken risks and become infected (McDonell, 1993). Thus, there are two classes of people with HIV infection: innocent victims who had no knowledge of their risk and are not held accountable (e.g., infected infants, hemophiliacs, and transfusion recipients), and those perceived as guilty for their contracting HIV (e.g., men who have sex with men, injection drug users, commercial sex workers, and the unmarried sexually active; McDonell, 1993). Blaming people with HIV for becoming infected, therefore, reflects a just world mentality.

Individuals who already suffer social discrimination confront further injustices in living with HIV–AIDS. Homophobia, prejudice against injection drug users, and dismay for people perceived as sexually promiscuous derail the potential power of public education efforts. Misinformation feeds prejudice, but it is not so easily corrected (Gallop et al., 1991; Mondragon et al., 1991). Widely held beliefs about HIV–AIDS, homophobia, and prejudices against addicts hinder policymakers from taking action to alleviate, rather than perpetuate, the problem (Herek, 1990).

Death and Dying

Western cultures typically hold negative views of death and dying. Death is associated with darkness, despair, and the unknown (Kalish, 1985). Fears of death influence the social and medical treatment of the terminally ill; people with HIV–AIDS experience these same prejudices. HIV infection reminds healthy people of their own mortality and ultimate finality. Thinking of individuals with HIV infection as inherently different helps one to maintain a safe distance from AIDS, providing a sense of protection from one's own vulnerability and mortality (Taerk et al., 1993).

Negative attitudes toward death, dying, and the terminally ill are therefore clearly linked to the social stigmas of HIV–AIDS and can have serious repercussions. Health-care professionals commonly avoid working with the terminally ill because they fear becoming attached to persons who they know will die. Nurses who lose multiple AIDS patients report experiencing significant emotional distress (Gordon, Ulrich, Feeley, & Pollack, 1993). Health-care providers must also deal with reactions of families and friends during periods of bereavement and grief (Weinberger, Conover, Samsa, & Greenberg, 1992).

EFFECTS OF HIV-RELATED STIGMATIZATION

Psychological Effects

Social stigmas can become a source of chronic stress for people living with HIV–AIDS. People who experience repeated acts of discrimination can become bitter, hostile, suspicious, and alienated. HIV-related stigmas therefore contribute to the anxiety, depression, and interpersonal distrust experienced by so many people living with HIV (Crandall & Coleman, 1992). Stigmatization also occurs across all phases of HIV disease and interferes with coping and adjustment (Crandall & Coleman, 1992).

During asymptomatic HIV infection, when there is minimal physical disfigurement, people with HIV are nonetheless perceived as discreditable. Threats of social isolation and discrimination may keep people from disclosing their HIV-infection status, therefore cutting off potential sources of social support. For example, individuals who do not disclose their HIV-seropositive status to others may still overhear derogatory remarks about people at risk for HIV and people with AIDS (Grossman, 1991). Crandall and Coleman (1992) found depression and anxiety were highest for people who had not disclosed their HIV-risk history to anyone. However, individuals who had gone completely public with their HIV status were also highly distressed. The researchers concluded that selective disclosure of HIV seropositivity to close and trusted confidants was related to the greatest degree of emotional adjustment.

Stigmas that people may internalize are another contributing factor to AIDS-related emotional distress. People with HIV infection commonly view their situation as a punishment and believe that HIV has contaminated all aspects of their life (Schwartzberg, 1993). Early in the epidemic Moulton, Sweet, Temoshok, and Mandel (1987) found that the degree to which people attribute the cause of HIV infection to themselves positively correlated with psychological distress and dysphoria. In contrast, attributing HIV infection to chance or to another person seems to lead one to experience less distress. Moulton et al. found that people with AIDS often feel guilty about contracting HIV and about the possibility that they might have infected others. Similarly, many HIV-seropositive men who contracted the virus through same-sex relations develop internalized homophobia, turning hatred and fear of homosexuality inward (Siegel, 1986). Wolcott, Namir, Fawzy, Gottlieb, and Mitsuyasu (1986) found that gay men with AIDS held negative attitudes toward their own homosexuality and toward disclosure of their sexual orientation. People who contract HIV through heterosexual contact or injection drug use may also internalize responsibility and blame, beliefs that can translate into self-reprehension.

Effects on Relationships

Loss of social support, isolation, and fear of abandonment are common in life-threatening illnesses. Although seeking social support is an important coping strategy (Leserman, Perkins, & Evans, 1992) and although social relationships critically influence emotional adjustment, many people with HIV–AIDS socially isolate themselves (McDonell, 1993). Similar to other stigmatized groups, people with HIV–AIDS may withdraw from social situations, increasing their emotional vulnerability. People with HIV infection often stop working and limit their participation in other social activities, cutting themselves off from others (Crandall & Coleman, 1992).

Not surprisingly, people with HIV infection are prone to disruptions in their most intimate relationships. In a study of HIV-seropositive gay men, Crystal and Jackson (1989) found that 31% had been rejected by at least one family member and that 38% had been abandoned by friends. In a related study, Pergami et al. (1993) found that 27% of HIV-seropositive women experienced changes in their social networks following notification of HIV infection and that nearly 66% suffered severe disruptions to their sexual relationships. H. A. Turner, Hays, and Coates (1993) found similar relationship conflicts in the lives of gay men with HIV infection, particularly among family members who were previously unaware of their sexual orientation. Accepting one's homosexual orientation opens up opportunities to discuss one's HIV-seropositive status and may, therefore, positively influence the availability of support.

As much as stigmas may affect available social supports, they also influence perceptions of received support. Perceiving that one lacks opportunities for support increases vulnerability to emotional distress and maladaptive coping (Green, 1993). Even for those who once had a socially supportive network, people with HIV–AIDS often find themselves removed from friends. It is therefore common for people with HIV infection to develop bonds among themselves, as a group with shared experiences and life challenges.

Effects on Families

AIDS affects multiple generations. The vast majority of children contracting HIV today become infected through perinatal HIV transmission. Thus, women are frequently the sole caregivers for their HIV-infected partner and their children. HIV-seropositive women, therefore, often bear the burden of a dual caregiver role (Hackl et al., 1997). Armistead and Forehand (1995) suggested that HIV infected women must manage multiple sources of stress, including decisions related to conception, disclosure of HIV status, and planning for the future. Women must also perform day-to-day parenting duties while managing other responsibilities in their lives. The fact that most HIV-infected mothers live in poverty only serves to extenuate these demands (Keogh, Allen, Almeday, & Temahagili, 1994). However, there is evidence that HIV-seropositive mothers develop poorer mother-to-child relationships and less effective parenting than noninfected mothers (Kotchick et al., in press).

Women with HIV must often care for their HIV infected children. Because HIV progresses at a much faster pace in children, they usually require extensive care early in their lives. The HIV infected mother is therefore often dependent on others for her own care as well as the care of her children (Flood, Hansen, & Kalichman, in press). The isolation that families with HIV–AIDS endure serves to further increase the distress and peril they face.

HIV-affected children, both infected and noninfected, constitute a rapidly growing population of orphans. By late 1993, an estimated 2.5 million children in the world had lost one or both parents to AIDS, and another 10 to 15 million orphans to AIDS are expected by the year

2000, over 90% of whom live in Africa (Merson, 1991). Improved prevention of perinatal HIV transmission and greater access to health care will likely serve to increase the number of orphans. Families often care for orphans to AIDS, but fears and stigma continue to shift orphans to nonfamilial caregivers (Foster, Makufa, Drew, Ashumba, & Kambeu, 1997). Children with HIV–AIDS suffer many of the same stigmas and discrimination as their parents, but children typically receive even less attention and support (Foster, 1996). Whether they are themselves infected or not, children of HIV-infected mothers experience significantly more difficulties in a variety of psychological domains, including child behavior problems and depression (Forehand, Steele, Armistead, Morse, Simon, & Clark, in press).

Health Effects

Stigmas present several potential adverse health-related outcomes. For one, the stress of social stigmas can have direct effects on health and wellness (Cole, Kemeny, Taylor, & Visscher, 1996). Concerns about discrimination and stigmatization are among the most common reasons why people avoid HIV-antibody testing (Kegeles, Coates, Lo, et al., 1989). Fear of harassment and job discrimination preclude opportunities for early medical interventions (Herek, 1990). HIV infection can result in loss of health insurance when it is deemed a preexisting condition. Although not entirely due to social perceptions of HIV disease, discontinued health-insurance benefits occur in a stigmatizing context and therefore join an accumulating array of adverse experiences. Stigmatization also originates from within the health professions, directly affecting the delivery of medical and mental health services. People with HIV often compare themselves to lepers in the health care system, facing impersonal attitudes of hospital staff and isolation within health care facilities (Frierson & Lippmann, 1987).

DISCRIMINATION

Discrimination against people with HIV–AIDS originates from the same fears and prejudices that give rise to other forms of stigma (Weiss

& Hardy, 1990). For example, foster parents of children with HIV infection fear contracting HIV and express concerns over rejection and
discrimination themselves should they take in an HIV-seropositive child
(F. L. Cohen & Nehring, 1994). Ridicule, violence, housing eviction, loss
of insurance, denial of health and dental care, loss of supportive services, and loss of employment are also very real consequences for those
who get too close to AIDS (Herek, 1990; Lyter, Valdiserri, Kingsley,
Amoroso, & Rinaldo, 1987). Discrimination is a common experience
for many HIV-seropositive gay men, injection drug users, school-age
children, and commercial sex workers. Crystal and Jackson (1989)
found that 11% of HIV-seropositive gay men had lost their housing
because of acts of discrimination. Gay men in the Chicago MACS cohort frequently reported discrimination that they attributed to their
HIV-seropositive status. For example, 6% of men in the cohort were
denied services by rental agents or bankers, 6% had been harassed by
the police, another 6% experienced physical violence or attempted violence, and 3% experienced work-related discrimination. Evidence for
the ill effects of AIDS discrimination comes from a survey of people
with HIV–AIDS that showed people who experienced more acts of
AIDS discrimination reported significantly less general life satisfaction
(Heckman, Somlai, Sikkema, Kelly, & Franzoi, 1997). The most destruc-
tive forms of discrimination involve employment, health care, and mental health services.

Employment Discrimination

It should be expected that HIV infection will be concealed from employers. Discrimination in the workplace against people living with
HIV–AIDS can include reduced responsibilities, isolation from coworkers and the public, or termination. Because places of employment
can be a major source of social contact, workplace discrimination
threatens one's sense of belonging. Although job termination on the
basis of illness is legal when physical limitations prohibit the performance of required duties, there is protection against discrimination for
disabled persons (Leonard, 1985; Terl, 1992). HIV–AIDS is included
under the Americans with Disabilities Act, which prohibits discrimi-

nation against "otherwise qualified" disabled individuals. However, laws and employment practices vary across states, and those who suffer illegal termination outside of high-AIDS-incidence areas usually lack adequate representation and advocacy.

People who have HIV and work in service-providing occupations are especially vulnerable to discrimination. Employers are no different from the general public and often hold irrational beliefs that HIV-seropositive employees will threaten the health of customers and clients. HIV-positive teachers, hairstylists, cooks, food servers, sales clerks, receptionists, and other service providers are among the most likely to endure employment discrimination. Even employers who know that HIV is not transmitted on the job may realistically fear that the public will not understand and that their business could be adversely affected if it became known that they had an HIV-seropositive employee. Like family members and friends, employers may fear HIV-related stigmas being displaced on them. To an even greater extent, HIV-seropositive physicians and other medical professionals must limit themselves to noninvasive procedures, and for some, like dentists, this is the equivalent of closing their practice. Despite universal precautions against HIV transmission and the fact that only a few providers have ever infected patients, the public fears dental and medical services from HIV-seropositive practitioners. A survey of adolescents, for example, found that teens hold a strong bias against receiving medical care from providers they perceive as being HIV seropositive (Ginsburg et al., 1995). However, stigmatization runs in the opposite direction as well, with health-care providers expressing discomfort about working with patients who are HIV seropositive.

Access to Care

A reality of AIDS is that some people can access treatments and others cannot. People living in developing countries are more likely to contract food- and water-borne diseases and lack access to even the most available and cheapest medicines, including PCP prophylaxis and antituberculosis drugs. Industrialized countries also have a clear gradation of treatment access. Antiretroviral therapies and AIDS care are expensive. The majority of U.S. adults and nearly all children with HIV infection receive medical care though public assistance, primarily the Ryan White Care Act. Inequities in accessing care are evidenced by a greater decline in AIDS-related deaths among men than among women, and among Whites than among minorities (CDC, 1997). In the case of differential access to care, discrimination is literally a life and death matter.

STIGMATIZATION BY MEDICAL PROFESSIONALS

Stigmas and prejudices propagated by health service providers are particularly troublesome. Studies over the past decade have shown that many medical professionals hold attitudes toward people with HIV mirroring those of society in general (Silverman, 1993). Medical staff often experience anxiety-like reactions to HIV-seropositive patients and feel reluctant to offer them treatment. Wallack (1989) found that 87% of physicians and nurses experience more anxiety when caring for AIDS patients than people with other illnesses. An AIDS-related phobia has been identified among physicians, nurses, and other caregivers and is characterized by fear, night terrors, and avoidance (Gordon et al., 1993; Horstman & McKusick, 1986; Silverman, 1993). Caring for people with HIV infection is reportedly more stressful than working with other equally serious medical disorders (P. Reed, Wise, & Mann, 1984; Silverman, 1993).

Several factors contribute to reluctance to provide health services to people with HIV–AIDS. In one study, Kegeles, Coates, Christopher, et al. (1989) found negative perceptions among health-care workers similar to those held by the general public. Willingness to provide services was clearly associated with fears of contracting HIV from patients, worrying about contact with hazardous materials such as syringes or surgical instruments, negative attitudes toward homosexuals and injection drug users, and death anxiety raised by caring for the terminally ill. Knox and Dow (1989) found that fears of contracting HIV infection and death anxiety can interrupt the delivery of health services to patients with HIV infection.

Because HIV is transmitted through blood, medical professionals who perform invasive procedures are the most fearful of becoming in-

223

fected. In one study, 60% of medical personnel expressed concerns over becoming HIV infected, with the greatest fear occurring among surgeons and emergency room physicians (Weinberger et al., 1992). Wallack (1989) found that 65% of hospital staff physicians and 63% of nurses felt at risk for contracting HIV even when following infection control guidelines. Concern over occupational HIV transmission among health-care workers is partially explained by distrust of technology, instrumentation, information, and health authorities (Gallop, Lancee, Taerk, Coates, & Fanning, 1992). Health care workers are aware that universal precautions reduce risk but do not guarantee protection against accidental HIV transmission (Taerk et al., 1993).

Exaggerated estimates of the relative risks of various medical procedures fuel fears over occupational HIV transmission (Gallop et al., 1991). Professionals may believe that HIV transmission occurs in ways that no one has ever become infected. Even highly knowledgeable medical professionals exaggerate the odds of contracting HIV (Gallop, Lancee, et al., 1992; Gallop, Taerk, Lancee, Coates, & Fanning, 1992). Risks related to medical accidents, particularly needle-stick injuries, are the product of three probabilities: the probability of the injury × the probability that the patient involved (source patient) is HIV seropositive × the probability of risk of HIV transmission associated with that type of accident. Using needle-stick injuries as an example, the odds of a piercing needle stick among health care professionals is less than 1 in 100 blood draws (McGuff & Popovsky, 1989); the probability of a patient having HIV infection varies with geographical location and medical specialty, but for example, the odds of a cardiac care patient in Seattle being HIV infected is less than 1% (CDC, 1992d); and the chance of HIV transmission occurring from a needle-stick injury with an HIV contaminated needle is also less than 1% (Marcus et al., 1988). Thus, the estimated probability of contracting HIV from an occupational needle-stick accident is a small fraction of 1%. Under most conditions, therefore, risks posed by medical accidents, even relatively common accidents like needle-sticks, are exceedingly low. The same factors that foster exaggerated risk perceptions in the general public cause medical professionals to overestimate their risk.

Paralleling discrimination outside of medical settings, factors un-related to fear of HIV transmission influence avoidance of patients with HIV–AIDS. Homophobia and negative attitudes toward injection drug users contribute to the resistance against working with HIV-seropositive patients (Bliwise, Grade, Irish, & Ficarrotto, 1991). In a survey of over 1,100 physicians, Gerbert, Maguire, Bleecker, Coates, and McPhee (1991) found over one third were uncomfortable caring for patients with injection drug addictions, reflecting sentiments toward drug users even without HIV infection. Like the general public, medical profes-sionals often view HIV–AIDS as a disease resulting from choice because of the behaviors associated with HIV transmission (Taerk et al., 1993). For example, nurses prefer to care for patients infected with HIV through blood transfusions as opposed to those infected through ho-mosexual activity (Gallop, Lancee, et al., 1992). Kegeles, Coates, Chris-topher, et al. (1989) also found that between 25% and 33% of health-care providers preferred to treat individuals infected with HIV through blood transfusions compared with HIV-seropositive gay men and in-jection drug users. Discomfort with HIV–AIDS patients is therefore closely associated with the socially sanctioned behaviors that result in HIV transmission.

In two early and widely replicated studies, Kelly, St. Lawrence, Smith, Hood, and Cook (1987a, 1987b) found that medical profession-als exhibited negative attitudes toward patients with HIV infection. Kelly et al. studied medical students (1987a) and physicians (1987b) using an experimentally controlled case vignette to manipulate char-acteristics of a patient independently, including the type of disease (AIDS or leukemia) and the sexual orientation of the patient (hetero-sexual or homosexual). There are several noteworthy aspects of the Kelly et al. (1987a, 1987b) case vignette. The early sections of the vi-gnette described the patient in positive and personal terms. The patient was a responsible and productive 32-year-old on an ambitious and suc-cessful career path. His leisure activities reflected middle- to upper-class interests, including skiing, sailing, and tennis. The vignette therefore set a context with which many of the medical-professional participants could identify. The onset of illness and the patient's declining health presented a tragic tone, but with the patient remaining courageous through difficult times. Thus, the patient's plight likely evoked sympathy. Following the positive description of the patient and his tragic illness, the patient's sexual orientation was introduced. The context of the vignette probably minimized attributions of blame to the patient and levels of discomfort treating the patient. The study results can therefore be taken as conservative estimates of stigmatizing attributions ascribed by health-care professionals early in the AIDS epidemic.

Using this case vignette with physicians, Kelly et al. (1987b) identified several negative attitudes held toward HIV-infected patients. Physicians believed AIDS patients were more responsible for their illness and less deserving of sympathy compared to leukemia patients. Physicians were also less willing to interact with AIDS patients interpersonally than they were with leukemia patients, even in situations as innocuous as casual conversations. Among medical students, Kelly et al. (1987a) found that negative attitudes toward AIDS correlated with homophobia; however, this association did not replicate in the sample of practicing physicians. Kelly et al. concluded that discomforts of medical-service providers ultimately limit interactions with HIV-seropositive patients, interfering with service delivery and quality of care—conclusions that have subsequently been empirically supported (McDonell, 1993).

Providers may also feel helpless and ineffective when dealing with HIV–AIDS, particularly when professionals have had minimal training and limited experiences with HIV infection (Weinberger et al., 1992). Minimal resources, limited support, and increased workloads associated with these difficult cases lead medical professionals to fear excessive stress and burnout (Bliwise et al., 1991; Silverman, 1993). Because most HIV-infected patients are uninsured they may pose a financial burden to health care professionals (Weinberger et al., 1992). Finally, providers have expressed concern over the possibility of spreading HIV infection to their friends and family should they become infected while on the job (Treiber et al., 1987). Early on, as many as two thirds of professionals reported that friends or family members are concerned about the risks of caring for HIV-seropositive patients (Blumenfield, Smith, Milazzo, Seropian, & Wormser, 1987).

AIDS stigmas, therefore, have the potential to interfere with professional service delivery (McDonell, 1993). For example, medical professionals frequently fail to discuss HIV-disease processes with their HIV-seropositive patients (Gerbert, Maguire, & Coates, 1990). In the Netherlands, the majority of physicians and nurses surveyed avoided invasive medical procedures with HIV-positive patients (Storosum et al., 1991). Medical students in the United States have preferred not to perform invasive procedures with HIV-seropositive patients, including routine blood draws (Imperato, Feldman, Nayeri, & DeHovitz, 1988). Likewise, medical students have also reported concerns about AIDS that influence their choice of specialty area, and they also believe they should have the right to refuse treatment to AIDS patients (Strunin, Culbert, & Crane, 1989). Another study found that 53% of hospital staff admitted that they have avoided performing procedures on patients with HIV infection (Wallack, 1989). Gerbert et al. (1991) showed that physicians feel a sense of responsibility for providing care, yet 50% would prefer not to work with AIDS patients if given a choice. Van Servellen, Lewis, and Leake (1988) reported that 23% of nurses surveyed would not accept AIDS case assignments. Blumenfield et al. (1987) found that nearly half of nurses surveyed indicated that they would transfer out of their current position if required to treat HIV-seropositive patients on a regular basis. Thus, AIDS stigmatizing attitudes translate to practices that compromise the quality of care offered to people with HIV–AIDS. Although studied to a lesser extent, similar types of fears and prejudice are observed among mental health professions.

STIGMATIZATION BY MENTAL HEALTH PROFESSIONALS

Unlike other health services, mental health professionals working in nonmedical settings do not incur any occupational risk for HIV infection. Nevertheless, fears and ignorance are no less common in the mental health field. Stigmatization of HIV-seropositive individuals here again stems from homophobia, prejudice against injection drug users, and death anxiety. In a study of hospital-based social workers, Dhooper,

Royse, and Tran (1987–1988) found 80% unwilling to accept clients with AIDS into their caseloads. Social workers feared contracting HIV infection from HIV-seropositive clients, suggesting widespread misinformation and prejudice. Dhooper et al. also found that social workers lacked empathy for HIV-seropositive clients and attempted to maintain distance from them. Fear of AIDS among social workers in the Dhooper et al. study correlated with homophobia; homophobic respondents were most afraid of contact with HIV-infected clients. Kegeles, Coates, Christopher, et al. (1989) surveyed a more heterogeneous sample of mental health professionals and found that they too avoided treating individuals with HIV–AIDS in their counseling practices.

Like physicians, clinical psychologists express generally negative attitudes toward people with AIDS relative to other medical patients (St. Lawrence, Kelly, Owen, Hogan, & Wilson, 1990). Using the same experimentally controlled case vignette used by Kelly et al. (1987a, 1987b), St. Lawrence et al. found that psychologists held AIDS patients more responsible for their illness and were less willing to see them in their practice relative to identical cases of leukemia patients.

Crawford, Humfleet, Ribordy, Ho, and Vickers (1991) surveyed clinical psychologists, counseling psychologists, and social workers in 13 U.S. cities using a case vignette modeled after the one used by Kelly et al. (1987a, 1987b). Mental health professionals were again hesitant to see clients they believed to have HIV infection, and they avoided contact with HIV-seropositive people. The study also replicated Kelly et al.'s findings, demonstrating that mental health professionals perceived people with AIDS as more responsible for their illness than patients with other medical conditions. Crawford et al. showed that negative attitudes toward AIDS were associated with homophobia, again replicating the Kelly et al. (1987a) medical student findings. Importantly, however, Crawford et al. (1991), St. Lawrence et al. (1990), and Kelly et al. (1987a, 1987b) used practically the same experimental case vignette in their respective studies. Thus, the findings were replicated but may not generalize to situations that differ from the case description. In addition, more recent research suggests that negative attitudes observed in earlier research may be dissipating. For example, Fliszar and

Clopton (1995) used a vignette modeled after the Kelly et al. (1987a) case and found clinical and counseling psychology graduate students were far more accepting of clients with AIDS than professionals in earlier studies. The study also showed, however, that many of the AIDS stigmas found in earlier studies prevailed in the more recent sample, including beliefs that people with AIDS are more responsible for their illness, more deserving of their condition, and more dangerous than leukemia patients.

In summary, AIDS stigmatization by mental-health professionals appears to mirror that of medical professionals and the general public. Professionals, like the general public, distrust sources of information about HIV transmission and commit cognitive errors when estimating the risks of HIV transmission. Thus, widely held social and cultural values fuel most negative attitudes toward people with HIV–AIDS. Fear of prejudice causes people to conceal things about themselves, such as sexual orientation and drug abuse. For similar reasons, people with HIV–AIDS do not always disclose their HIV-positive status to others.

DISCLOSURE

People affected by stigmatized medical conditions, especially when symptoms are not visible, often hide their diagnoses from others (Kleck, 1968). The social context of AIDS creates an environment of shame and secrecy that fosters concealment when one has HIV. Individuals may hide their HIV serostatus from others for fear of straining friendships and potentially damaging already stressed family relationships (Herek, 1990). Siegel and Krauss (1991) identified four considerations among HIV-seropositive gay men that influenced disclosure of their HIV status: fears of rejection, the wish to avoid pity, the wish to spare loved ones' emotional pain, and concerns about discrimination. Concealing one's HIV serostatus can also be part of a larger effort to maintain as much normalcy as possible in one's life. The sections below overview the issues of disclosing HIV-seropositive status to health care providers, families, and friends. Issues concerning disclosure of HIV serostatus to sex partners, however, are discussed in chapter 7.

Disclosure to Providers

People with HIV–AIDS may not disclose their HIV serostatus to providers for fear that they will be refused services or suffer other forms of discrimination. Such concerns are supported by the negative attitudes and beliefs about AIDS held by providers, as reviewed above. In a survey of HIV-seropositive men who had seen a physician or dentist for care not associated with their HIV condition, Marks, Mason, and Simoni (1995) found that 21% of men had not disclosed their serostatus to any such providers. Of men who had not disclosed to providers, 28% stated that they believed the physicians or dentists would refuse to treat them if they knew they were HIV infected. Indeed, Marks et al. reported that 11% of their sample had been refused treatment. Choosing not to communicate one's HIV condition can risk misdiagnoses, improper treatment, and adverse drug interactions. In this case, not disclosing one's HIV serostatus can be life threatening

Disclosure to Friends and Family

Concealing HIV infection decreases the availability of social support (Herek, 1990). Stress caused by efforts to conceal a positive HIV serostatus is partially due to the necessity of structuring interactions to minimize risks of disclosure. Selective disclosure of HIV infection tends to divide one's world into those who know and those who do not know. Living a "double life" can involve lying about recurrent illnesses, hiding medications, and covering up symptoms (Siegel & Krauss, 1991). In a study of Hispanic men with HIV infection, Marks, Richardson, Ruiz, and Maldonado (1992) found disclosure of HIV status to be a highly selective process and that disclosures increased as HIV disease advanced. In this study, men disclosed to their sexual partners and close friends more often than to their families. Disclosure of HIV serostatus and communicating about HIV infection with friends and family can lead to greater satisfaction with the social supports one receives (H. A. Turner et al., 1993).

Considerable differences exist in patterns of disclosure in various types of relationships. For example, Mason et al. (1995) found that Latino and White men disclosed their HIV serostatus to their mothers more often than to their fathers. In addition, Caucasian men were more likely to disclose to parents than were English-speaking Latinos, who in turn were more likely to disclose than Spanish-speaking Latinos. In related research, Simoni et al. (1995) found that HIV seropositive people were about equally as likely to disclose to their mothers and fathers. However, for both men and women, disclosure to friends was far more frequent than disclosure to family.

HIV-seropositive parents can find it painful to disclose their serostatus to their children. For one, parents fear that their children will suffer harm from stigmatization of having a parent with HIV–AIDS (Armistead & Forehand, 1995; Pliskin, Farrell, Crandles, & DeHovitz, 1993). Families have expressed concerns about word getting out about an HIV-seropositive family member, more so because of sanctions placed on risk behaviors rather than on HIV–AIDS itself. Mothers of hemophiliacs, for example, fear that AIDS stigma will be placed on their sons even when the latter are not HIV infected. Likely related to these fears, mothers of HIV-seropositive hemophiliacs report greater emotional distress in comparison to mothers of HIV-seronegative hemophiliacs (W. A. Brown, 1996). Parents are more likely to disclose their HIV status to older children and when the HIV-infected parent becomes seriously ill (Armistead, Klein, Forehand, & Wierson, 1997). The social baggage of AIDS, particularly attitudes toward HIV-transmission-related behaviors, also complicates familial disclosure. Disclosing that one is HIV positive can mean simultaneously coming out with one's sexual orientation, sexual history, or drug use history.

As people approach the later stages of HIV infection, hiding their HIV serostatus becomes increasingly difficult. Greater frequencies of medical visits, a mass of medications, deteriorating health, changes in appearance, and occupational disability can force disclosure (Crandall & Coleman, 1992). AIDS therefore threatens to uncover a life-style that may have been hidden for years, leading to a cycle of emotional distress and loss of social support. People with HIV–AIDS will be least likely to disclose when doing so carries high personal expense. Thus, the best way to promote disclosure of HIV serostatus is to remove the stigmas and threats of discrimination that prohibit disclosure in the first place.

CONCLUSION

The expanding AIDS crisis has brought new fears and prejudices against people living with HIV–AIDS. As the number of people needing medical services increases, HIV infection will place even greater demands on an already burdened health care system, again exacerbating negative attitudes toward HIV–AIDS (Herek, 1990). Education is the first line of defense against the epidemic of HIV-related stigma. Even brief education programs can successfully reduce negative attitudes toward HIV–AIDS and remove unfounded fears of contracting HIV infection (Bliwise et al., 1991; Gallop, Taerk, et al., 1992; Riley & Greene, 1993). Crawford et al. (1991) found that mental health professionals who received AIDS education held less negative attitudes and more often accepted people with HIV–AIDS. Including discussions with HIV-seropositive public speakers or using videotapes of patient interviews can also help ease concern and increase comfort (Gallop, Taerk, et al. 1992).

Although necessary, education alone may be insufficient to eliminate HIV-related stigmas. Education efforts with medical students, for example, have shown little effect on misperceptions of risk and negative attitudes (Imperato et al., 1988). Education does not stop people from blaming HIV-seropositive individuals for having become infected (Herek, 1990). Homophobia and prejudice against injection drug users also persist despite AIDS education. As the epidemic spreads among inner-city ethnic minorities, new dimensions of stigma that are based on racial and socioeconomic discrimination will emerge. Public and professional distrust in information from authorities about the "truth" of HIV–AIDS will ultimately thwart education efforts. Providing factual information about routes of HIV transmission to families with an HIV-seropositive member had little effect on dispelling anxieties about casually contracting HIV infection (Frierson et al., 1987). Thus, removing social stigmas attached to HIV infection will require greater change than offered by unidimensional education programs. What seems necessary to dispense AIDS stigmas are more sweeping social changes in attitudes toward groups most affected by AIDS. Removing stigmas increases opportunities for social support and eliminates the distress caused by blame and condemnation.

PART THREE

Sexual, Psychological, and Social Adjustment

I told my comrades that human life, under any circumstances never ceases to have a meaning, and that this infinite meaning of life includes suffering and dying, privation and death. . . . They must not lose hope but should keep their courage in the certainty that the hopelessness of our struggle did not detract from its dignity and its meaning.

(Victor Frankl, 1963, pp. 131–132)

Like some rabid animal, AIDS picked me up by the scruff of my neck, shook me senseless, and spat me out forever changed. I am today a totally different person than I was when the decade and the epidemic began. AIDS has been a cosmic kick in the ass—a challenge to finally begin living fully.

(Michael Callen, 1990, p. 2)

7

Sexual Adjustment

The sexuality of people living with HIV–AIDS has only recently been open to discussion. Despite research showing that many people who test HIV seropositive continue to practice unsafe sex, interest in HIV-related sexual issues was confined to primary prevention with at-risk populations. There are many reasons why the sexuality of people living with HIV–AIDS was ignored for so long. First, there is little attention given to the sexual adjustment of people with chronic illnesses in general. Avoiding sexuality in chronic illness may stem from preconceived notions about the chronically ill and discomforts that many people experience when asking questions about sex. In addition, once a person is diagnosed with HIV, there are many issues of greater importance that must be dealt with, including managing a life-threatening condition, accessing care, and gaining support.

There was also hesitance to research the sex lives of people living with HIV–AIDS because such information could conceivably be used against people living with HIV. Calling attention to the sexual behavior of people who are living with HIV–AIDS could promote beliefs that blame infected people for their condition. A lag in information about the effects of HIV on sexuality has therefore arisen from a discomfort in dealing with sexuality and the tendency to ignore the sexuality of people with chronic illness, as well as from genuine concerns for people with HIV–AIDS. Unfortunately, failing to address sexual issues for much of the first decade of AIDS has led to a virtual dearth of information that would be useful in helping people who experience difficulties adjusting to HIV–AIDS sexually.

This chapter overviews the issues of sexual adjustment to HIV–AIDS. Learning that one is HIV infected has profound effects on an individual, including on their sexuality. Although there are aspects of sexual adjustment that are clearly associated with emotional and social functioning, the nature of AIDS suggests that there are unique issues of direct relevance to sexuality, sexual practices, and sexual relationships.

HIV AND SEXUALITY

Sexuality is complex, encompassing cognitive and emotional processes, behavioral expressions and experiences, and relationships. Various aspects of one's sexuality interact with the effects of living with HIV–AIDS (see Table 7.1). Sexual history, sexual self-concept, and sexual functioning, for example, play important roles in sexual adjustment to HIV–AIDS.

Sexual History

On the basis of what is known about people most likely to become HIV infected, many people living with HIV–AIDS were likely sexually abused as children and adults. Sexual abuse is an enormous social problem in its own right, with over 100,000 cases of sexual abuse entering child protective services each year and more than 27% of women and 16% of men reporting being sexually abused prior to age 18 (Finkelhor, 1986). Community-based research suggests an even greater problem, with high rates of child-sexual-abuse histories found in adolescent victims of sexual assault (Muram, Hostetler, Jones, & Speck, 1995) and adolescents receiving mental health inpatient care (L. K. Brown, Kessel, Lourie, Ford, & Lipsitt, 1997). Substantial evidence shows that adoles-

Table 7.1	
Aspects of Sexuality That Interact With HIV–AIDS	
Aspect of Sexuality	Relationship to HIV–AIDS
Sexual history	Preexisting sexual experiences and events are exacerbated by AIDS (i.e., child sexual abuse and risk behavior history).
Sexual self-concept and sexual self-esteem	Negative effects of stigmas and self-defacement; adverse reactions to sexually transmitted infections.
Sexual functioning	Loss of sexual interest, depression, reduced sex drive, illness, medication side-effects, hypogonadism.
Sexual behavior	Continued sexual-transmission risk behavior, substance use during sex, disinhibition, psychopathology.
Disclosure to partners	Adverse consequences inhibit disclosure; stress from pressure to disclose.

cents and adults who were sexually abused as children are at greater risk for HIV infection than adolescents who did not experience abuse (Berenson, San Miguel, & Wilkinson, 1992; Lodico & DiClemente, 1994; Rosenfeld & Lewis, 1993). These findings are consistent with research showing that both men and women who were sexually abused as children are vulnerable to HIV–AIDS as adults (Cunningham, Stiffman, & Dore, 1994; Doll et al., 1992; Zierler et al., 1991). Bartholow et al. (1994), for example, found that gay and bisexual men who were sexually abused as children were more likely to report an array of HIV-risk associated sexual- and substance-abuse behaviors, paralleling the effects of child sexual abuse in women (Zierler et al., 1991). It should not be surprising that sexual abuse is associated with subsequent vulnerability to HIV–AIDS given the long-term trauma caused by sexual abuse and its relationship to a plethora of mental-health problems in adulthood.

There are numerous other sexual history factors that may have contributed to initial risks for HIV that carry over and affect the sexuality of people living with HIV–AIDS, including homophobia, commercial sex work, drug addiction, and past sexual partners. In particular, an individual's sexual history can be the source of feeling guilty or ashamed. Many of the sexual problems that people with HIV–AIDS experience cannot, therefore, be solely attributed to having HIV. However, testing HIV positive surely interacts with sexual histories, complicating the sexual adjustment process.

Sexual Self-Concept

People who sexually contract HIV are vulnerable to all of the social maladies common to having any sexually transmitted infection, especially guilt, self-blame, and shame. Guilty feelings can stem from self-degradation, which can include beliefs that one is contaminated, damaged, or dirty. It is therefore not surprising that many people with HIV–AIDS disassociate themselves from their sexuality (Gochros, 1992). Sexual self-images and self-esteem are also affected by perceptions of physical attractiveness. Although the later stages of AIDS are often accompanied by body disfiguring illnesses, such as HIV wasting syndrome and skin diseases, viewing oneself as sexually undesirable can occur much earlier in the HIV disease process. Internalized AIDS stigmas and negative images of AIDS become incorporated into one's sexual self-schema. The damage caused by these images is immediate and appears to persist for some time following receipt of an HIV-positive test result (Hankins, Gendron, Tran, Lamping, & LaPointe, 1997).

Sexual Functioning

Despite the fact that sexual satisfaction is an important aspect of quality of life for people living with HIV–AIDS (Tindall, Forde, Goldstein, Ross, & Cooper, 1994), people living with HIV frequently experience a loss of interest in sex. Diminished sexual interest can be coincidental with physical illness or depression. Sexual disinterest can also be an independent result of having HIV (D. C. Turner, 1995). Gochros (1992), for example, described living with HIV as an antiaphrodisiac, principally because of the associations of HIV and images of illness and death.

Loss of sexual desire and diminished sexual performance can result from the HIV disease process. Testosterone deficiency or hypogonadism, for example, is frequently observed in HIV-seropositive men and is related to diminished sexual desire (Poretsky, Can, & Zurnoff, 1995; Wagner, Rabkin, & Rabkin, 1995). Indeed, testosterone replacement therapy can effectively treat hypoactive sexual desire disorder in men living with HIV–AIDS. Rabkin, Wagner, and Rabkin (1996), for example, found that HIV-seropositive men who received testosterone treatment for depression significantly increased their sexual interest, erectile functioning, and sexual satisfaction. In addition, men who continued in treatment reported sustained improvement, whereas 80% of men who entered a placebo control arm of the study relapsed to lost sexual interest.

Women living with HIV infection also experience a loss in sexual desire, with more than one third of women with HIV meeting the diagnostic criteria for hypoactive sexual desire disorder (Goggin, Engelson, Rabkin, & Kotler, 1997). Goggin et al. found abnormal hormone levels in women with HIV–AIDS that paralleled those observed in men; there was not an association between testosterone-related hormones and decreased sexual desire in women. Thus, in contrast to men, loss of sexual desire in women seems more closely related to fear of rejection, lacking a sex partner, fatigue, relationship problems, and fear of infecting partners. Although it is common for women with HIV to experience reduced sexual desire (G. Brown & Rundell, 1990; Meyer-Bahlburg et al., 1993), Hankins et al. (1997) reported that nearly all women with HIV infection experience a period of sexual adjustment that lasts approximately 8 months, after which sexual activity typically resumes.

In addition to hypoactive sexual desire, men and women living with HIV can experience other sexual dysfunctions as a consequence of HIV infection. For example, men may experience erectile dysfunction and women orgasmic dysfunction because of the anxiety, distraction, or discomfort with sex (Hankins et al., 1997). Painful intercourse (dyspareunia) and accompanying spasms that narrow the vaginal opening have also been reported in women who test HIV seropositive (Catalan et al., 1996). Difficulty ejaculating despite maintaining an erection and prolonged stimulation can also occur in situations where a man fears that he may infect his partner. Rosser, Metz, Bockting, and Buroker (1997) found that more than half of HIV-seropositive gay and bisexual men experienced negative effects of HIV on their sexual functioning, including fear of sex and loss of erection. In a study of gay men and hemophiliacs, Jones, Klimes, and Catalan (1994) found that HIV-seropositive men frequently reported delayed ejaculation. Although psychological and social factors clearly play a role in sexual dysfunction, many sexual problems have their origins in organic disturbances. Tindall et al. (1994) showed that nearly half of HIV-seropositive gay and bisexual men experience some form of sexual dysfunction, but that sexual problems were far more common in the later stages of HIV disease.

SEXUAL BEHAVIOR

It is more likely that people with HIV–AIDS will refrain from sexual intercourse than they will practice frequent acts of unprotected sex. Still, a sizable minority of people living with HIV–AIDS continue to practice high-risk sexual behavior despite the pressures placed on them to take steps to protect their sex partners, including potential social and legal sanctions for placing partners at risk (Bayer, 1996). In a relatively brief period of time, research has investigated the sexual behaviors and sexual contexts of people living with HIV–AIDS. Across several studies with diverse populations, as many as half of men and women living with HIV infection report practicing unprotected sexual behaviors that pose high risk for HIV transmission (Kwitkowski & Booth, in press; Metsch, McCoy, Lai, & Miles, in press). Although most people report unprotected sex in monogamous relationships with an HIV infected partner, unprotected sex outside of such contexts is also extremely common. Studies with men who have sex with men, substance abuse populations, and women have found similar behavioral patterns of continued sexual risk behavior.

Men Who Have Sex With Men

The majority of studies investigating continued unsafe sex practices following testing HIV positive have been conducted with gay and bisexual men. In general, studies find that approximately one third of both HIV-seropositive and seronegative gay and bisexual men report recent unprotected anal intercourse (Lemp et al., 1994). Darrow et al. (in press), for example, found that 39% of HIV-antibody-positive men reported current practice of unprotected anal intercourse and the majority of these men did so outside of long-term relationships. In a study of self-identified gay and bisexual men recruited through advertisements in newspapers and community outreach to gay bars and social organizations, 39% of men reported engaging in unprotected anal intercourse in the 3 months prior to participating in the study (Kalichman, Kelly, & Rompa, 1997). None of the men in this study reported using condoms every time that they had anal intercourse, and condoms were used by HIV-seropositive men during an average of only 39% of anal intercourse occasions. Among the 33 HIV-seropositive men in this study who reported engaging in unprotected anal intercourse, one third reported unprotected acts with only one partner, one third reported two partners, and one third had engaged in unprotected anal sex with three or more men. Of HIV-seropositive men engaging in unprotected anal intercourse, 55% did so outside of exclusive sexual relationships. Among seropositive participants reporting any unprotected anal intercourse in the past 3 months, over 50% reported that at least one unprotected anal intercourse partner was not known to be HIV seropositive, 20% reported that their most recent sex partner was HIV seronegative, and 49% stated that their most recent partners' HIV serostatus was unknown.

In another study of gay and bisexual men who participated in an HIV risk-reduction intervention delivered by telephone, Kalichman, Roffman, & Picciano (1997) reported that HIV-seropositive men engaged in significantly more unprotected anal intercourse than their seronegative counterparts. A similar pattern was observed for differences between groups on unprotected anal sex acts occurring only with nonprimary partners; seropositive men reported more unprotected anal sex with nonprimary partners. However, differences between seropositive and seronegative men on frequencies of unprotected and protected anal sex with primary sex partners were not significant.

Heterosexuals and Injection Drug Users

Heterosexually identified men who have HIV infection engage in similar rates of continued risk behavior as observed in gay and bisexual men. For example, Singh et al. (1993) reported that 29% of HIV-positive injection drug users had engaged in unprotected sex in the previous 6 months. In a survey of homeless men living in Atlanta, Kalichman, Belcher, et al. (1998) found that among 32 HIV-seropositive men, 13% had used injection drugs in the previous 3 months, nearly 50% gave someone money or drugs in exchange for sex, 33% received money or drugs from someone for sex, 33% reported having sex with a man, and 50% had multiple female sex partners in that same time period. HIV-seropositive substance abusing men also report high rates of sexual risk behaviors with multiple partners in a relatively short span of time (Kalichman, 1995).

Women

In a community survey of people living with HIV, Heckman, Kelly, and Somlai (in press) found that 54% of women were currently sexually active with male partners. Nearly one third of the sexually active women never or rarely used condoms during vaginal intercourse. Kalichman (in press) found that 41% of HIV-seropositive women had engaged in unprotected vaginal intercourse, 10% practiced unprotected anal intercourse, and 20% practiced unprotected penile−oral intercourse in the 6 months prior to the study. Most concerning was the 12% of women that reported practicing unprotected intercourse with more than one male partner in that time period. Kalichman and Nachimson (1998) also found that half of women indicated that they experience difficulty maintaining safer-sex practices and 46% experience difficulty disclosing their HIV status to sex partners. Substance use was also common among HIV-positive women, with 57% reporting alcohol use, 38% marijuana use, and 42% cocaine use.

Contextual Factors

A review of the scientific literature suggests that there are a number of plausible correlates of continued risk behavior among seropositive people. Studies of continued sexual risk behavior have concentrated on frequencies of high- and low-risk sex acts as well as predictors of sexual risk practices. Identified risk correlates among seropositive men and women include the following: relationships, economic conditions, emotional states, substance use, and psychological control and behavioral disinhibition. In addition, self-disclosure of HIV serostatus is an important stressor for seropositive individuals and has direct implications for their own and their partner's risks. The following sections briefly review the empirical literature of risk-associated factors among people living with HIV infection.

Relationships

The relationship contexts within which sexual behaviors occur are an important aspect of understanding continued risky sex in HIV-seropositive individuals. In many cases, unprotected sex occurs with another seropositive partner, posing no risk for new HIV infections. However, the risks in such cases are significant for re-infection with a more virulent or drug resistant variant of HIV. In addition, risks of co-infection with other sexually transmitted pathogens must be considered given the potential synergistic effects of viral infections in activating HIV. Co-infection and re-infection, for example, may accelerate the course of AIDS. The risks of unprotected sex posed to seropositive people and their partners are of growing concern.

HIV-seropositive individuals who have sexual relationships with uninfected partners are not at risk for infecting them unless they practice unprotected intercourse. Fisher, Kimble, Misovich, and Weinstein (in press) found that more than half of HIV-seropositive men who have sex with men had practiced unprotected sex with a partner known to be HIV seronegative or of unknown HIV serostatus. Fisher et al. also showed that 43% of men who engaged in unsafe sex did so with anonymous partners. In contrast, several studies suggest that unsafe sex is more frequent in primary relationships than in casual relationships (Doll et al., 1992), including serodiscordant relationships (Remien, Carballo-Dieguez, & Wagner, 1995). Fisher et al. (in press) indicated that seropositive men in relationships used condoms during 23% of their insertive and 33% of their receptive anal-intercourse experiences. HIV-infected individuals may also negotiate safety in their relationships by selecting seroconcordant sex partners regardless of whether they practice safer sex (Kippax et al., 1993).

Economic Conditions and Survival Sex

HIV-seropositive men and women may engage in unprotected sex for money, drugs, or to meet other survival needs. The economic conditions that existed before one becomes HIV infected do not improve by becoming infected. Among seropositive men attending substance-use support groups, for example, Kalichman, Greenberg, and Abel (1997) found that 24% had exchanged sex for money or drugs. Kalichman, Belcher, et al. (1998) found that nearly one third of HIV-seropositive men engaged in sexual commerce and survival sex. Kalichman and Nachimson (1998) also found that 18% of HIV-seropositive women were involved in commercial sex work.

Emotional Distress and Coping

Depression, anxiety, and hostility correlate with high-risk sexual practices among HIV-seropositive men (Kennedy et al., 1993). Seropositive men and women seeking HIV-prevention services who continue to practice unprotected intercourse are more depressed than their HIV-seropositive counterparts who only practice safer sex (Kelly, Murphy, Barh, Koob, et al., 1993). Kalichman, Roffman, et al. (1997) also observed more symptoms of psychoticism and anxiety among seropositive men who practiced unprotected anal intercourse compared to men who denied unsafe sex behavior.

Seropositive men who practice risky sex use fewer behavioral coping strategies to deal with stress when compared with men who consistently practice safer sex (Folkman, Chesney, Pollack, & Phillips, 1992; Robins et al., 1994), and HIV-seropositive men who continue high-risk sex have a lower capacity for coping with sexual risk-producing situations than do lower-risk men (Kalichman, Roffman, et al., 1997). Depression and coping deficits may precipitate engaging in unprotected sex as is the case for some HIV-seronegative individuals. Similar associations between life stressors, emotional distress, and sexual risk behavior are also observed in HIV-seropositive women (Kalichman, 1998), but there have been fewer studies of women than of men.

Substance Use

Alcohol and drug abuse are commonly associated with unprotected sexual behaviors. Research with HIV-serodiscordant couples has shown that substance use plays a significant role in failure to use condoms (Kennedy et al., 1993). High-risk sex among people with HIV is related to using illicit drugs to help them cope with stressful situations related to HIV infection (Robins et al., 1994). In a study of HIV infected adolescents with hemophilia, King, Delaronde, Dinoi, and Forsberg (1996) found that alcohol and other drugs were used by about 30% of teens in their efforts to cope with having HIV–AIDS, and more than half had used alcohol or drugs in conjunction with their most recent sexual experience. Seropositive men and women seeking mental health services and prevention services continue practicing sexual risk behavior that is directly connected to alcohol and other drug use (Kalichman, Kelly, et al., 1997; Kelly, Murphy, Barh, Koob, et al., 1993). In prevention intervention studies, for example, seropositive men who engage in unprotected anal intercourse report greater use of nitrite inhalers than do men who only practice safer sex behaviors. In addition, seropositive men who practice unprotected anal intercourse indicate that their sex partners more frequently use alcohol and nitrite inhalants (Kalichman, Kelly, et al., 1997), demonstrating the relationship context of substance use. A majority of HIV-seropositive men in an Atlanta survey also reported past and current use of alcohol and drugs. Kalichman, Belcher, et al. (1998) found that 72% of seropositive men recently drank alcohol, 81% recently used cocaine, and 69% reported that their drug of choice was cocaine. The study also found that 43% of seropositive women reported use of drugs other than alcohol in the previous 6 months. The prevalence of cocaine abuse among seropositive people is particularly noteworthy, given the close association between crack cocaine and HIV infection in at-risk populations (Eldin et al., 1994).

Psychological Control and Behavioral Disinhibition

A number of mental-health problems are associated with high risk for HIV infection, including manic episodes, hypersexuality, and serious personality disorders (Kalichman, Carey, & Carey, 1996). However, the more subtle nuances of personality dispositions may also have profound influences on sexual practices. Gold, Skinner, and Ross (1994), for instance, showed that HIV-infected gay men who continued to practice unsafe sex were inclined to seek adventures and excitement, suggesting a propensity toward sensation seeking in relation to continued HIV transmission risk behaviors.

Persistent and pervasive thoughts about sex that are linked to strong desires and urges can be indicative of psychosexual disturbances. Sexual preoccupations that encompass cognitive and affective processes characterized by excessive sexual–erotic ideation relate to excessive sexual acting-out behavior. It is therefore plausible that these same attributes contribute to continued sexual risk practices after testing HIV seropositive. Kalichman, Greenberg, et al. (1997) reported that HIV-seropositive men who report multiple unprotected sex partners express greater sexual preoccupation and disinhibition than men with one or no unprotected partners. These findings suggest that some HIV-seropositive people who continue to engage in high-risk sex experience mental-health problems related to sexual acting out.

Disclosure to Sex Partners

To the degree that sex partners are placed at risk, people with HIV are obligated to inform them of their HIV status (Bayer, 1996). However, many people with HIV do not tell unprotected sex partners that they have tested HIV seropositive, and most people with HIV–AIDS do not know their partner's HIV serostatus (Dawson et al., 1994). HIV-seronegative or unknown-HIV-serostatus sex partners are least often informed because of fears of rejection and abandonment (Marks, Richardson, Ruiz, & Maldonado, 1992). Unsafe sex is therefore more likely to occur with partners who are unaware that their partner is HIV infected, whereas condoms are used quite frequently when a sex partner is known to be HIV infected (Wenger, Kusseling, Beck, & Shapiro, 1994).

There are numerous social barriers that inhibit disclosing one's HIV serostatus to sex partners. Perry et al. (1994) found that nearly one third of HIV-positive men and women had not disclosed their HIV serostatus to past or present sex partners. Similarly, Stein et al. (1997) showed that 40% of sexually active seropositive people had not disclosed their serostatus to all of their sex partners. In a study of HIV-seropositive gay men, half had kept their HIV-seropositive status a secret from at least one partner (Marks, Richardson, & Maldonado, 1991). Although 69% of men with one sex partner disclosed their HIV status, only 18% of men with five or more partners had disclosed to at least one. The likelihood of self-disclosure of HIV infection therefore decreases in relation to the number of partners. In addition, men who disclosed their HIV-seropositive status to HIV-seronegative sex partners tended to engage in safer sex practices, whereas those who disclosed to HIV-positive partners were more likely to practice unprotected intercourse.

Disclosure of HIV serostatus is associated with having to disclose other aspects of one's life. Kalichman, Roffman, Picciano, and Balan (in press) found that bisexual men who had disclosed their same sex behavior to partners were more likely to disclose their HIV serostatus. In another study, Mason, Marks, Simoni, Ruiz, and Richardson (1995) found that men who were open about their sexuality were also more open about their HIV serostatus. Importantly, Mason et al. found that English-speaking Latino men disclosed their HIV serostatus to a greater extent than did Spanish-speaking men; acculturation was an important factor in Latino men's disclosure of their HIV infection status.

One may not tell all of his or her partners they are infected because disclosure of HIV infection is usually a selective process. Higgins et al. (1991) showed that HIV-infected gay men tend to disclose their serostatus to sex partners they feel most emotionally invested in, as opposed to more casual partners. The study found that 96% of men told exclusive and long-term sex partners that they were HIV positive, whereas only 44% disclosed to regular but not exclusive partners, and none disclosed to casual and anonymous sex partners. Among people receiving primary care for HIV–AIDS, Stein et al. (1997) found 21%

had not disclosed to exclusive partners and 12% had not disclosed to a spouse. Selective disclosure was also demonstrated in a study of HIV-seropositive Hispanic men that found intimate partners were most frequently informed of the Hispanic participants' HIV infection (Marks, Bundek, et al., 1992). Similarly, the majority of gay men sampled from four U.S. cities informed their regular sex partners of their HIV serostatus, and their relationships tended to last longer than those of men who did not disclose (Schnell et al., 1992).

People who do not disclose their positive serostatus to sex partners, however, do not necessarily put their partners at risk because they may practice safer sex. For some, removing risks for HIV transmission can alleviate the burden of informing sex partners. Taking responsibility to protect partners from HIV infection, whether through disclosure of one's serostatus or otherwise, weighs heavily on most people living with HIV.

Many people who learn that they are HIV infected experience conflicts in their intimate relationships. A study of HIV-seropositive women, for example, showed that relationship partners were more likely to react with anger and emotional withdrawal than were family members and friends (Simoni et al., 1995). Of women who disclosed to partners, one in five were abandoned by their partner, confirming the reality of their fears. However, other studies suggest that disclosure does not inevitably lead to abandonment. For example, Schnell et al. (1992) showed that 82% of HIV-positive men had disclosed their HIV status to sex partners and that most men who did disclose reported stronger relationship bonds as a result. It is unfortunately not known which relationship characteristics best predict positive outcomes and how long partners maintain their support. Fears of abandonment, violence, and other harsh reactions may serve self-protective functions and likely interfere with disclosing to partners, particularly among women.

SEXUAL ADJUSTMENT COUNSELING

Recognition of a problem and understanding its nature are the predecessors of developing targeted intervention strategies. Because sexual adjustment to HIV has only recently been the subject of such under-standing, it is not surprising that there are few counseling and inter-vention models available to address the sexual needs of people living with HIV–AIDS. Sex has been dealt with in the context of general coping interventions, offering the possibility of indirectly affecting sex-ual adjustment. Support groups for people living with HIV infection, for example, may address issues of sexuality and sexual behavior within a broader range of topics. For example, Hedge and Glover (1990) in-cluded safer sex as one of ten topics in informational support groups for HIV-seropositive men and women. Messeri et al. (1994) examined 22 HIV–AIDS-related support groups and found that sexual behavior and behavior changes to protect sex partners were rarely included among topics discussed. Support groups may, however, help people liv-ing with HIV infection maintain safer sexual practices and reinforce individuals for making positive behavioral changes (Greenberg, John-son, & Fichtner, 1996).

Counseling interventions deigned to help people cope and adjust to being HIV seropositive have also included measures of sexual risk behavior as part of their outcome evaluations. Coates, McKusick, Kuno, and Stites (1989), for example, conducted a stress-management pro-gram for HIV-seropositive men in San Francisco that included system-atic desensitization, relaxation training, health habit changes, diet, ex-ercise, and learning self-management skills for stress reduction. The intervention was delivered in eight 2-hour sessions plus a full day re-treat. Using a pretest and posttest study design, the program reduced participants' number of sex partners. In another study, Kelly, Murphy, Bahr, Kalichman, et al. (1993) examined sexual behavior outcomes from a cognitive–behavioral coping-skills group intervention that included relaxation training, cognitive-restructuring exercises, and rational problem-solving skills. The study found that the cognitive–behavioral group intervention, as well as a more traditional support group and individual counseling, showed evidence of reducing sexual risk behav-iors in seropositive men.

Interventions specifically designed to address sexual risk behavior among seropositive people have only recently been reported. Cleary et al. (1995) reported the evaluation of a six-session structured intervention aimed to reduce high-risk sexual practices among HIV-seropositive men and women. The intervention used educational and skills building techniques and was delivered in a health-care setting. Compared with a community referral condition, the structured intervention failed to demonstrate significantly different changes in sexual risk behaviors. However, of the 135 participants assigned to the intervention, only 51 (38%) actually attended one or more of the group sessions. Thus, 62% of people assigned to the intervention never received any of its content, failing to provide a valid test of the intervention and likely explaining the lack of differences between conditions. Cleary et al. reported that people with HIV were reluctant to attend the groups, possibly because of concerns about confidentiality, inconvenience, and opportunities to access alternative sources of support. These findings contrast with other studies that have successfully enrolled and intervened with HIV-seropositive men. Unlike Cleary et al.'s study, which was conducted in a clinic, other interventions conducted in community settings rather than where people receive their medical care have proven successful (Coates et al., 1989; Hedge & Glover, 1990; Kelly, Murphy, Bahr, Kalichman, et al., 1993). Although there has not yet been a formal evaluation of an intervention to address the sexual needs of people living with HIV–AIDS, the emerging literature offers some guidance for the development of such treatments. Research thus far suggests that sexual risk reduction interventions of HIV-seropositive people should include elements to reduce stress, normalize sexuality, boost self-esteem, improve relationships, and build self-efficacy for safer sex and serostatus disclosure.

Emotional Adjustment and Coping With Stress

Counseling programs that specifically address the sexual needs of people living with HIV must attend to the more general concerns that cause emotional distress in people living with HIV–AIDS. Studies showing that sexual acting out can be used as a coping mechanism in dealing with the stress of having HIV and the link between stress and sexual dysfunction underscore the importance of stress reduction for sexual adjustment. Thus, sexuality should not be treated as a unidimensional issue, but rather sexuality should be placed in a context of the total person.

Normalizing Sexuality

Testing HIV positive can have devastating effects on perceptions of sex and acceptance of one's sexuality. Of course, this is especially true for people who believe they contracted HIV sexually. Redefining one's sexuality after HIV infection can include clarifying sexual values and establishing new parameters for attaining sexual satisfaction. It can take months after testing HIV positive for a person to reinitiate sexual interactions, and in many cases sex remains less than accepted even when people are sexually active (Hankins et al., 1997). Thus, similar to other negative attitudes regarding AIDS, people with HIV likely internalize culturally held negative perceptions of sex. Interventions can focus on challenging these beliefs and establishing a sense of sexual normalcy.

Sexual Self-Esteem and Sexual Self-Concept

Guilt and shame are common aftereffects of sexually transmitted infections, including HIV. People with HIV–AIDS often harbor adverse feelings toward themselves, resulting in diminished self-esteem. Rebuilding self-esteem, and for many people establishing a positive self-image for the first time, is a long process and requires a considerable commitment. Counseling can help by providing opportunities to experience one's positive attributes and actively disputing negative images and internal messages. Secrecy and stigma in AIDS promote negative feelings about having HIV infection. Connecting to other people with HIV–AIDS, volunteering to assist others in greater need, and taking active steps to regain control of one's life can all lead to positive experiences of the self and ultimately result in bolstered self-esteem.

Attending to Relationships

Many sexual problems play out in relationships, and many relationship issues can lead to sexual problems. Any comprehensive approach to sexual adjustment must therefore attend to sexual relationships. People with HIV–AIDS may benefit from examining relationship values and exploring the factors that have gone into partner selection. In some cases, partners may have predated the HIV diagnosis, having sustained their ties through extraordinarily difficult times. Feeling betrayed is likely when one is infected in a relationship, particularly when a partner did not disclose their HIV serostatus. Needless to say, there are multiple adverse consequences in relationships where a person contracts HIV from someone other than their primary partner. In contrast, relationships may grow after having tested HIV positive, so that people enter into the relationship with an idea of what may be in store. Whether the relationship commenced before or after HIV testing and no matter if only one or both partners are HIV seropositive, the strain of HIV on relationships will surely spill over and affect relationship and sexual satisfaction. In addition, relationships are influenced by the same factors as individuals, particularly AIDS stigmas and blame, and should therefore be dealt with in terms of their effects on the relationship.

Managing Sexual Risk

People with HIV infection who practice unsafe sex may place themselves and their partners at risk for serious health problems. However, seropositive and seronegative individuals may be misinformed about the potential risks of HIV re-infection and sexually transmitted disease co-infection. Therefore, a major part of sexual risk reduction for people with HIV is education about risks and realities. The effect of being infected with multiple strains of HIV is poorly understood, but it is clear that antiretroviral drug resistant strains of HIV can be transmitted to sex partners, seriously compromising the potential benefits of an entire class of medications. It is also well established that co-infection with other disease causing agents can accelerate the rate of HIV disease.

Another point of confusion concerns the perceived infectivity of people taking protease inhibitors and people who have undetectable viral loads. Although reductions of HIV in blood are paralleled by reductions in semen (Vernazza et al., 1997), an undetectable viral load does not mean the virus is absent and the necessary dose for HIV infection is unknown. In addition, viral load is quite unstable, so a person may have an undetectable viral load one day but could have quite a different reading just days later without any way of knowing. Thus, clarifying these issues through information materials and educational counseling will at least inform people of their actual risks.

Sexual risks are also closely related to substance abuse in people with HIV just as substances and sex are connected when people are at risk but uninfected. Drug and alcohol treatment is therefore an important dimension of care for people living with HIV–AIDS who are substance abusive. In addition to the indirect effects of drug and alcohol treatment on unsafe sex practices, the direct connection between substance use and the risky sexual encounter can be addressed in counseling by raising awareness of the substance abuse and identifying problem-solving strategies to break the link between substance use and sexual behaviors.

Building Safer Sex Self-Efficacy

Self-efficacy is developed through a variety of techniques that include modeling and practicing specific behaviors under conditions that offer optimal chances for receiving reinforcement. Health-related behavior programs that are based on social cognitive theory generally target four interactive determinants of behavior (Bandura, 1997). First, behavior change requires accurate information to increase awareness and knowledge of risks associated with specific risk-producing practices. Second, people must possess social and self-management skills to allow for effective action implementation. Third, behavior changes require enhancement of skills and the development of self-efficacy, usually accomplished through modeling, guided practice, and corrective feedback on skill performance. Finally, behavior change entails creating supportive reinforcements for behavior changes (Bandura, 1997). Theories of HIV-risk behavior change have integrated these same social cognitive principles as necessary components for risk behavior change (Catania, Kegeles, et al., 1990; Fisher & Fisher, 1992). Thus, interventions built on cognitive–behavioral principles integrate information, attitudinal change to enhance motivation, development and reinforcement of behavioral skills, and self-efficacy to implement behavior changes.

Models for sustaining long-term behavioral changes that are based on social–cognitive principles will be an important dimension of HIV-risk-reduction interventions for HIV-seropositive people. Factors associated with continued sexual risk behavior among seropositive men and women overlap with those that predict sexual risk behavior lapses among seronegative persons (Abid & Coates, et al., 1991; Ekstrand, 1990; Hart et al., 1990; Kelly et al., 1991; Stall, Heurtin-Roberts, McKusick, Hoff, & Lang, 1990). Marlatt and Gordon's (1985) relapse prevention model also offers a framework for building self-efficacy for sexual risk reduction interventions for seropositive individuals. In this model, self-efficacy to reduce risk leads to effective coping responses in risky situations and the enactment of behavioral skills for HIV risk reduction. In contrast, diminished self-efficacy results in ineffective coping with high-risk situations, an increased likelihood of lapsing to unsafe sex and therefore violating sexual abstinence, and reducing coping capacity for future risky situations. Marlatt and Gordon's relapse prevention model offers a number of strengths for designing HIV-risk reduction interventions for seropositive people. First, social pressures placed on seropositive individuals to remain sexually safer suggest that those who are engaging in sexual risk behavior are to some degree lapsing to unsafe sex (Kelly et al., 1991). Second, emotional distress observed in HIV-seropositive individuals who practice unsafe sex taxes an already overwhelmed person and may further promote ineffective coping. Finally, unexpected reductions in high-risk behaviors observed in general relaxation and coping interventions for seropositive men may be explained by the role of coping skills and enhanced sense of self-efficacy in managing risk producing situations (Coates et al., 1989; Kelly, Murphy, Bahr, Kalichman, et al., 1993). These findings suggest that the application of self-efficacy enhancement and building training for relapse prevention will be important for HIV-risk-reduction interventions for HIV-seropositive people.

Safer Disclosure Skills

The stigmas of AIDS and the behaviors associated with HIV risks have resulted in significant barriers to disclosing one's HIV infection status. Supporting people to make effective decisions as to whether, when, and how to disclose their HIV serostatus can occur in psychological interventions. Counseling can provide a safe place for considering the relative costs and benefits for disclosing to specific people under specific circumstances. Selective decision making should be considered for disclosure to sex partners, but it should also be recognized within a broader context of challenges in disclosing to health-care providers, family, children, friends, employers, and others. In individual and group counseling sessions, role plays can be used to build self-efficacy for disclosure in a safe environment. Disclosure decision making should include an assessment of risks for disclosing at a particular place and time, allowing for feedback on options to disclosure. The potential for violence and abandonment in response to disclosure should be considered along with strategies for managing such situations. A goal of disclosure decision-making skills building is for people to feel confident in critically deciding if, how, with whom, when, and under what circumstances they can effectively disclose their HIV status. People can be encouraged to explore their own situations where disclosure may be safest and most likely to succeed.

A Model for HIV Risk Reduction for People Living With HIV–AIDS

Adapted from Ozer and Bandura (1990), social cognitive theory posits that enhancing self-efficacy for managing life stress, including risk-producing situations, leads to effective coping responses. Figure 7.1 presents a model of self-efficacy enhancement for sexual risk reduction that is based on social cognitive theory. In this model, reducing emotional distress and activating risk reducing behavioral skills facilitates coping with sexually risky situations. Enacting coping responses that result in reduced emotional distress empowers people to manage stressful situations, including coping with sexual risk producing situations. Self-efficacy operates through similar paths with other interpersonal

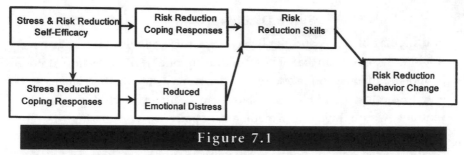

Figure 7.1

Model of self-efficacy for skills enhancement that is based on social cognitive theory.

and self-protective behaviors (Bandura, 1997; Ozer & Bandura, 1990). Coping self-efficacy has also been associated with health-related outcomes among HIV-seropositive men (Benight et al., 1997). Thus, interventions that use behavioral skills enhancement techniques to build self-efficacy offer great promise for sexual risk reduction interventions for people living with HIV–AIDS.

CONCLUSION

The absence of sexual issues in AIDS research is striking when one examines the literature concerning coping and adjustment in people living with HIV–AIDS; such a void is also apparent in the prevention arena. The vacuum of information on AIDS-related sexuality has affected the content of interventions and services. The gap between what we know and what we need to know in order to develop effective programs for addressing sexual issues in HIV is now being filled by an active research agenda. However, as has been the case for many other problems, the lag of research means delays in providing answers for services. As research and practice experiences accumulate there should be a parallel improvement in sexual adjustment intervention services for people living with HIV–AIDS.

8

Coping, Adjustment, and Social Support

M ost people adjust soon after testing HIV seropositive, and most adapt well to the challenges of HIV infection and AIDS. Coping, however, is complicated by multiple and competing demands placed on many people living with HIV–AIDS, particularly those who face discrimination, poverty, domestic violence, and substance abuse. *Coping*, defined here as the thoughts and behaviors specifically used to manage HIV infection (Lazarus & Folkman, 1984), is therefore a function of specific strategies for managing external and internal demands, particularly those experienced as most threatening.

In her now classic research with people facing life-threatening illnesses, S. E. Taylor (1983) proposed the Cognitive Adaptation Model, which I have adapted here to provide a structure for describing HIV-related emotional adjustment. According to S. E. Taylor, there are three themes that emerge in efforts to adapt to life-threatening illnesses: searching for meaning; attempting to regain mastery or control over illness; and enhancing self-esteem. The adjustment process is not, however, always rational and can hinge on distorting reality in the service of self-preservation. Achieving emotional equilibrium and stability are the ultimate goals of finding meaning in suffering, gaining a semblance of control over the uncontrollable, and boosting one's sense of self (S. E. Taylor, 1983; S. E. Taylor & Brown, 1988).

Models of cognitive and behavioral coping have also helped explain adjustment to HIV infection. In their widely applied model, Lazarus and Folkman (1984) identified seven basic types of coping: self-control; cognitive escape–avoidance; behavioral escape–avoidance; distancing; planful problem solving; social support seeking; and positive reappraisal. In general, these types of coping strategies comprise two clusters of coping behaviors: problem-focused coping and emotion-focused coping (Lazarus & Folkman, 1984; Wolf et al., 1991). Problem-focused coping includes thoughts and behaviors that actively seek problem resolution. In contrast, emotion-focused coping strategies are geared toward alleviating immediate emotional distress without directly confronting the source.

Examples of illness-related problem-focused coping include seeking information about the disease, calling others for help, and seeking medical advice and effective treatments. Problem-focused coping strategies are similar to confrontational coping behaviors (Feifel, Strack, & Nagy, 1987) and to the fighting spirit that has been observed in some cancer patients (Greer, Morris, & Pettingale, 1979). People facing serious illnesses also use emotion-focused coping strategies. Selective ignoring, wishful thinking, blaming others, focusing on the positive, distancing, avoidance, and acceptance are examples of emotion-focused coping used in response to chronic illnesses. Adjustment to HIV infection can therefore be conceptualized as the product of coping behaviors that are used in the service of finding meaning, establishing a sense of control, and enhancing self-esteem. Together, these themes and strategies offer a framework for understanding how people emotionally adjust to living with HIV–AIDS (see Figure 8.1).

MEANING, CONTROL, AND SELF-ESTEEM

As noted previously, S. E. Taylor (1983) described three themes in cognitive adaptation to chronic and life-threatening illnesses: meaning, control, and self-esteem. These dimensions also play important roles in adjustment to HIV infection.

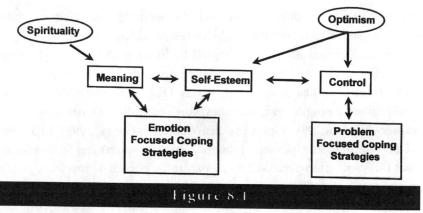

Spirituality, optimism, and themes of adapting to terminal illness in relation to emotion-focused and problem-focused coping.

Meaning

Meaning is derived through efforts to understand adversity and human suffering. Perceptions of how one contracted HIV and beliefs about its implications provide such a sense of meaning. In searching for meaning, individuals attempt to answer the question "Why me?" The need to achieve a sense of meaning is apparent in holocaust survivors, combat veterans, victims of violence, and survivors of natural disasters (Schwartzberg, 1993). Similarly, searching for meaning is part of how cancer patients try to understand having cancer. Because the exact cause of cancer is unknown, meaning may be derived through either internal attributions (e.g., hereditary factors), external and uncontrollable attributions (e.g., accidents or trauma), or external and controllable attributions (e.g., exposure to toxins, stress, smoking, or diet; S. E. Taylor, 1983). Meaning in terminal illness is also influenced by many cultural and personal factors (Kleinman, 1988; Moos & Tsu, 1977). A sense of meaning is not universally achieved by the terminally ill (S. E. Taylor, 1983). However, when achieved, meaning can bring a discovery of beneficial, self-affirming attitudes toward life in general and a new sense of self-knowledge and positive regard (Moos & Tsu, 1977; S. E. Taylor, 1983).

One way that people with HIV–AIDS experience meaning is

through conscious efforts to live each day to its fullest. What may have once seemed a monumental problem may suddenly appear trivial and irrelevant in a new life context framed by living with HIV. People living with HIV–AIDS commonly experience personal growth as a result of their condition. Learning that one has HIV can raise self-awareness, build inner strength and resiliency, and consolidate core beliefs and values (Borden, 1991; Viney, Crooks, Walker, & Henry, 1991). In a study of HIV-seropositive gay men, for example, Schwartzberg (1993) found that HIV was often perceived as a catalyst for personal growth. A greater appreciation for loved ones, reprioritizing values and time commitments, and becoming more forgiving and less self-centered are common by-products of learning that one is HIV seropositive. Schaefer and Coleman (1992) also found that gay men with HIV infection gained a sense of meaning, purpose, and value after testing HIV positive. Relationships, self-discovery, aesthetic appreciation, and contributing to the lives of others are all potential sources of meaning for people living with HIV–AIDS.

Control

Control is gained by mastering the challenges of living with HIV–AIDS. A sense of control buffers the effects of stressful life events and can lead to active coping behaviors that in turn improve one's health. On the other hand, feeling that a chronic illness can be controlled can develop from the successful use of coping strategies or from a generally optimistic style, where the world is viewed as a positive place (S. E. Taylor, Helgeson, Reed, & Skokan, 1991). There may, however, be a third set of factors causing both a sense of control and emotional adjustment, such as available social supports or access to medical care (S. E. Taylor et al., 1991). Nevertheless, believing that a chronic illness can be controlled is essential to the adjustment process, even when such perceptions are illusory (Lazarus & Folkman, 1984; Somerfield & Curbow, 1992).

The perceived source of control is also important. Control can be attributed to oneself, powerful others, God, or chance. More generally, a sense of control can originate through perceptions of internal resources and external forces. Internal control, or personal control, stems from beliefs about one's own actions that can change the course of HIV disease. In contrast, external control involves beliefs that powerful external agents or forces control the course of HIV infection (Reed, Taylor, & Kemeny, 1993). Internal and external sources of perceived control are described in reference to HIV–AIDS in the following sections.

Internal Control

Perceiving that one has personal control over stressful life events helps to reduce emotional distress. For example, perceptions of control over the course of disease are associated with better adjustment in women with breast cancer (S. E. Taylor, Lichtman, & Wood, 1984), people with chronic arthritis (Affleck, Tennen, Pfeiffer, & Fifield, 1987), and people with HIV infection (Remien, Rabkin, Williams, & Katoff, 1992). It appears that the greater the uncertainty posed by a medical condition, the more important is the sense that the condition can be controlled. Perceived control over an illness is also associated with hope for longer survival and improved quality of life (Rabkin, Williams, Neugebauer, Remien, & Goetz, 1990). The mental health benefits of perceiving internal control over chronic illness are well established. S. E. Taylor et al. (1991), for example, showed that perceived personal control plays a causal role in reducing psychological distress in chronic illness.

In contrast, beliefs in control over chronic illness can become maladaptive in some people, particularly when such beliefs create a false sense of hope (Burish et al., 1984). Still, most evidence suggests that feelings of control reestablish themselves even in the midst of deteriorating health, where perceived control persists despite situations becoming increasingly uncontrollable. The need to maintain personal control can drive the choice of coping strategies. For example, perceived personal internal control was associated with positive coping behaviors in a large study of gay men in San Francisco (Folkman et al., 1996). Using path analysis, Folkman et al. showed that perceptions of control give rise to a constellation of HIV-related coping strategies. A sense of control among HIV-seropositive men led them to become more involved in their own treatment, such as through planful problem solving, advice and information seeking, and positive appraisals. Similar findings were reported in a sample of long-term AIDS survivors (Remien et al., 1992).

Perceived personal control can directly affect health by influencing the selection of coping strategies. For example, efforts to remain adherent to complicated medication regimens are one way of taking personal control that may be expressed as an active coping strategy. Practicing problem-focused coping can offer feedback to enhance a sense of personal control over HIV–AIDS.

In an unusual example of how coping strategies can increase a sense of control, Schneider, Taylor, Hammen, Kemeny, and Dudley (1991) found that suicidal thoughts linked to AIDS-related events can function as a means of coping. Schneider et al. showed that suicidal ideations may alleviate emotional distress and do not always emerge from despair. Contemplating suicide helped some individuals continue functioning with a greater sense of internal control in relation to their future. One of Schneider et al.'s participants illustrated these findings by stating, "I think that thinking about suicide as an alternative is a way for me to cope, or deal with the 'what would I do' question if I were to develop AIDS" (Schneider et al., 1991, p. 785). This is not to suggest that all suicidal ideations serve to achieve a sense of control over HIV infection; rather this study illustrates the powerful need for control that many people experience and the subtleties by which control needs can be expressed.

The need to control one's own health decisions and physical functioning is observed at all stages of HIV disease: when people first seek HIV antibody testing (Siegel & Krauss, 1991), as they enter early HIV infection (Pakenham, Dadds, & Terry, 1994; Reed et al., 1993), and during later stages of AIDS (S. E. Taylor et al., 1991). Control is exerted over symptoms, illnesses, the general course of HIV disease, or a combination of disease processes. S. E. Taylor et al. (1991) found that gay men in the Los Angeles Multicenter AIDS Cohort Study (MACS) held a sense of control over day-to-day symptoms, health maintenance, and medical treatment. Feeling in control of HIV-related symptoms can sustain coping and emotional health (Reed et al., 1993), particularly among individuals who suffer moderate to severe symptoms (S. E. Taylor et al., 1991). Perceptions of control may motivate actions to suppress HIV-related symptoms, such as increased relaxation and sleep, improved self-care, and stress reduction (Reed et al., 1993).

External Control

Studies of people with chronic illnesses show that perceived external control interacts with illness-related factors to influence emotional adjustment. Taylor and her colleagues (S. E. Taylor et al., 1984, 1991) have shown that women who believe that external forces control the course of their breast cancer are better adjusted when they have more favorable prognoses. In contrast, women who believe that others control the course of breast cancer are not well adjusted when their prognosis is poor. Ascribing control to powerful others therefore only enhances adjustment when there is hope for a positive outcome. Affleck et al. (1987) found that arthritis sufferers who believe physicians control their daily symptoms experience greater emotional distress, but those who believe that physicians control the course of their illness are better adjusted. Thus, whether perceived external control positively or negatively affects emotional well being depends on illness status and its expected outcomes.

Believing that medical professionals control the course of HIV infection is also related to poorer psychological adjustment (e.g., Kelly, Murphy, Bahr, Koob, et al., 1993), particularly at later stages of HIV infection (Reed et al., 1993; Remien et al., 1992). People with HIV infection who believe others control their health and medical care are less well adjusted when compared with those who ascribe little control to external sources (S. E. Taylor et al., 1991). It is typical for traditional medical care to stifle beliefs in internal control while reinforcing the perceived control of powerful others. Giving up control of treatment decisions to providers can be a source of significant stress, particularly when a physician is reluctant to treat people with HIV–AIDS or lacks AIDS expertise (Reed et al., 1993). Therefore, as in recurrent cancer, HIV infection with a poor prognosis coupled with beliefs that external forces control one's demise will naturally lead to dysphoria.

Self-Esteem

Enhancing self-esteem is a central part of adjusting to any chronic illness. Self-enhancement is achieved by pulling oneself up from illness experiences by either focusing on the positive or by comparing oneself with others who are worse off (S. E. Taylor, 1983). Taylor found that cancer patients tend to compare themselves with others who are doing worse rather than better than themselves to build up their self-esteem. Downward social comparisons enhance the sense of self by focusing on one's positives relative to other's negatives. Unfortunately, little research has examined self-enhancement processes in coping with HIV infection. Although people with HIV may experience diminished self-esteem, conclusions must be held until more research is available.

The need to achieve a sense of meaning, control, and self-esteem influences the selection of coping strategies that either directly address the illness and its related problems or attend to emotional responses (Fleishman & Fogel, 1994; Folkman, Lazarus, Dunkel-Schetter, DeLongis, & Gruen, 1986; McCrae & Costa, 1986; Pearlin & Schooler, 1978). Problem-focused and emotion-focused coping are quite different but both strive to achieve the same end. The particular coping strategies that an individual with HIV infection may use at a given time is determined by multiple factors, including stage of illness, personal coping history, and perceived available coping resources. For example, men living in urban gay communities have access to resources that facilitate active coping with HIV infection such as support groups, information forums, and state-of-the-art treatments (Neugebauer et al., 1992). In contrast, people with HIV infection who live in rural areas lack such resources (Bozovich et al., 1992). There is evidence that men and women, ethnic groups, and HIV risk groups differ in their use of various coping strategies (Billings & Moos, 1981, 1984; Fleishman & Fogel, 1994). Thus, it should be expected that people will vary in their capacity to cope with the challenges of HIV–AIDS.

PROBLEM-FOCUSED COPING

Problem-focused coping consists of behavioral and cognitive strategies aimed at solving problems and resolving conflicts. The application of problem-focused coping generally stems from beliefs that one's actions will influence the problem, that is, a sense of internal control (Scheier & Carver, 1987). Directly confronting symptoms by seeking medical care is a common example of problem-focused coping in chronic illness (e.g., Feifel et al., 1987). Mobilizing against a chronic disease has positive effects on one's emotional well-being (Wolf et al., 1991), global psychological adjustment, subjective health (Namir, Wolcott, Fawzy, & Alumbaugh, 1987), and to some degree physical health (Mulder & Antoni, 1992). People with HIV infection frequently engage in action-oriented, problem-focused coping behaviors, often with positive results (S. E. Taylor & Aspinwall, 1990). People who have an active, "fighting spirit" style of coping with HIV may experience health benefits (Leserman, Perkins, & Evans, 1992; Solano et al., 1993). Being able to cope effectively varies over the duration of HIV infection and is often a function of changes in health status (Chidwick & Borrill, 1996). However, the relationships between coping and health are correctional; with improved health people feel better and have more energy to engage in activities that in turn promote their health and a sense of well-being.

Examples of problem-focused coping include trying to learn more about HIV infection, focusing on healthy changes in life-style, and gaining access to new therapies (Fleishman & Fogel, 1994; Longo, Spross, & Locke, 1990). In response to a coping inventory, HIV seropositive men and women frequently endorsed active, problem-focused coping strategies in response to the challenges of living with HIV–AIDS (Kalichman, 1995). As shown in Table 8.1, problem-focused coping strategies were commonly reported, with over half of respondents endorsing five of the seven listed strategies. Similarly, long-term survivors with AIDS frequently use active coping strategies (Remien et al., 1992). Consistent with theories of coping, actively coping with HIV–AIDS can encompass increased involvement in medical treatment, information seeking, life-style changes, and social activism.

Medical Involvement

Becoming active in one's medical care can facilitate adjustment to HIV infection (Storosum, Van den Boom, Van Beauzekom, & Sno, 1990).

Table 8.1

Problem-Focused Coping Strategies Endorsed by Persons With HIV Infection

	% Endorsing Item	
Coping Strategy	Men	Women
Knew what had to be done so I doubled my efforts to make things work	77	80
Talked with someone to find out more about the situation	86	72
Got professional help	72	74
Made a plan of action and followed it	80	77
Talked with someone who could do something concrete about the problem	79	74
Changed something so things would turn out all right	84	79
Came up with a couple of different solutions	76	79

Seeking treatments, becoming informed about possible treatment side effects, identifying opportunities to enroll in clinical trials and experimental treatments, exploring complementary therapies, and developing alliances with medical professionals are all examples of how people can become involved in their care (Remien et al., 1992; Siegel & Krauss, 1991). In addition, participating in research and AIDS clinical trials offer additional benefits beyond receiving a potentially effective treatment including altruism, increasing a sense of control, and fostering hope (Robiner et al., 1993).

Information Seeking

Finding and using pertinent information are among the greatest needs expressed by people who are chronically medically ill (Felton & Revenson, 1984) and by people with HIV infection in particular (D. Miller & Pinching, 1989). Namir, Wolcott, Fawzy, and Alumbaugh (1990) found that 85% of HIV-seropositive gay men had tried to find out more information about their illness. Kalichman (1995) also found that 62%

of HIV-positive men and women indicated that they had talked with others about ways to access information.

A large number of information services have been established to meet the information needs of people with HIV–AIDS. Federal, state, and local health departments, as well as activist and grass-roots organizations, for example, have produced brochures, booklets, newsletters, and Internet websites for people with HIV infection. For people who are not information seeking, however, the rapid pace of AIDS can be stressful. Developments in new treatments for HIV infection and HIV-related opportunistic illnesses can be overwhelming, particularly for those who have recently tested positive.

Life-Style Changes

Coping can take the form of changing life-styles to promote healthy habits. Namir et al. (1990) found that 81% of HIV-seropositive people began eating more healthily and taking vitamins in response to testing HIV positive. Individuals with HIV also report resting more and reducing their use of alcohol and drugs (Siegel & Krauss, 1991). Aerobic exercise is another common change in life-style that can buffer stress (LaPerriere, Schneiderman, Antoni, & Fletcher, 1990). Changes in life-style boost a sense of control in a similar fashion as other problem-focused coping strategies. Although such changes improve both emotional and physical well-being, there is little evidence that healthy life-style changes significantly alter the clinical course of HIV infection.

Social Activism

Although only 7% of HIV-seropositive people are politically active, those who are activists benefit from greater emotional adjustment (Namir et al., 1990). In addition, those who are not themselves activists may vicariously benefit from knowing others who are. Activism was perhaps the first form of problem-focused coping in AIDS, encouraging people to do what they could about a problem with an unknown cause. Today, political activism remains an important part of AIDS, including as a means of coping.

In summary, taking action against HIV–AIDS through problem-focused coping occurs in response to aspects of the disease that appear controllable, such as medical care, health-behavior changes, social relationships, and public policies. Forestalling the onset of or curing opportunistic illnesses can increase involvement in treatment, information seeking, and healthy changes in life-style. However, when problem-focused coping strategies are unsuccessful, or at least perceived as unsuccessful, or when active coping is applied to uncontrollable aspects of HIV–AIDS, efforts to cope may be shifted to emotion-focused strategies (Somerfield & Curbow, 1992).

EMOTION-FOCUSED COPING

Emotion-focused coping strategies such as denial, acceptance, avoidance, escape, distancing, use of distractions, and positive reappraisal do not directly intervene with the source of stress (Lazarus & Folkman, 1984). Chronic medical patients benefit from certain emotion-focused coping strategies (e.g., Derogatis, Abeloff, & Melisaratos, 1979). One model of coping with terminal illness almost exclusively relies on emotion-focused coping. Kübler-Ross (1969, 1975, 1981) described five stages of adjustment to terminal illness and loss: *denial,* experience and expression of *anger, bargaining* with external forces perceived as controlling the course of illness, *depression* in the face of continued deterioration, and *acceptance.* Given that emotion-focused coping is most effective when a person has little control over the course of illness (S. E. Taylor & Aspinwall, 1990), it is not surprising that Kübler-Ross' coping model is centered on emotion-focused strategies. Consistent with Kübler-Ross, Kalichman (1995) found that people with HIV–AIDS commonly engage in denial, acceptance, avoidance, and distractions as coping strategies. Table 8.2 presents the percentages of HIV-seropositive people in Kalichman's study that endorsed eight emotion-focused coping strategies.

Denial

Denial can be used as a coping strategy throughout the experience of living with HIV–AIDS. People may avoid getting tested for HIV antibodies despite high-risk histories or even symptoms of having HIV–

Table 8.2		
Emotion-Focused Coping Strategies Endorsed by Persons With HIV Infection		

	% Endorsing Item	
Coping Strategy	Men	Women
Turned to work or substitute activity to take my mind off things	78	67
Looked for the silver lining; tried to look on the bright side of things	87	83
Told myself things that helped me to feel better	87	83
Didn't let it get to me; refused to think too much about it	74	70
Wished that I could change what happened or how I felt	93	87
Daydreamed or imagined a better time or place than the one I was in	79	76
Wished the situation would go away or somehow be over with	85	80
Reminded myself how much worse things could be	87	86

AIDS (Lyter, Valdiserri, Kingsley, Amoroso, & Rinaldo, 1987; Siegel, Levine, Brooks, & Kern, 1989). Following receipt of an HIV-positive test result, some may engage in denial by believing that HIV infection is not the cause of AIDS (Chuang, Devins, Hunsley, & Gill, 1989). Still others do not believe that their test results were correct, choosing to either get retested or to just go on as if they were not tested in the first place (Siegel et al., 1989). HIV infection may also be denied by misattributing symptoms to non-HIV-related causes (Weitz, 1989). Although denial may recur over the course of HIV infection, few long-term survivors with AIDS use denial as a coping strategy (Rabkin, Remien, Katoff, & Williams, 1993). Leserman et al. (1992) found that gay men with AIDS who used denial experienced a greater frequency of negative moods, particularly anger.

Acceptance and Resignation

Realistic acceptance was proclaimed by Kübler-Ross (1969) as the final common pathway in coping with terminal illness. Kübler-Ross described acceptance as a state of calm, relatively void of negative and positive emotions. According to Kübler-Ross, however, acceptance is not necessarily a constant state, but rather fades in and out over the course of illness. Studies show that acceptance and resignation are most common in diseases that have little chance for cure or long-term remission (Feifel et al., 1987). Griffiths and Wilkins (1993) found that individuals diagnosed with HIV infection for five years or longer accepted their condition. Long asymptomatic periods of HIV infection may facilitate acceptance of impending illness (Nichols, 1985). More than half of people in one study had accepted their being HIV seropositive and believed that nothing could be done to help them (Kalichman, 1995).

Accepting one's HIV infection is not, however, necessarily associated with emotional well being. Reed et al. (1994) found that realistic acceptance of HIV did not predict how well a person emotionally adjusted to having HIV–AIDS. Reed et al. also found that individuals who were resigned to dying of AIDS lived a shorter period of time. These findings suggest that personal acceptance of future debilitation, loss of functioning, and death may predict poorer emotional adjustment to AIDS. Acceptance and resignation are contrary to the confrontational styles of coping and fighting spirit that seem to characterize problem-focused coping. Perhaps because AIDS brings multiple opportunistic illnesses, each of which may be successfully treated, AIDS patients believe, and with good reason, that they can live longer if they can survive opportunistic illnesses one at a time. Pushing past an opportunistic illness could mean making it to yet another new treatment and ultimately living for the cure.

Cognitive Coping

Emotion-focused cognitive coping strategies strive to achieve a perspective that protects against realities of HIV or seek meaning from being HIV positive. People with HIV–AIDS often adopt a life view that facilitates emotional well-being (Wolf et al., 1991). Examples of cognitive adaptation strategies include meditation, self-hypnosis, and mental imagery (Namir et al., 1987). Planning for the future and focusing on positive thoughts about the future are also common strategies. Fleishman and Fogel (1994) found that concentrating on how things could be worse and looking on the brighter side of situations may protect against depression. Kalichman (1995) found that 62% of HIV-seropositive men and women had rediscovered what was important in their lives after learning they had HIV–AIDS.

Avoidance

Avoidance as a coping strategy occurs relatively frequently early in asymptomatic HIV infection as compared with later symptomatic phases (Kurdek & Siesky, 1990). Like other medical conditions, avoidance coping in HIV–AIDS leads to increased emotional distress and dysphoria (Nicholson & Long, 1990; Vedhara & Nott, 1996). HIV-seropositive women, ethnic minorities, and injection drug users are more likely to use avoidance coping strategies relative to their White gay male counterparts (Fleishman & Fogel, 1994; Leserman et al., 1992). Avoidance coping can include simply trying to forget about being HIV positive, canceling medical appointments and avoiding treatment, and refusing to even discuss HIV–AIDS.

Distraction

Distraction is related to the avoidance strategies discussed above but appears to be more likely to promote emotional health (Namir et al., 1990). In one study, 38% of HIV-seropositive men and women stated that they had gone on vacation to cope with HIV, and 44% turned to work or some other activity to distract themselves from thoughts of HIV (Kalichman, 1995). People with HIV infection report going out with friends, treating themselves to something special, thinking about things other than AIDS, and enjoying movies, theater, and music as a means of distraction (Remien et al., 1992). Unfortunately, opportunities to divert attention away from being HIV positive diminish as HIV disease advances. Loss of employment and dwindling social relationships also cut into the number of available distracting activities. People with

HIV–AIDS must often give up their pets and even hobbies, such as gardening, because of risks of exposure to disease-causing microbes.

Other Emotion-Focused Strategies

Substance use offers a temporary reprieve from the stress of HIV–AIDS. Alcohol and drug use is common in gay communities and particularly frequent among men at risk for HIV infection (Ostrow, 1994), and the close association of crack cocaine to HIV in heterosexuals is well established. Given the close connection of substance use and the HIV epidemic, it is not surprising that so many people with HIV–AIDS rely on alcohol and other drugs for coping. Binge drinking and periods of rampant sexual acting out can be extreme expressions of denial or desperate attempts to escape. Less self-destructive, however, emotion-focused coping can include wishful thinking and intellectualization. Like all emotion-focused coping strategies, these activities are used for the purpose of immediate relief.

OPTIMISM AND SPIRITUALITY

Thus far, emotional adjustment to HIV–AIDS has been considered the product of being able to derive meaning, enhance self-esteem, and control AIDS through various coping strategies. However, one's world view strongly influences each of these coping dimensions, as well as has direct effects on emotional adjustment. Thus, optimism about the future and maintaining spiritual beliefs may both serve as sources of coping in their own right. In relation to the model of coping presented in Figure 8.1, optimism can foster a sense of control and build self-esteem, whereas spirituality is more closely connected to the search for meaning.

Optimism

People facing chronic illness can gain inner-strength by looking toward the future with hope and optimism (Peterson, Seligman, & Vaillant,

1988; S. E. Taylor et al., 1992). For example, people with coronary heart disease who are optimistic about their recovery have fewer symptoms than do more pessimistic patients (Scheier et al., 1989). People with HIV–AIDS who are optimistic have a greater sense of control and are more inclined to use problem-focused coping (S. E. Taylor et al., 1992). Knowing that one has HIV can evoke a sense of optimism about not developing AIDS, especially when effective treatments are accessible. Like internal control, optimism enables one to use problem-focused coping strategies (Pakenham et al., 1994; Rabkin et al., 1990). Optimism and hope both build expectations that something positive lies ahead, enhance confidence about the future, and result in positive appraisals about one's life (Rabkin et al., 1990).

Advances in anti-HIV treatments have reestablished hope for ultimately controlling HIV–AIDS. Of course, people with an inclination toward thinking positively may be most likely to benefit from this renewed hope. Indeed, such optimism can have far-reaching effects. For example, treatment optimism is an important factor in medication adherence, so people who believe they will profit from treatment are more likely to follow treatment regimens (Mehta, Moore, & Graham, 1997). A positive outlook can motivate other health behaviors and therefore indirectly influence general health and wellness.

In addition to HIV-specific optimism, a more global style of positive thinking, or *dispositional optimism*, may reduce fears and promote problem-focused coping (S. E. Taylor et al., 1992). Dispositional optimism can actually reduce emotional distress, alleviate worries and concerns about AIDS, decrease perceptions of risk of developing AIDS, and increase use of problem-focused coping (S. E. Taylor et al., 1992). Long-term survivors with AIDS demonstrate a psychological resiliency that is characteristic of dispositional optimism (Hardy, 1991). Rabkin, Remien, et al. (1993), for example, found that long-term survivors with AIDS were able to state their goals clearly and to see positive things in their future. Thus, thinking positive, optimism, and hope compose a constellation of attitudes that contribute to the emotional welfare of people with HIV–AIDS, particularly among people at later stages of infection.

Spirituality

People with HIV–AIDS express a wide range of religious beliefs and diverse spiritual practices, including maintaining long-held faith as well as inquiring into new spiritual outlets (Winiarski, 1991). Once again, like other chronic illnesses, existential and spiritual issues emerge out of questioning how the tragedy of AIDS could happen to anyone (D. Grant & Anns, 1988). Spiritual beliefs and practices are common means of coping that relate to finding positive meaning (Folkman, 1997). Thus, spiritual experiences serve to guide individuals in their search for meaning.

Unlike other life-threatening illnesses, however, HIV infection is associated with behaviors that are sanctioned by many traditional religious institutions (Warner-Robins & Christiana, 1989; Weitz, 1989; Yates, 1991). People with HIV–AIDS may encounter reprehension rather than support when seeking spiritual guidance. Thus, it is not uncommon for individuals with HIV infection to seek new and alternative means of spiritual expression. For example, Carson (1990) found that gay men with AIDS do not achieve spiritual well-being as a result of participating in formal religions, but rather through their personal responses to existential crises. In another study of gay men with HIV infection, Somlai and Kalichman (1994) found that men who were ambivalent toward formal religious doctrines developed new and alternative outlets for spiritual expression, particularly practices with immediate and tangible benefits such as body therapy, meditation, and rituals.

For many people, facing a life-threatening illness requires them to call upon their religious beliefs, particularly for persons who were religious before they became ill. HIV infection can serve as a catalyst for spiritual growth, including a return to religious beliefs, deepening of existing spirituality, and developing new dimensions to one's spirituality (Schwartzberg, 1993). A consistency of spiritual practices is commonly observed in HIV-seropositive people, with more than half of participants in one study indicating that they frequently prayed, 40% reporting they had found new faith, and 62% hoping that a miracle would happen in relation to being HIV positive (Kalichman, 1995). People with HIV–AIDS who have stronger spiritual beliefs often experience greater emotional adjustment (Somlai et al., 1996). Formal and informal religious practices may therefore provide a means of support that cannot be attained in other ways.

Spiritual practices potentially provide multiple sources of comfort, including feeling connected to a higher power and the social support that can be gained from a spiritual community. Religiosity and spirituality can both reduce the burdens of caregiving for partners of HIV-positive persons who may also be HIV seropositive themselves. Social support, whether through participation in spiritual practices or otherwise, constitutes an important dimension of adjustment to HIV.

ENHANCING COPING CAPACITIES

Coping with HIV is enhanced by applying the coping theories reviewed above. The following suggestions are offered for building stronger coping capacities for people living with HIV–AIDS.

People with HIV infection should be empowered to chart their own course of health care and medical treatment. Living with HIV–AIDS can lead to a sense of fatalism, effectively halting plans for the future. People with HIV may therefore be encouraged to exert control over their responses to HIV disease, seek the latest treatments, and become active participants in their medical care. Asking questions and developing treatment alliances with providers is an important task for people with HIV. Clinical trials and complementary therapies offer opportunities to become engaged in one's own treatment and such actions have possible effects on emotional adjustment as well as physical health (Robiner et al., 1993).

Anticipating physical declines can facilitate coping. It is important for people with HIV–AIDS to recognize that their needs for coping and support will change over the course of HIV disease. Fatigue, weakness, symptoms, and treatment side effects interfere with emotional well-being at earlier stages and physical disability impedes coping at the later stages of AIDS. Recognizing these changes before their onset creates opportunities to build a safety net of coping supports in advance of physical deterioration.

275

The availability of multiple coping strategies facilitates emotional adjustment. Therefore, individuals with a broader range of coping options will be more effective at managing stress. Cancer patients who use multiple coping strategies adjust better than those with narrow coping repertoires (Dunkel-Schetter, Feinstein, Taylor, & Falke, 1992; S. E. Taylor & Aspinwall, 1990). Diversity and flexibility in coping allows the replacement of ineffective coping responses with new strategies, increasing the chances that coping will meet the needs of a given situation.

Distractions from HIV–AIDS can be emotionally healthy. HIV infection can completely consume a person. Relationships are often lost and the ability to actively participate in life diminishes as HIV progresses. HIV infection usually leads to physical decline resulting in disability, unemployment, and restricted social activities. Opportunities for distractions from HIV–AIDS become harder to access as HIV infection advances. Thus, new and creative means of distraction should be established at various stages of illness.

As the HIV epidemic progresses and more people die of AIDS, psychological numbing, complacency, and hopelessness may replace a fighting spirit. People with HIV infection should be encouraged to look toward future developments in treatment to sustain their hope and their will to endure. Advances in antiretroviral therapies have brought new hope, but its durability is uncertain. Breakthroughs in preventing, treating, and curing HIV-associated opportunistic illnesses are also occurring at an astounding pace. Thus, hope that people will live longer with a higher quality of life can become the focus of encouragement and support for people living with HIV–AIDS.

Denial is maladaptive when it interferes with medical treatment decisions and when it deters proactive health decisions. There are numerous ways that denial is used in coping with HIV–AIDS. For example, some people believe that HIV is not the cause of AIDS or that the HIV-antibody tests have a high false-positive rate. Unfortunately, such beliefs diminish motivations to seek early interventions. Realistic optimism, on the other hand, can increase treatment seeking and promote proactive health decisions, as well as other problem-focused coping strategies. It may therefore be necessary for people with HIV–AIDS to deny their condition for a brief time, but ultimately facing their HIV infection will lead them to actively engage in the care system. Substance use as a means of avoidance is common, where alcohol and other drugs are used as an escape from daily life stressors including HIV infection. Like other acts of denial, substance abuse can provide a temporary escape from the emotional trauma of HIV–AIDS. Prolonged substance abuse, however, interferes with adaptive coping, and disrupts social relationships. Eliminating substance use as a means of coping requires adopting alternative coping behaviors that meet immediate needs.

SOCIAL SUPPORT

Interpersonal relationships can help prevent and alleviate the emotional distress associated with chronic and life-threatening illnesses (Cobb, 1976). Social support refers to the number and types of contacts a person has, the functional aspects of relationships, and the perceived quality or adequacy of support (Green, 1993). In relation to chronic illness, each of these dimensions of social support tends to vary with the different stages of disease (Broadhead et al., 1983). Social support can facilitate coping, enhance self-esteem, and foster a sense of belonging (Linn, Lewis, Cain, & Kimbrough, 1993; Wolf et al., 1991). Unfortunately, the chronically ill often lack adequate social support at times when it is most needed. Depression and anxiety are associated with chronic illness and can limit relationships, distancing people from potential sources of support (Shinn, Lehmann, & Wong, 1984; H. A. Turner, Hays, & Coates, 1993).

Two types of conceptual models of health-related social support have been described: (a) models that emphasize the main effects (or direct effects) of support and (b) models that view social support as a buffer of stress. Main-effects models posit that social support directly increases health through providing information, enhancing self-esteem, or restoring a sense of internal control (S. Cohen, 1988). Stress-buffering models, on the other hand, state that when a person is under duress, social support increases information, emotional well-being, or tangible resources that in turn affect health outcomes (S. Cohen, 1988).

In addition to the functional aspects of support, the structure of support has important health implications. Structural aspects of support include the frequency of social contact, the relationships that serve as sources of support, the opportunity to reciprocate support, and the integration of individuals into a supportive network (Stowe, Ross, Wodak, Thomas, & Larson, 1993). Individual differences in perceived support, personality dispositions, and the match between available support and individual needs ultimately determine the effects of social support (Lakey & Cassady, 1990). Figure 8.2 summarizes the structural and functional dimensions of social support. Independent of or in combination with various coping strategies, social support plays important roles in the emotional adjustment to HIV infection.

Structurally, having a spouse or domestic partner, frequencies of social contacts, formal and informal group memberships, and numbers of close friends influence emotional adjustment. Functionally, it is the content of social relationships that affects adjustment. Social support fosters a sense of purpose or meaning and promotes health behaviors,

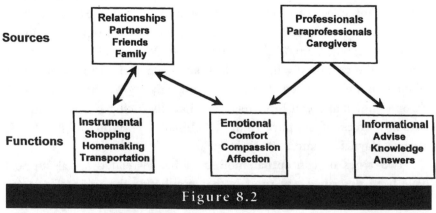

Figure 8.2

The sources and functions of social support.

including treatment seeking and treatment adherence (House, Landis, & Umberson, 1988). Social support may also affect perceptions of stressful events and coping (Mulder & Antoni, 1992; O'Leary, 1990). Thus, there is considerable evidence that the structural and functional dimensions of support are both important factors in promoting emotional adjustment to HIV–AIDS.

Structure of Social Support

Like many aspects of AIDS, information about the structure of social support has come from studies of primarily White, middle-class, gay and bisexual men. This bias in the literature may be particularly troublesome here because social networks of gay men are qualitatively different from those of heterosexuals (Kurdek, 1988), and gay communities have extended support to people with AIDS to a greater degree than other communities.

Gay communities themselves are heterogeneous, however, with differences in social support occurring among subgroups of gay and bisexual men. Ostrow et al. (1991) found that African American gay men benefit less from social support and report less affirming social relationships than do White men. The social networks of women also differ from those of men. Smith and Rapkin (1996) found that men and women clearly differ in the sources from which they gain social support. Men are more likely to rely on partners and traditional family members, whereas women have a broader array of supports, including partners, family, and friends. However, gay, bisexual, and injection drug using HIV-seropositive men depend on friends for support to a greater degree than family. Johnston, Stall, and Smith (1995) showed that because HIV positive men rely on friends for support, multiple losses to AIDS threaten what might otherwise be stable supportive networks.

There are many sources of isolation for people with HIV–AIDS, including depression, fear that others will discover one is infected, and concerns of transmitting HIV to others. Even before learning their HIV serostatus, however, many HIV-positive people compartmentalize their social networks (R. B. Hays, Chauncey, & Tobey, 1990). For example, gay men commonly have two sets of friends, gay and heterosexual, and two sets of family members, those who do and do not know their sexual orientation. Parsing relationships is also common to injection drug users and women living in poverty (R. B. Hays, Catania, McKusick, & Coates, 1990). Although partitioning relationships leads to fewer social contacts, the actual number of contacts per se is less important in emotional adjustment than is the quality of contacts (R. B. Hays, Chauncey, et al., 1990; Namir, Alumbaugh, Fawzy, & Wolcott, 1989). Thus, relationships form the conduit through which support flows, and the sources of support can be many, including relationship partners, friends, family, and professionals (Pearlin, Mullan, Aneshensel, Wardlaw, & Harrington, 1994).

Relationship Partners

Relationship partners are a primary source of social support (Bor, Prior, & Miller, 1990; R. B. Hays, Chauncey, et al., 1990; Kurdek, 1988). As in other chronic medical conditions, support from a spouse or committed relationship partner is an important aspect of receiving stable social support for HIV–AIDS. Unfortunately, support offered by relationship partners is often threatened by HIV–AIDS. In particular, sexual relations and pair bonding can deteriorate when one or both partners are HIV seropositive (Gochros, 1992). Agle, Gluck, and Pierce (1987) found that hemophiliacs often experience sexual relationship problems, with over half of those studied feeling concerned about potentially transmitting the virus to their partners. Similar issues arise for other groups of people with AIDS. Sexual relationships can be strained by declines in health, as well as by fears of transmitting the virus. In addition to caregiving, burdens are placed on partners who are HIV seropositive. Folkman, Chesney, Cooke, Boccellari, and Collette (1994) showed that depression is common in HIV-seropositive gay men who provide care to their partners. The stress of HIV infection can ultimately end long-term relationships (Hart, Fitzpatrick, McLean, Dawson, & Boulton, 1990), leaving friends as the primary source of social support.

Friends

People with HIV–AIDS typically rely on friends and peers for social support. Friends are the main source of social support for gay and bisexual men as well as injection drug users (Namir et al, 1989; Stowe et al., 1993). Empathy, accessibility, shared values, and common cultures are offered by friendships.

Integration into a community that is sensitive to the needs of people with HIV–AIDS increases the size of one's HIV-positive support network. As the HIV epidemic expanded, community-based organizations emerged to bring people with HIV infection together. Peer support and volunteer programs serve the dual functions of providing services and acting as a source of support for those who volunteer. Relationships formed among people with HIV are grounded in common experiences that completely circumvent the barriers of ignorance and stigmatization often found in people who have not been affected by AIDS.

Family

Family relationships offer a stable source of support during chronic illness, despite the disruptions that illness causes to family continuity (Sales, 1991). Stigmas that predate AIDS, such as homophobia and racism, can create insurmountable obstacles to accessing family support. For example, early in the epidemic Donlou, Wolcott, Gottlieb, and Landsverk (1985) found that HIV-seropositive gay men did not perceive their families as helpful in their efforts to cope with HIV–AIDS. Family estrangement and rejection can be deeply rooted. R. B. Hays, Chauncey, et al. (1990) found that HIV-seronegative as well as HIV-seropositive gay men perceived their partners and siblings as the least supportive people in their lives. However, Hays et al. also reported that 92% of gay men with fully diagnosed AIDS sought help from family members, a higher number than both asymptomatic HIV-seropositive and HIV-seronegative gay men.

Families may assume greater responsibilities for caregiving, particularly at the later stages of AIDS (Takigiku, Brubaker, & Hennon, 1993). Family caregivers experience significant emotional distress, with over three quarters of parents experiencing symptoms of depression and just as many siblings having recurrent thoughts of death and dying (Bumbalo, Patsdaughter, & McShane, 1993; McShane, Bumbalo, & Patsdaughter, 1994). Parents experience distress from the uncertainties of HIV disease and from witnessing its devastation over a long period of time (Agle et al., 1987; Siegl & Morse, 1994; Takigiku et al., 1993). Caregiver stress is obviously compounded when the parent is also HIV seropositive and he or she is caring for an HIV-infected child (Reidy, Taggart, & Asselin, 1991). Dual patient and caregiver roles in HIV infection can exacerbate stress because HIV-seropositive parents tend to have limited coping resources and are often socially isolated (Hackl, Kalichman, & Somlai, 1995). Thus, family support contributes to the adjustment of individuals with HIV infection, but caregiving comes at an emotional cost to families.

Professional Caregivers

Significant demands are placed on professionals who provide care for people with chronic illnesses. In addition to the usual stress of working with the terminally ill, HIV infection carries added burdens of social stigmas, prejudices, and negative biases (Adelman, 1989; George, Reed, Ballard, Colin, & Fielding, 1993; Silverman, 1993). Like other chronically ill patients, people with HIV–AIDS often express anger toward professional caregivers (Dilley, Ochitill, Perl, & Volberding, 1985). Paraprofessionals and volunteers who offer support may experience similar types of angry reactions (R. L. Miller, Holmes, & Auerbach, 1992). Caregivers of people with HIV infection are therefore in need of support themselves (Land & Harangody, 1990; Reidy et al., 1991). Unfortunately, the nature of professional caregiver relationships restricts reciprocity of support that can help sustain supportive relationships (R. B. Hays, Catania, et al., 1990).

Disclosure, Reciprocity, and Loss

People can receive social support without disclosing their HIV status, but to receive support specific to issues of living with HIV–AIDS, individuals must disclose. Barriers to serostatus disclosure include fears of rejection, violence, and social isolation. The risk for losing support comes at a time of increased needs for social support. Disclosures of HIV infection by parents to children are inhibited by fears of rejection and by the desire of parents to protect their children (Pliskin, Farrell,

Crandles, & DeHovitz, 1993). The potential costs of rejection and abandonment for disclosing one's HIV status are therefore pitted against the potential benefits of gaining support.

Opportunities to reciprocate support are another important dimension to feeling supported. Providing social support to others can buffer stress to an even greater extent than receiving support. For example, reciprocity can decrease hostility and depression in people with HIV infection (R. B. Hays, Cantania, et al., 1990). Many people with HIV–AIDS seek opportunities to support others by joining support groups or volunteer organizations. The rewards of helping others have been documented in AIDS service volunteers (R. L. Miller et al., 1992).

Relationships are disrupted as a result of unemployment, rejection, and deaths of friends. The shrinking size of social networks naturally attenuates available social support (Zich & Temoshok, 1990). Illnesses and deaths of relationship partners, friends, and acquaintances further reduce opportunities to gain and reciprocate support (H. A. Turner et al., 1993). For those who have been hit hardest by AIDS, particularly gay men and the inner-city poor, relationship losses have been devastating. Entire segments of gay communities have been lost, resulting in a depletion of available support for individuals living with HIV–AIDS (R. B. Hays, Chauncey, et al., 1990). Paradoxically, by becoming connected to a supportive network, such as through an AIDS service organization, activism, or a support group, a person risks losing even more relationships (J. L. Martin & Dean, 1993).

In summary, relationships with committed partners, friends, peers, family members, and professional helpers form a structure and context for social support. Ethnic, cultural, and gender differences in social networks, and AIDS stigmas, create barriers to support, isolating people who may need support most. To gain and reciprocate support, HIV-seropositive individuals must recognize and reduce the risks of disclosure.

Supporting People in Rural Areas

Although most cases of AIDS in North America have been reported in larger cities, many people with AIDS move to rural areas and there are increasing numbers of new HIV infections outside of major cities. People living in rural communities do not have access to many AIDS social supports, including health and social services. People with HIV–AIDS living in rural areas experience less life satisfaction, less family support, more loneliness, and perceive greater stigma towards AIDS than people living in cities (Heckman, Somlai, Kalichman, Franzoi, & Kelly, in press). People with HIV–AIDS living in small towns and rural communities have lower levels of health-related quality of life, including emotional, social, and physical well-being (Heckman, Somlai, Otto-Salaj, & Davantes, in press). The effects of living with AIDS in a rural community can therefore lead to social isolation with all of the ill effects that follow.

Functions of Social Support

Feeling supported requires more than merely having contact with people. Traditional models of social support encompass three functions that buffer stress and promote mental health: emotional, informational, and instrumental support. Emotional support is delivered through affection, comfort, and encouragement and results in positive effects on self-esteem, feelings of self-worth, and a sense of belonging (H. A. Turner et al., 1993). Informational support, such as advice or updating knowledge, may help people interpret, comprehend, and cope with HIV infection. Finally, materials, assistance, and services offer practical help, composing an instrumental dimension of support (S. Cohen & Willis, 1985). All three types of support promote emotional and social adjustment in people living with HIV–AIDS.

Emotional Support

Emotional support, like emotion-focused coping, does not directly address matters that affect HIV-related disease processes. Emotional support does, however, enhance emotional well-being by fostering hope and optimism (Rabkin et al., 1990; Zich & Temoshok, 1990). Emotionally supportive behaviors, such as expressing concern, providing encouragement, and serving as a confidant, are often the most beneficial actions received by HIV-positive people (R. B. Hays, Magee, & Chauncey, 1994).

A specific need for emotional support identified by people with HIV–AIDS is physical contact (Wolcott, Namir, Fawzy, Gottlieb, & Mitsuyasu, 1986). When touch is avoided it clearly communicates fear and distance. In contrast, touch symbolizes acceptance and understanding. Having a confidant is another type of emotional support that promotes emotional well-being (Ostrow, 1989; Ostrow, Grant, & Atkinson, 1988; Remien et al., 1992). Emotional support can result from simply enjoying the companionship of another person. Thus, intimate relationships, friendships, support groups, and professional helping relationships potentially provide emotional support.

Informational Support

Uncertainties about HIV infection and the rapid development of new treatments can cause an urgent need to keep up with new information. Accurate information can lead to realistic expectations about the course of illness and effectiveness of treatments, which may in turn facilitate emotional adjustment (Linn et al., 1993). People with HIV infection may seek information about their prognosis, health care and treatment options, insurance coverage, and so forth (R. B. Hays et al., 1992). Seeking information promotes a sense of control and is therefore considered a problem-focused coping strategy (R. B. Hays et al., 1992). The value of informational support has led to a proliferation of information networks, newsletters, and internet services.

Instrumental Support

Practical assistance with everyday needs can help to reduce distress in ways that emotional and informational support cannot (Belkin, Fleishman, Stein, Piette, & Mor, 1992). In some circumstances, instrumental support can have greater benefits than either emotional or informational support (Namir et al., 1989). For example, assistance with shopping and housework are particularly important at later stages of AIDS. The availability of practical assistance can relieve stress caused by physical limitations. As is the case for other aspects of HIV–AIDS, needs for and the availability of instrumental support change over the course of HIV infection. Thus, social support must be understood in the ever changing context of health.

Social Support Over the Course of HIV Infection

After initially testing HIV seropositive, individuals tend to be in a crisis, where emotional and informational supports are most needed (Coleman & Harris, 1989). Unfortunately, fears, stigmas, and attitudes toward sickness, death, and AIDS make emotional support unavailable to many people who have just tested HIV positive. Posttest counselors and AIDS service providers usually offer the first line of support in the experience of having HIV. After the initial receipt of test results, and as HIV infection progresses, the need for multiple types of support from multiple sources also increases (Lennon, Martin, & Dean, 1990).

Fatigue, diminished self-esteem, physical disability, and illnesses restrict the ability to establish long-term supportive relationships. Becoming ill therefore creates barriers to accessing support even when it is available. R. B. Hays et al. (1992) found that satisfaction with informational support positively influenced emotional adjustment, but satisfaction with support depended on the number of HIV symptoms that one had. Gay men who experience HIV symptoms and who have limited informational support were more depressed relative to men with few symptoms and high informational support. Thus, informational support may buffer the stress associated with developing symptoms (R. B. Hays et al., 1992). The associations between social support and illness suggest that individuals who are most in need of support are most inclined to be dissatisfied with the support that they receive (H. A. Turner et al., 1993).

Decreased availability of social support at later stages of HIV–AIDS can give rise to anger, resentment, hopelessness, and depression (Zich & Temoshok, 1987, 1990). When HIV leads to hospitalizations, disabilities, unemployment, and fatigue, social support diminishes and people become increasingly isolated. Support networks eventually shrink from AIDS deaths. Sources of support are also lost to emotional exhaustion and an inability to deal with anticipatory loss (Namir et al., 1989). People with AIDS must therefore seek support from multiple sources and find ways to replenish support as HIV infection advances.

CONCLUSION

Despite the overwhelming complexity of AIDS, people diagnosed with HIV infection frequently exemplify the best of how people can manage under extraordinary circumstances. Resiliency in coping with HIV–AIDS parallels that of persons who have cancer, survive a violent crime, or who have other traumatic, life-redefining experiences. Even people who lack basic resources, such as people living in poverty, oppressed minority groups, people addicted to drugs, the persistently mentally ill, and the homeless, seem to adjust surprisingly well to the early stages of HIV infection. However, as HIV disease progresses, symptoms emerge, and the need for medical care increases, these same people may very well require the greatest assistance in managing HIV over the long haul. Unfortunately, most of our coping theories hinge on cognitive processes that in many ways assume that more basic survival needs have been met, which of course is often not the case. AIDS poses daunting challenges to even the most resourceful individuals. Before the emotional needs of people living with HIV–AIDS can be approached, it is therefore essential that social services be available to meet basic needs such as providing shelter, meals, employment, and medical care.

9

Counseling and Psychotherapy

The demands of living with a chronic, stigmatized, life threatening illness bring many people with HIV–AIDS to seek mental health services. A survey of 472 caregivers of people living with HIV–AIDS in Los Angeles and San Francisco showed that 93% of the people with HIV–AIDS had sought some form of supportive service (Wight, LeBlanc, & Aneshensel, 1995). In addition, 20% had attended HIV–AIDS support groups, 22% received emotional support from a volunteer agency, and 29% had been treated in individual or group psychotherapy. These data testify to the need and use of psychological and social services for people affected by HIV–AIDS.

Interventions specific for persons with HIV are available in many communities, particularly larger metropolitan areas. Support groups and other avenues for receiving social support are among the most available services for people with HIV–AIDS. In addition, there are growing numbers of counselors and psychotherapists offering services to people affected by HIV–AIDS. This chapter overviews mental health assessment, social support interventions, counseling, and psychotherapy for people with HIV–AIDS.

ASSESSMENT AND TREATMENT PLANNING

Several aspects of HIV disease must be considered in the assessment and evaluation of HIV-seropositive people. Emotional reactions are to be expected as a chronic illness like HIV infection progresses. The problem becomes sorting through the illness symptoms and medication side effects that often overlap with somatic symptoms of emotional distress. Overlapping symptoms of HIV infection and emotional reactions to HIV infection pose particular problems when assessing depression and anxiety. For example, 7 of the 21 items on the Beck Depression Inventory (BDI; A. T. Beck & Steer, 1993) directly parallel symptoms of HIV infection. Symptom overlap occurs for problems in concentration and decision making, changes in physical appearance, increased difficulty in social and occupational functioning, sleep disturbances, fatigue, loss of appetite, and excessive weight loss. Worrying about physical health and physical attractiveness, declining sexual interests, and excessive guilt, also co-occur with HIV disease processes. Similarly, the *DSM-IV* (American Psychiatric Association, 1994) diagnostic criteria for several clinical syndromes rely heavily on vegetative symptoms. For example, to meet criteria for a diagnosis with major depression, a person must exhibit five of nine symptoms, five of which overlap directly with symptoms of HIV disease: significant weight loss, insomnia, fatigue, diminished ability to think or concentrate, and psychomotor retardation. Diagnostic criteria for dysthymia reflect similar overlapping physical symptoms with HIV infection.

In a study that investigated symptom overlap, Kalichman, Sikkema, and Somlai (1995) found that people with HIV infection who scored above the clinical cutoff on the BDI reported significantly more HIV symptoms than did nondepressed people, although depressed and nondepressed participants did not differ in their number of AIDS-defining conditions or T-helper cell counts. Specifically, 82% of depressed HIV-seropositive people had persistent fatigue and 57% reported night sweats, compared with 47% and 15% of nondepressed people, respectively. Physical signs of depression that overlap with HIV symptomatology are particularly important in clinical assessment because sleep disturbances and loss of appetite are among the most common symptoms of depression in people with HIV–AIDS (Ritchie & Radke, 1992). Hintz, Kuck, Peterkin, Volk, and Zisook (1990) also found that HIV-seropositive individuals have more disturbed sleep patterns and suppressed appetites than depressed HIV-seronegative individuals. In a factor analysis of several measures, HIV symptoms have been found to correspond more closely with measures of depression and anxiety than with immune status and AIDS-related conditions (Kalichman et al., 1995). Although potentially attributable to depression, somatic symptoms are poor diagnostic indicators of depression unless overlapping HIV symptoms are accounted for. Table 9.1 summarizes HIV symptoms that overlap with symptoms of depression and anxiety that are commonly included in assessment instruments.

Psychological assessment can be made more specific to emotional distress by decomposing instruments into cognitive, affective, behavioral, and somatic domains. For example, Kertzner et al. (1993) modified the Hamilton Rating Scale for Anxiety for use with people with HIV by omitting items pertaining to somatic distress. Unfortunately, altering some standardized instruments limits their potential clinical usefulness because norms are rendered invalid and scores from idiosyncratically derived item subsets have unknown psychometric properties. Alternatively, it is possible to examine symptom responses by

Table 9.1
**Overlapping Symptoms of Depression and Anxiety
With HIV Infection**

Distress Symptom	HIV-Related Symptom
Fatigue and lethargy	Malaise
Suppressed appetite	Weight loss
Muscle aches	Muscle aches
Insomnia; Increased sweating	Night sweats
Gastrointestinal distress	Diarrhea
Headaches and dizziness; Memory lapses	Neurological disturbances

conducting content analyses of scales. For example, after scoring a scale according to standardized procedures and using available normative data to interpret a score, the scale can be inspected item by item to determine the amount of symptomatology accounted for by subsets of items, a common clinical practice that becomes essential in assessing people with HIV infection. The case example presented in Table 9.2 illustrates the importance of item-level analyses by focusing on the symptom comorbidity of the BDI.

Taken from a study of HIV-positive men and women (Kalichman et al., 1995), a participant scored 18 on the BDI where the clinical cutoff for depression is 15. Responses shown in Table 9.2 indicated that 11 of the 18 scored points were accounted for by symptoms of depression that overlap with symptoms of HIV infection. Thus, an elevated depression score for this person was partially accounted for by physical and behavioral symptoms of depression that overlap with HIV infection. However, these physical symptoms, of course, did not occur in isolation of cognitive and affective depression. On a separate index of HIV-related symptoms and illnesses, this same person indicated that he or she had persistent fatigue for at least 2 weeks, unintentionally lost at least 10 pounds, had diarrhea for at least 2 weeks, had muscle aches and cramps, and had been diagnosed with two AIDS-defining conditions, lymphoma and HIV wasting syndrome. Thus, interpreting this person's BDI at face value would lead to erroneous conclusions. Instead, the cognitive and somatic items should be sorted and scored separately using procedures described by A. T. Beck and Steer (1993).

Psychological tests that do not include physical symptoms can reduce the potential problems of disease-distress overlap. For example, the Hospital Anxiety and Depression Scale was developed to avoid physical symptom overlap in medical illnesses and may be useful in assessing people with HIV–AIDS (Zigmond & Snaith, 1983). Another strategy is to assess clinical constructs that are closely associated with depression and anxiety but do not reflect physical symptomatology. For example, the Beck Hopelessness Scale correlates with measures of depression, predicts suicidal intentions, and does not include any physical symptoms (A. T. Beck, Kovacs, & Weissman, 1975). Similarly, assessing lone-

---

Table 9.2

Item Responses on the Beck Depression Inventory by a Person With Advanced HIV Infection

Beck Depression Inventory Item	Scored Points
I feel sad	1
I feel discouraged about the future	1
I do not feel like a failure	0
I don't enjoy things the way I used to	1
I don't feel particularly guilty	0
I don't feel I am being punished	0
I am disappointed in myself	1
I don't feel I am any worse than anybody else	0
I don't have any thought of killing myself	0
I don't cry anymore than usual	0
I get annoyed or irritated more easily than I used to	1
I am less interested in other people than I used to be	1
I make decisions about as well as I ever could	0
I am worried that I am looking old or unattractive	1
I have to push myself very hard to do anything	2
I don't sleep as well as I used to	1
I get tired from doing almost nothing	2
My appetite is not as good as it used to be	1
I have lost more than 10 pounds	2
I am worried about physical problems such as aches and pains; or upset stomach; or constipation	1
I am less interested in sex than I used to be	1

NOTE: Items that overlap with HIV-related symptoms are in italics.

liness, guilt, and anger provides valuable information concerning negative affective states without reliance on concurrent HIV-related symptomatology. Corollary assessments may be used in combination with depression and anxiety inventories to examine the convergent verification of other test results.

Other emotional reactions to HIV infection require similar considerations. Suicide risk fluctuates during HIV infection, and motivations
to attempt suicide differ over the course of the disease. That is, a person
may be at risk for suicide when learning they have HIV and, again,
when they feel unable to cope with impending illness. However, people
at later stages of AIDS may contemplate suicide to terminate their pain
and avoid suffering. Therefore, hopelessness and despair are the most
likely impetus for attempting suicide early in the course of HIV, and
exerting personal control to avoid suffering may emerge as reasons for
suicide later in HIV infection. Periodic assessments of suicidal risk, as
well as other aspects of emotional distress, such as hostility, life satisfaction, and quality of life are therefore important in the clinical assessment of HIV-positive people.

Another factor to consider in assessing HIV-related depression is
the potential for neurocognitive deficits to contaminate psychological
test results. As described in chapter 5, lethargy, poor concentration,
psychomotor slowing, and other neuropsychological symptoms must be
sorted out from overlapping symptoms of depression. Clinically assessing people with HIV–AIDS will also require evaluating scores against
existing norms; populations most affected by HIV have been the most
underrepresented in normative samples. Culture and gender differences
in symptom expression and subpopulation base rates may confuse the
conclusions drawn from clinical assessments. These issues underscore
the importance of collecting convergent and divergent assessment instruments when evaluating people with HIV infection.

SOCIAL SUPPORT INTERVENTIONS

Among HIV-seropositive people's most frequently unmet needs are
those for affiliation and support. Smith and Rapkin (1996) found that
39% of people with HIV–AIDS have at least some unmet support needs
and 22% reported their support needs have gone completely unmet.
Social support interventions for individuals affected by HIV–AIDS can
provide multiple types of support including emotional, informational,
and instrumental support. The most accessible social support interven-

tions for people living with HIV–AIDS have thus far included support groups, volunteer programs, and hospice services.

Support Groups

Support groups for people living with HIV infection and their caregivers are similar to those developed for other medical populations. Support groups can foster interpersonal relationships between group members, potentially benefiting people with HIV infection (Adelman, 1989; DiPasquale, 1990). There are nearly 2,000 support groups listed by the U.S. National AIDS Hotline. Wight et al. (1995) found that 22% of people with HIV–AIDS and 16% of their caregivers attend support groups, making groups among the most used services for people affected by AIDS.

In one of the few systematic evaluations of a support group for HIV-seropositive substance abusers, Greenberg, Johnson, and Fichtner (1996) examined the process and outcome of group attendance. Studying 100 HIV-seropositive men and women, 93% of whom were African American, Greenberg et al. found that the group process consisted of a "rap session" format, where group members took turns sharing experiences, expressing emotions, and narrating stories of their recovery and AIDS-related situations. The groups were facilitated by volunteers and were conducted in a private home. The researchers coded a total of 2,230 verbal exchanges and found that 22% of speaking turns concerned issues of drug abuse and abstaining from drugs. Not surprisingly, members who more frequently attended groups reported less use of substances and a greater likelihood of remaining drug free than did those who attended less often. The outcomes for participants, therefore, lined up well with the self-directed purpose of the groups.

Of course, support groups are not for everyone. Willingness to participate in a group requires one to reach out to others. People with HIV infection who do not attend support groups differ from those who do attend support groups in their experience of emotional distress and use of coping strategies. Kalichman, Sikkema, and Somlai (1996) found that people who attend support groups experience less anxiety and less depression than people who do not attend groups. However, people who attended support groups also knew they were HIV infected for a significantly longer period of time, and time since testing positive accounted for the differences in emotional well-being. Thus, with time, people who live with HIV become increasingly well adjusted and more socially connected. However, there were differences between attendees and nonattendees in general coping strategies; not attending groups meant a stronger tendency to use avoidant coping strategies than was used by people attending support groups, and these differences were not accounted for by the duration of knowing one's HIV status. For people living with HIV–AIDS who are attracted to groups, support groups function well in meeting both emotional and informational support needs.

Emotional Support

Support groups can help people with HIV infection achieve a sense of emotional balance. Being a part of a group can help foster hope, create opportunities to gain insights from others, allow for emotional catharsis, and create interpersonal connectedness (Buck, 1991). Mathews and Bowes (1989) identified five dimensions of effective HIV-related support groups: (a) sharing common experiences, (b) providing group cohesiveness, (c) reinforcing hope, (d) helping others, and (e) learning from others' experiences. Sadovsky (1991) suggested that support groups deal with fears and prejudices, coordinate community services, encourage independence and hope, allow for focusing on self, and promote informed choices.

Bringing people with common life experiences together in a group creates a potentially supportive environment and mutual understanding (Adelman, 1989; O'Dowd, 1988). Support groups also provide opportunities to deal with immediate crises. Problem solving can occur naturally in group settings because group members offer suggestions from their diverse backgrounds and experiences (Adelman, 1989; Gamble & Getzel, 1989). The goals of support groups may include fostering an environment for exchanging coping strategies and reinforcing effective coping behaviors (Buck, 1991). Support groups allow people to share their concerns and serve as a vehicle for developing and reinforcing coping strategies. However, for many people, support groups are most valued when they offer something tangible that people can take with them, such as friendships or new information.

Informational Support

Support groups channel informal and formal information to group members. Some groups focus exclusively on delivering and exchanging information, providing a forum for people with HIV infection to share experiences, knowledge, and ideas (Hedge & Glover, 1990). Knowledgeable group leaders can become primary sources of information for people who attend support groups. In addition, outside experts may be invited to attend groups as guest speakers and present current information on such topics as infectious diseases, new treatments, optimal use of medications, adherence to treatment regimens, nutrition, insurance, living wills, social services, returning to work, and so forth.

There are several models available for information-based support groups. Coleman and Harris (1989) conducted a psychoeducational support group to meet five specific information needs, which included information pertaining to HIV disease, management of health problems, health care and health insurance concerns, nutrition and its role in HIV infection, and issues of sexuality and intimate relationships. Similarly, Hedge and Glover (1990) described an informational support group that focused on general health, stress, diet, medications, the medical and legal systems, relationships, safer sex, complementary therapies, and life-style changes brought about by HIV infection. The information content of sessions and the information needs of group members vary during the course of HIV infection. In a support group, people receive information in the context of emotional support, with opportunities to share information with others, therefore reciprocating support. The mix of receiving and reciprocating support makes groups particularly effective venues for enhancing social support.

Structure and Format of Support Groups

Support groups vary widely in their structure and format. Groups may have limited numbers of sessions or groups may go on indefinitely. Groups can have a set agenda or groups may evolve over time. Support groups may be open with regard to allowing new members to join, or groups may be closed to new members. Formatting groups as either open or closed requires choosing between the benefits of infusing the fresh perspectives offered by open groups versus the benefits of trust and fostering confidentiality in a closed group (Hedge & Glover, 1990; Land & Harangody, 1990).

Another issue is group composition. Mixing members who recently tested HIV seropositive with those who have been seropositive for a long time, versus limiting groups to individuals at a particular stage of HIV infection influences the issues addressed by the group. The types of support needed after an initial diagnosis differ from those during symptomatic illness (Watson, 1983). Bringing people who have recently been diagnosed together with long-term survivors in the same group allows the newly diagnosed to gain emotional and informational support from those who have "been there" and are surviving HIV infection. On the other hand, the newly diagnosed may not be ready to encounter a person with advanced AIDS. Decisions regarding group composition therefore shape many of the issues that arise in group sessions. Other decisions include whether to mix groups or keep them homogeneous with respect to gender, sexual orientation, and modes of having contracted the virus. Although homogeneous groups are considered more effective (Buiss, 1989; S. H. Levine, Bystritsky, Baron, & Jones, 1991), there are benefits to group diversity. Professional versus peer facilitators, cofacilitators versus a single facilitator, whether to invite outside speakers, and the degree to which group members and leaders should be matched for gender, ethnicity, and HIV status are issues that require careful consideration (Coleman & Harris, 1989; Gambe & Getzel, 1989).

One study reported interviews that focused on the experiences and perceptions of support groups for people with HIV infection (Kalichman, 1995). All of the interview participants who had known they were HIV seropositive for more than a few months had attended at least one support group offered by AIDS service organizations. It was almost universal that the emotional tone of support groups influenced participant satisfaction. Groups were preferred that focused on positive attitudes and hope, rather than expression of negative feelings and sharing the perils of HIV infection. Information exchange was another critical factor in the effectiveness of support groups. Information shared by fellow support group members was considered among the greatest benefits of a group. One woman illustrated this sentiment, stating the following:

> I can't sit in a group and listen to a lot of sadness. Some people do that; they would rather whine about it. When I get together with my HIV-positive friends, we talk about new drugs that have come out or something like that. I think it is a little more beneficial; hopeful that we can go out and do something.

Emotional support is therefore gained from the feeling of not being alone. Groups can foster friendships and opportunities for activities or social events.

With respect to group composition, Kalichman (1995) found that the majority of gay men and heterosexual women felt comfortable coming to a mixed group and believed that diversity was a good thing. However, heterosexual men and injection drug users felt that their issues were different from those of gay men and heterosexual women and preferred separate groups. Views on mixing groups with people of different stages of HIV infection seem to depend on the stage of illness of the person asked. People early in the course of HIV infection felt that they could benefit from the experience of people who had been HIV seropositive longer. For example, one man who had been HIV positive for 5 years stated, "There is a lot of support in seeing someone who has survived a long time with HIV and hear their stories." On the other hand, those at later stages of HIV infection believed that the newly diagnosed could offer emotional support and encouragement, but to a lesser degree than other people who have been dealing with HIV–AIDS for some time. For example, one man who had been HIV seropositive for 8 years stated,

> From newly diagnosed guys in the group I can learn about their fears, about their jobs, and about things they are going through.

299

But I don't have to worry about a lot of that stuff anymore. I've been there. I get most of my support from other guys in the group who are at about the same stage of HIV. Learning what they do to cope with things on a daily basis, or maybe that their doctor allows me to take some new information to my doctor and say let's try this.

Support Groups for Caregivers and the Bereaved

Groups can also meet the support needs of caregivers and people bereaved from AIDS. Caregiver support groups allow members to express and reconcile feelings related to caregiving (Frost et al., 1991). Support groups for caregivers are therefore geared toward sustaining emotional well-being to enable caregivers to continue their work (Kelly & Sykes, 1989). Like groups for people with HIV infection, caregiver support groups require addressing multiple losses. Helping people with HIV infection means dealing with issues of death and dying (Bennett & Kelaher, 1993; Killeen, 1993). Goals for professional caregiver support groups may include stress reduction to prevent burnout, reinforcing values that promote continued work with HIV seropositive clients, enhancing and maintaining compassionate care, and establishing professional boundaries with clients while fulfilling caregiver responsibilities (Grossman & Silverstein, 1993). Although there are few empirical studies of caregiver support groups, there is evidence that support provided to professionals who care for HIV-seropositive clients effectively buffers stress and improves their quality of care (George, Reed, Ballard, Colin, & Fielding, 1993).

Support groups may be developed specifically to prevent and manage caregiver burnout. AIDS caregivers, like caregivers for people with other chronic diseases, are particularly prone to emotional exhaustion. Risk for burnout is greatest in emotionally charged, personal service professions. Nurses caring for AIDS patients experience similar stress and burnout as oncology and geriatric nurses (Kleiber, Enzman, & Guzy, 1993). Work loads, organizational support, beliefs about occupational risks for infection, and coping resources influence resilience against burnout in AIDS care (Bennett, Miller, & Ross, 1993; Van Servellen & Leake, 1993). Support groups therefore offer a means for facilitating coping with the stress of caring for people with HIV–AIDS (Barbour, 1994).

The death of a person to AIDS results in bereavement similar to that found in loss from other chronic illnesses. Support groups assist survivors in rebuilding their lives (Adelman, 1989). Needs for support during bereavement are well recognized. Lennon, Martin, and Dean (1990) found that grief reactions were greatest among those who had cared for a friend dying of AIDS who did not have their own support system. In addition, one third of the men in Lennon et al.'s study indicated that they did not receive adequate instrumental support when providing care for their friend and were not receiving emotional support while grieving.

There have been few systematic studies of support groups for individuals who have suffered AIDS-related losses. In one small pilot study, three men and four women who suffered a personal loss because of AIDS participated in a support group that was based on cognitive and behavioral coping strategies (Sikkema, Kalichman, Kelly, & Koob, 1995). A nine-session support group focused on identifying and expressing emotions, developing adaptive coping strategies, increasing feelings of support, reducing emotional distress, and avoiding maladaptive coping behaviors. Sikkema et al. found that the support group significantly reduced depression, grief reactions, anxiety, somatization, and other symptoms of distress. The group participants benefited from focusing on specific rather than global stressors, support offered by fellow group members, and their own emotional expression. Although it was based on a small sample without a control group, the study showed evidence for the potential value of support groups and other group interventions for those who suffer AIDS-related losses.

VOLUNTEERING

AIDS service organizations that provide support to people with HIV infection rely on volunteers, many of whom are HIV seropositive themselves (Adelman, 1989; Siegel, 1986). For example, programs may designate a buddy to provide one-to-one support for individuals with HIV infection. Buddy volunteer programs provide both companionship and physical assistance. Buddy programs and peer counseling are also available to assist people through the HIV antibody testing process. One study found that 14% of people with HIV–AIDS use buddy support programs (Wight et al., 1995). Volunteers visit and call to offer emotional support as well as provide instrumental support by shopping, cleaning, cooking, and providing transportation (Lennon et al., 1990; Velentgas, Bynum, & Zierler, 1990). When individuals with HIV infection themselves volunteer to help others, they may gain support by joining a network of fellow volunteers as well as the reciprocity of support offered by these relationships. Volunteer experiences can increase self-esteem, perceived internal control, and a sense of personal worth.

Volunteering for AIDS organizations can serve to meet the support needs of volunteers as well as benefit those who receive services. Omoto and Snyder (1995) found that AIDS volunteers who received greater social support in their lives tended to volunteer for shorter periods of time. Having less support on the other hand, predicted longevity of volunteering. People with more extensive social networks may experience time conflicts, and the emotional strain of volunteering can interfere with other relationships. For those who stay in volunteer roles, however, volunteering and its associated relationships sustain volunteers, particularly those who have less extensive social networks.

PALLIATIVE CARE AND HOSPICE

Hospice is an interdisciplinary approach to caring for the terminally ill for whom recovery is unlikely and a prognosis is stated in months or weeks (V. Moss, 1990). Hospice care emphasizes quality rather than quantity of life, holistic approaches to pain control that include psychological and spiritual pain, and the involvement of family and others in the care of the patient (Benjamin & Preston, 1993). Caregivers are a central part of hospice care, and many hospice programs offer primary-caregiver relief and respite care. Another important aspect of hospice is its emphasis on palliative care, a specialized form of care for patients with advanced progressive diseases where curative treatments are no longer feasible (Butters, Higginson, George, & McCarthy, 1993; Mansfield, Barter, & Singh, 1992). Hospice care therefore integrates psychological, social, and medical approaches to address the unique issues of the terminally ill (Cassileth et al., 1985).

The progressive nature of HIV infection places it within the scope of the hospice mission. Unfortunately, many traditional hospices have been unwilling to accept AIDS patients (Mansfield et al., 1992). The reluctance to care for people with AIDS is primarily due to conflicts between features of HIV disease and eligibility for hospice care. For example, people with AIDS often do not have a family member or friend willing to serve as a primary caregiver, a necessity for hospice home care (Benjamin & Preston, 1993). Moreover, AIDS has a largely unpredictable course, with sudden changes and reversals of life-threatening conditions. These characteristics of AIDS set it apart from other chronic illnesses serviced by most hospice programs. Thus, hospices have been started to care for people with AIDS exclusively (Mansfield et al., 1992; Sadovsky, 1991). In general, AIDS hospice care does not differ much from non-AIDS hospice; both emphasize pain control and quality of life. However, AIDS hospice care can attend to the special needs of people with AIDS. The same may be said for other psychological services, where the structure and mechanisms of care are not that different but the therapeutic context and treatment are tailored to address AIDS-related needs.

PSYCHOTHERAPY

A growing literature is demonstrating the benefits of psychotherapy for people living with HIV–AIDS. Clinical studies, although few in number, have shown promise for both individual and group therapy. In addition, several conceptual models of psychotherapy have now been described for use in HIV–AIDS. Thus, clinical studies as well as clinical experiences have revealed common themes in HIV–AIDS psychotherapy. In the following sections, cognitive-behavioral, interpersonal, psychodynamic, and other approaches to HIV–AIDS-related therapy are explored and a discussion of the common themes that arise in therapy for people with HIV—AIDS is presented.

Cognitive—Behavioral Approaches

Cognitive—behavioral therapy has successfully helped clients adjust to chronic illness. Stress management, cognitive restructuring, behavioral self-management skills, and coping-effectiveness training have been the basis for several interventions with HIV-positive people. For example, Coates, McKusick, Kuno, and Stites (1989) described group therapy that consisted of eight 2-hour weekly sessions and emphasized instruction in systematic relaxation, health habit change such as smoking and alcohol reduction, increasing rest and exercise, and other stress-management skills. Coates et al. reported several benefits of participating in the group. Similar cognitive—behavioral group therapies with HIV-positive clients have been effective in reducing emotional distress and enhancing quality of life (e.g., Emmot, 1991; Lamping et al., 1993; Mulder et al., 1992). Antoni et al. (1991) enrolled gay men into a cognitive—behavioral therapy intervention prior to notification of their HIV-antibody test results and tested for difference in adjustment between seropositive and seronegative men. Antoni et al. (1991) based their treatment on cognitive—behavioral therapy that included the following: behavioral stress management, relaxation skills training, self-monitoring of environmental stressors, stress reappraisal, active coping, enhancing self-efficacy, and expanding social networks. This multifaceted therapy produced significant reductions in emotional distress among men who subsequently tested HIV positive. Antoni et al. (1991) concluded that therapy buffered post-HIV-test-notification depression and increased a sense of personal control among men who tested HIV positive.

Similar results were reported in ten 90-minute sessions of cognitive—behavioral stress management compared to a waiting-list control group (Lutgendorf et al., 1997). Gay men who received the cognitive—behavioral treatment demonstrated reductions in anxiety and dysphoria relative to the control group. The declines in distress measures occurred in the context of already low levels of distress at baseline.

The reductions in depressed mood occurred in men who were not clinically depressed. Although there were no differences between groups on HIV-related health markers, there was a difference in herpes simplex virus antibodies, offering modest evidence for immune benefits of the treatment.

Kelly, Murphy, Bahr, Kalichman, et al. (1993) also tested an intensive cognitive–behavioral therapy group for depressed HIV-positive clients. They randomly assigned 68 HIV-positive (non-AIDS) men with heightened depressed mood to one of three experimental treatment conditions: (a) a cognitive–behavioral treatment group, (b) a social support group, or (c) an individual psychotherapy comparison condition. They described the cognitive–behavioral condition as follows:

> The cognitive–behavioral groups focused on the use of cognitive and behavior strategies to reduce maladaptive anxiety and depression. Each session had a behavioral or skill training theme and the sessions involved teaching participants the skill, group discussion of potential uses and benefits of the skill, and weekly review of success in implementation. Skill areas included modification of cognitions that exacerbate anxiety or depression, progressive muscle relaxation, imaginal and cue-controlled relaxation, disclosure of serostatus and safer sex practices if sexually active, and establishment of a network of socially supportive relationships. Participant questions, concerns, and problems in implementation of change were handled from a cognitive problem-solving perspective. Most sessions also included at-home practice assignments. (p. 1681)

Results of the study showed that both group interventions positively affected group members relative to the individual therapy control condition. However, the social support group appeared to have the greatest benefit over a 3-month follow-up period. Of the social support group participants, 86% demonstrated clinically significant improvement on an index of distress severity, whereas 66% of the comparison condition showed clinical deterioration, regressing below baseline levels. Although members of the cognitive–behavioral group demonstrated a pattern of clinical change that was intermediate between the social support groups and the control condition, cognitive–behavioral group participants did decrease their use of illicit substances to a greater degree than the other two groups.

Kelly, Murphy, Bahr, Kalichman, et al. (1993) concluded that the two group models provided different types of support with different outcomes. Whereas the social support group allowed more time for emotional support and therefore emotion-focused coping, the cognitive–behavioral group emphasized problem-focused and active coping skills training. Because the interventions did not differentiate between controllable and uncontrollable circumstances to which coping strategies are applied, and because emotion focused coping seemed more effective, it is likely that problem-focused coping was applied to uncontrollable problems (Chesney, Lurie, & Coates, 1995). Thus, the results of Kelly et al.'s study speak to the importance of fitting coping strategies to the controllability of problem situations.

In another clinical trial, Eller (1995) examined the effects of two cognitive and behavioral stress reduction techniques, guided imagery and progressive muscle relaxation. Most interesting, the treatments were brief and focused on the two stress techniques. The guided imagery treatment consisted of a single 21-minute audiotape that was used over a 6 week period. Similarly, the progressive muscle-relaxation treatment was a 12-minute audiotape also used daily for 6 weeks. Both conditions were compared to a standard of care control group. Despite testing only a small number of participants, the study demonstrated reductions in depression for both treatment conditions. Thus, even quite minimal cognitive–behavioral therapy has shown promise in treating HIV-infected people. Below is a brief description of cognitive–behavioral techniques used with HIV-positive clients.

Relaxation and Stress Reduction

Standard relaxation exercises have been effective in reducing stress in people with HIV–AIDS (Antoni et al., 1991; Eller, 1995). Tension-relaxation procedures combine focused attention with neuromuscular tension reduction to produce a response incompatible with anxiety. Alternatively, guided imagery relaxation techniques can be used and may be preferable for individuals with medical ailments. If imagery is used in relaxation training, however, it is important that clients not confuse it with spiritual or alternative healing imagery, which have their own potential benefits. Like all behavioral skills training, relaxation requires a thorough assessment, homework assignments, self-monitoring, practice, and feedback. It is helpful to suggest daily practice in a designated place and time. Audiotape recordings of relaxation instructions are often helpful, and scripts for relaxation skills are widely available.

Cognitive Restructuring

Reframing and reappraising stressful life events can reduce emotional distress and increase a sense of personal control. Techniques for cognitive restructuring are described by proponents of self-instruction training (Meichenbaum, 1977), cognitive therapy (A. T. Beck, 1976), and rational—emotive therapy (Ellis, 1962). In general, cognitive restructuring involves identifying maladaptive thoughts or self-statements, therapist modeling of adaptive behavior, and reinforcing messages that guide adaptive coping. Cognitive restructuring can help people reappraise their current health status, reframe illness symptoms, and maintain a realistic outlook on their illness. Thus, cognitive therapy techniques are commonly applied to work through denial, particularly maladaptive denial (Schmaling & DiClementi, 1991).

Health-Related Life-Style Changes

HIV-seropositive people often require assistance to change health-related behaviors, including reducing practices that have adverse health effects (e.g., poor nutrition, tobacco use, alcohol and drug use, etc.), increasing behaviors that enhance fitness (e.g., rest, exercise, medication adherence, etc.), and eliminating sexual and drug-use behaviors that risk HIV transmission and reinfection. Changes in life-style are conceptually broader than the narrow behavior changes that are often the focus of health-behavior interventions. Life-style changes typically focus on clusters of health related behaviors rather than on any one behavior. Techniques such as keeping daily diaries and other self-monitoring devices, structuring daily activities, and reinforcing steps toward behavior change can help initiate and maintain health-behavior change.

Coping Effectiveness Training

Coping effectiveness training is a group-based approach that emphasizes fitting coping strategies to specific problem situations. Chesney, Folkman, and Chambers (1996) described coping effectiveness training that consisted of ten 90-minute sessions, with an additional day-long retreat between the fourth and fifth sessions. The training included six central elements: (a) appraisal of stressful situations, (b) problem and emotion focused coping, (c) determining the fit between coping strategies and controllable versus uncontrollable stressful situations, (d) maximizing use of social support, (e) training in maintenance of stress reduction through effective coping, and (f) effectively using a series of workbook exercises. The training emphasizes both problem-focused and adaptive emotion-focused coping strategies with an attempt to fit specific coping strategies to specific situations. Thus, coping effectiveness training offers a specific and well defined approach to enhancing coping capacities that can be applied across a variety of stressful situations.

Interpersonal Therapy

Interpersonal psychotherapy focuses on helping clients relate changes in their moods to external events and subsequent changes in social roles (Markowitz et al., 1995). This school of therapy focuses on the here-and-now and offers the client a comfortable space to reflect and self-examine. Treatment is time limited in interpersonal therapy. Markowitz and his colleagues (Markowitz, Klerman, & Perry, 1992; Markowitz, Klerman, Perry, Clougherty, & Josephs, 1993) reported treatment outcomes for 23 HIV-seropositive clients who received an average of 16 sessions of individual, interpersonally oriented psychotherapy. Markowitz et al. (1993) encouraged and supported clients to become involved in their medical care, prevent HIV transmission, tailor their work and social activities to changes in physical functioning, and adhere to medical treatments. Again, therapy emphasized the here-and-now and framed illness as an opportunity to examine relationships, values, goals, and other important issues. Markowitz et al. (1993) emphasized exploring options and reinforcing hope. The results of evaluations taken over the course of therapy found that clients showed declines in depressed mood and other signs of emotional distress, thus providing evidence to support the use of interpersonal therapy in treating people with HIV.

In a randomized clinical study, Markowitz et al. (1995) compared interpersonal therapy with a time-contact matched supportive therapy control group. Results showed that after 16 weeks of treatment, individuals who received interpersonal therapy demonstrated less emotional distress than individuals assigned to the control condition. Despite the fact that this study only included midcourse of treatment and immediate posttreatment assessments, it is among the very few controlled studies that demonstrate efficacy of individual psychotherapy for people living with HIV–AIDS.

Psychodynamic Perspectives

There is little research investigating the efficacy of treating people with HIV–AIDS from a psychodynamic perspective. Indeed, there is little reason to believe that psychodynamic approaches will apply differently for people living with HIV–AIDS. However, clinicians have written extensively on transference and countertransference in psychotherapy with people affected by AIDS. Cadwell (1997) for example, describes transference as emerging from four core issues, death and dying, disease, sexuality, and injection drug use. Of particular importance are when these core issues arise in the context of therapeutic relationships where the client and therapist share experiences such as when a gay therapist has a gay client or has lost someone to AIDS. Cadwell notes that many characteristics including gender, age, ethnicity, and life circumstances can be powerful influences on the therapeutic process. Barrett (1997) described similar transference and countertransference issues in psychotherapy with AIDS affected clients. As expected in any treatment context, vigilance against personal issues encroaching on the therapeutic process must be kept in check throughout the therapeutic relationship.

Humanistic–Client-Centered Psychotherapy

There is evidence that humanistic psychotherapy for AIDS affected clients is effective in both individual and group formats. For individual therapy, Markowitz et al. (1995) used a multisession client-centered therapy condition as a control group. Although not delivered as it would be in typical clinical practice (W. A. Brown, 1996), Markowitz et al. found that client-centered therapy improved symptoms of depression although not to the same extent of interpersonal therapy. In a humanistic group treatment also used as a clinical study control condition described above, Kelly, Murphy, Bahr, Kalichman, et al. (1993) found improvements in the mental health of depressed clients that exceeded those of clients in a cognitive–behavioral treatment.

Group Therapy

There are several lines of evidence that suggest people with HIV infection and AIDS can benefit from group psychotherapy. Not to be confused with support groups, therapy is conducted by trained therapists rather than peer facilitators, and therapeutic techniques are an integral part of the group experience (Beckett & Rutan, 1990). Group therapy does encompass similar features of traditional support groups, including disseminating information and fostering supportive relationships, but it goes beyond the group experience by focusing on therapeutic techniques. HIV-related group therapy has been based on models designed for other chronic illnesses. S. H. Levine et al. (1991), for example, described a psychotherapy group that treated six clients with symptomatic HIV infection. The primary focus of the group was humanistic psychotherapy, but it included providing accurate HIV-related information, instruction in adaptive coping strategies, and working through losses and anticipatory grief. S. H. Levine et al. stated that the treatment was centered around a supportive atmosphere that reduced HIV-related fears, addressed relationship issues, and built social supports. Like other evaluations of group therapies, Levine et al. found that clients in the group experienced less emotional distress as a result of being in the group.

Psychopharmacological Treatments

Depression is often considered a normal reaction to having been diagnosed with HIV infection, keeping many clinicians from considering drug treatments (Walker & Spenger, 1995). Failing to consider drug treatment for depression is unfortunate, however, because medications have been effective in treating depressed HIV-seropositive clients. Markowitz, Rabkin, and Perry (1994) reviewed clinical trials of antidepressant medications in HIV infection and found that three controlled studies of imipramine demonstrated the efficacy of this drug with HIV-positive individuals. Similar results were reported with other antidepressants as well as stimulants used to treat depression. On the basis of their review, Markowitz et al. (1994) concluded that using antidepressants with HIV-seropositive clients is supported by the available research. In one study, Rabkin, Rabkin, Harrison, and Wagner (1994) conducted a double-blind placebo controlled trial of imipramine to treat depressed people with HIV infection. Imipramine was found to reduce depression at a significantly greater rate than the control condition, and there was no evidence for adverse immune reactions to the drug. This study extended previous research that suggested safety and efficacy of imipramine in depressed HIV-positive people (Rabkin & Harrison, 1990). Elliott et al. (1998) showed that imipramine and paroxetine, a short-half-life selective serotonin reuptake inhibitor, were both effective in treating HIV-positive depressed people. Additional research with Prozac has shown positive treatment of depression in people with HIV–AIDS (Judd, Mijch, & Cockram, 1995; Rabkin, Rabkin, & Wagner, 1994). Testosterone replacement therapy has also shown promise in treating depression in HIV-seropositive men (Wagner, Rabkin, & Rabkin, 1996). Thus, psychopharmacologic treatment can be a safe and effective adjunct to counseling and therapy for depression in HIV-infected people.

Of concern, however, are the potential drug interactions between some psychoactive drugs and antiretroviral therapies. For example, monoamine oxidase inhibitors are not recommended for use in combination with other drugs (Capaldini, 1997). As discussed in chapter 3, protease inhibitors can interact with psychopharmacologic agents that share the same metabolic pathway. Finally, many drugs used to treat people with HIV–AIDS can themselves cause depression, including zidovudine (AZT), acyclovir, and alpha-interferon (Capaldini, 1997). Use of antidepressants with people living with HIV–AIDS, therefore, requires careful monitoring for adverse side effects and drug interactions.

Flexibility in AIDS-Related Psychotherapy

Experts in psychotherapy with people living with HIV–AIDS have suggested that a key element to success is throwing away preconceived recipes for therapy and establishing a flexible stance. Winiarski (1991), for example, suggested that therapists adapt their roles to meet the needs of people with HIV. Winiarski's idea of bending the frame of psychotherapy to work within the unique demands of living with AIDS has been echoed by several subsequent authors. Eversole (1997) recommended reconceptualizing the role of psychotherapists in treating people with HIV. For example, clinicians might consider conducting sessions at a client's home when they are too ill to come in and try to provide basic medical information to clients rather than only referring them to medical providers. Kain (1996) concurred with the importance of bending frames of reference in treating people with HIV–AIDS.

THEMES IN PSYCHOTHERAPY

Populations most affected by AIDS present an array of mental health challenges. People may seek services to cope with the emotional turmoil of AIDS, deal with loneliness and isolation, or manage their fears of illness and death. People with HIV–AIDS will also seek help with issues of returning to work and managing relationships. Counselors and therapists can provide accurate information, clarify medical treatment decisions, address spiritual issues and financial concerns, and assist in meeting other immediate needs. Figure 9.1 presents themes commonly encountered in psychotherapy with HIV-seropositive clients, each of which is discussed below.

Information Needs

It is outside of the role of mental health professionals to provide detailed biomedical information or medical advice to clients. However,

AIDS-Related Themes in Counseling & Psychotherapy

- ► **Need for Information**
- ► **Changing Behavior & Life-Style**
- ► **Serostatus Disclosure**
- ► **Relationships**
- ► **Thoughts of Suicide**
- ► **Neuropsychological Concerns**
- ► **Symptoms and Illnesses**
- ► **Substance Abuse**
- ► **Bouncing Back to Good Health**
- ► **Self-Image**
- ► **Spirituality**
- ► **Letting Go of Attachments**

Figure 9.1

Common themes in HIV–AIDS counseling and psychotherapy.

counselors and therapists can disseminate psychologically relevant information and can serve as a valuable information resource. Beliefs that are based on inaccurate information cause anxiety, and simply correcting misinformation can alter such beliefs (Schmaling & DiClementi, 1991). Therapists need a basic understanding of HIV disease to recognize misinformation when they hear it. Numerous hotlines and Internet websites are readily available to assist therapists as well as their clients in answering questions and clarifying concerns. Physicians and public health officials can also serve as information resources. Armed with information, mental health professionals can educate their clients about psychological issues related to HIV infection, and psychological reactions to medical symptomatology. For example, educating clients about the overlapping symptoms of depression, HIV infection, and medication side effects can help lead to better understanding and improved emotional adjustment (Markowitz, Klerman, & Perry, 1993).

Behavior and Life-Style Changes

Changing health-compromising habits and adopting health-promoting behaviors can both improve general wellness and enhance a sense of personal control. Counseling can help clients alter their behaviors that have potentially detrimental health effects. For example, cognitive and behavioral techniques for smoking cessation are widely available and can be integrated into counseling (Royce & Winkelstein, 1990). Aerobic exercise promotes fitness and a sense of internal control. Exercise can also reduce depression and anxiety and increase self-esteem (LaPerriere, Antoni, et al., 1990; Pfeiffer, 1992). Health psychology offers a rich literature to guide treatments for sleep disorders, improve nutrition, maintain weight, adhere to treatment regimens, and help with other problems common to HIV infection.

The benefits of health-behavior change are many, but it is important that clients not be misled to believe that such changes reverse the course of HIV infection. There is no conclusive evidence that behavior changes have clinically significant effects on the progression of HIV infection. Clients who stop smoking or start exercising, but whose health falters may blame themselves for starting too late or not doing enough. However, because changes in health behavior will not accelerate HIV disease processes but can improve general well-being, clients should be encouraged to make such changes with expectations that are realistic.

Dealing with Serostatus Disclosure

Disclosing HIV seropositivity is among the greatest challenges facing people with HIV–AIDS. Disclosure can result in rejection, abandonment, and even violence. However, disclosure is also necessary to gain HIV-specific support and to inform sexual and injection drug use partners, dental and medical providers, and others. Disclosure to children can be particularly difficult and requires an understanding of children's ability to comprehend the complexity of AIDS. In some cases, a counselor and therapist may be the only person that a client had told about their HIV serostatus. Disclosure of HIV should be approached with clients on a person-by-person, case-by-case basis. Weighing the potential costs and benefits of disclosing must be evaluated in terms of options for how and when to disclose. Role-plays and rehearsal can take place in therapy, where the therapist helps troubleshoot potential adverse responses to the disclosure (Landau-Stanton, Clements, & Stanton, 1993). The potential for rejection, abandonment, and even abuse should be directly dealt with in counseling, and systems for managing those risks should be in place before disclosing. When clients are unable to bring themselves to disclose to sexual and injecting partners, therapy can offer a vehicle for disclosure by way of couples sessions. The therapist then knows that the partner has been told and can provide support to both the client and their partner. Therapists can also assist in problem solving, mediating interpersonal conflicts, and clarifying relationship issues.

Relationships

Family conflicts often predate HIV infection and can become exacerbated after a family member tests HIV seropositive (Bor, Perry, & Miller, 1989). AIDS fears and AIDS stigmas add to the isolation that many HIV-positive clients experience before becoming infected. Long-term partnerships are also disrupted by HIV infection, and clients with HIV–AIDS are often kept away from children. Issues of disclosing to partners, maintaining safer sexual relations, fears of future illness, and anticipatory loss are among the many consequences AIDS poses to relationships (Slowinski, 1989). Counseling and therapy may therefore involve working through relationship issues and, when appropriate, including partners, family members, and children in treatment.

Multiple Losses

People with HIV experience multiple losses, including loss of health, abilities, activities, and relationships. Grief work is therefore a central theme in HIV-related psychotherapy. Working through grief can involve emotional catharsis and explorations of meaning. Multiple losses can cause bereavement overload, in which a person does not have time to grieve before suffering their next loss. In addition, the accumulation of losses can cause the loss of self, in which a person no longer fully recognizes their own identity (Kain, 1996). Rituals and tangible exercises can help bring finality to loss, reestablish a sense of stability, and help a person move forward.

Recurrent Risk for Suicide

Risk for suicide in HIV-positive clients has two distinct contexts. Consistent with other clinical problems, suicidal ideations should be expected in conjunction with hopelessness and clinical depression. In another instance, however, clients may view suicide as a reasonable solution to their pain, particularly at later stages of disease. Monitoring suicide risk is therefore an ongoing process that requires reinterpretation over the course of HIV infection. HIV-seropositive clients are reminded of their mortality and may consider suicide in response to the deaths of others, the onset of symptoms, hospitalizations, anniversaries of HIV testing, and the deaths of friends (Spector & Conklin, 1987). Counselors must clarify their values concerning hastened death and partner-assisted hastened death so that they can remain nonjudgmental when dealing with these serious issues.

Neuropsychological Effects of HIV Infection

Cognitive changes in relation to HIV infection require continued reassessment. Even minor signs of cognitive deficiencies can be the cause of great concern for people with HIV–AIDS. Because many people do not experience neuropsychological impairment even late in the course of AIDS, clients should be reassured that cognitive deficits are not inevitable. If neuropsychological symptoms are confirmed, counselors and therapists can assist clients in adapting to cognitive decline or visual impairment. Examples of interventions may include maintaining home environment safety, use of time management techniques, and breaking down difficult tasks into smaller steps (Mapou & Law, 1994). Lapses in memory can be addressed by using reminders such as lists, notebooks, and calendars. Clients should be encouraged to be patient with themselves because completing complex tasks may require more time than in the past.

316

Issues of Medical Management

Counseling and therapy can help clients address medically related concerns, including access to care, adherence to treatment, and life-and-death issues. Specific interventions are available to assist in adherence to medical treatments. Medication side effects can often be managed with relaxation techniques, cognitive restructuring, and problem focused coping. HIV-seropositive clients can also be helped to clarify their wishes for terminal care, such as life support options and resuscitation. Haas et al. (1993) found that 62% of people with AIDS had not discussed preferences for life-sustaining care and advanced directives with their physicians even though 72% of them wanted to do so. Counselors and therapists can help clarify such issues by using problem solving techniques to address barriers and role-plays to practice communicating desires for terminal care with physicians. Terminal care should be discussed early in the course of HIV infection because illnesses can increase difficulty in decision making (Dilley, Shelp, & Batki, 1985).

Substance Abuse Treatment

Injection drug use can be particularly difficult to treat because of the strong addictive qualities of injected drugs and the social context in which injection drug use occurs. All types of substance use including alcohol, can serve as avoidance coping strategies, raising the risk for engaging in a multitude of health-compromising behaviors. Denial is symptomatic of substance abuse disorders and can permeate coping responses to HIV–AIDS. Working through denial can therefore become a central focus of therapy with substance abusing clients. In addition to substance abuse treatment per se, counseling can assist HIV-seropositive clients who are motivated to stop using substances by helping them replace drug use with more adaptive coping strategies.

Bouncing Back

Antiretroviral therapies as well as the prevention and treatment of opportunistic illnesses have more than doubled the AIDS survival time since the start of the epidemic. Many people have prepared themselves for death only to find themselves rebounding to better health. Readjusting to improved health can mean returning to work, going back to school, starting new relationships, and making long-term plans for the future. Many people therefore begin a second life agenda and require skills to assist their reentry into work, school, and other pre-HIV activities (Rabkin & Ferrando, 1997). Resume writing seminars, job-interviewing skills workshops, and other preparatory services are now offered by many AIDS service organizations. Counseling can help people adjust to the life redefining process of getting off disability and going back to work. Many people will also require support for managing issues of medical insurance, disability benefits, disclosing HIV serostatus to employers, and readjusting to work schedules.

Successfully responding to antiretroviral therapies can cause people to reassess their identity as a person living with HIV–AIDS. Many people may feel that they have wasted years preparing to die when they suddenly find themselves contemplating a longer life. Returning to work can cause as much, or more, stress as does going on disability. People must manage their medication schedules, medical appointments, and fluctuations in health status while working. Many people who respond positively to HIV therapies will experience subsequent treatment failures, introducing another iteration of stress associated with returning to disability. Counseling and therapy therefore provides an opportunity for testing the realities of returning to work and planning strategies for managing these stressors.

Self-Esteem and Self-Image

Working through life's issues to achieve goals can itself be a self-enhancing process. Because people with life-threatening illnesses may have special needs to enhance their self-esteem (S. E. Taylor, 1983), counseling and therapy can help people attain self-acceptance. One therapeutic technique that is useful in this regard is the life review, where clients are guided through a self-examination of life transitions (Landau-Stanton et al., 1993). Chronic illness can prompt one to reflect upon the past to gain a sense of closure. Therapy can provide structure and support the life review process. For example, the life review may be framed in terms of a time line, starting with earliest memories and moving through each stage of life, recorded on a chart or in a journal. Life reviews can be useful in helping clients recognize their capacities, recurring patterns, and ability to overcome obstacles (Borden, 1989).

Spirituality

Clients with HIV–AIDS are frequently estranged from formal religious institutions and may subsequently have unmet spiritual needs. Therapists can help clients clarify their spiritual values and identify spiritual needs. Developing strategies for exploring traditional and nontraditional spiritual practices should be addressed directly in counseling. Therapy can, therefore, be used as a means of problem solving the barriers that people confront in meeting their spiritual needs (Haburchak, Harrison, Miles, & Hannon, 1989).

Redefining Quality of Life

An individual's needs and abilities change as a function of HIV infection. Adjusting the goals, focus, and course of therapy becomes increasingly important as HIV infection progresses (Coreless et al., 1992; Perry & Markowitz, 1986). In particular, quality of life must be continuously evaluated and redefined over the course of HIV infection. Changes in pain, health status, physical functioning, social relationships, and energy contribute to fluctuations in quality of life (Wachtel et al., 1992; Wu et al., 1991). When activities are disrupted and abilities are impaired, counselors can help explore new activities that match current abilities and reframe quality of life to fit current functioning. Volunteering to help others, rediscovering hobbies and interests, taking time for oneself, and focusing on relationships are examples of ways to enhance quality of life.

Attachments and the Need to Let Go

Professionals who treat people suffering from life-threatening illnesses experience a great deal of stress. Terminal illness can bring hopelessness, fear of death, spiritual crises, and recognition of one's own mortality.

Boundaries between client and therapist are blurred by the universality of death, especially when therapists themselves have not worked through these issues. A clear sense of one's own views on death and dying enables helping professionals to better serve their HIV-positive clients.

ETHICAL ISSUES

Privacy and trust are essential to effective counseling and psychotherapy. Therapists, however, are obligated to break confidentiality under certain circumstances. Issues of duty to protect are therefore among the greatest ethical and legal challenges facing helping professionals (Adler & Beckett, 1989; Ginzburg & Gostin, 1986; Melton, 1988; Sherer, 1988). Perceptions of dangerousness and identifying third parties who may be at risk bring up issues raised by the widely noted case of *Tarasoff v. Regents of the University of California* (1976).

For *Tarasoff* to apply, there must be a foreseeable danger to an identifiable party as a result of a client's planned actions (Knapp & VandeCreek, 1990). The *Tarasoff* ruling set a standard for professionals to use reasonable care to protect intended victims when danger is reasonably predicted (Melton, 1988). The relationship between AIDS and *Tarasoff* is highlighted by the fact that communicable diseases have long been considered a valid reason to break professional confidentiality to prevent the spread of illness (Silva, Leong, & Weinstock, 1989). In fact, *Tarasoff* itself was based on court decisions ruling that physicians have a duty to act to protect when they know patients with infectious diseases threaten others (Knapp & VandeCreek, 1990). Thus, the application of *Tarasoff* in cases of AIDS is grounded in public health law.

The relationship between AIDS and *Tarasoff* is not, however, quite so clear-cut. *Tarasoff* is usually associated with a direct verbal threat (Kermani & Weiss, 1989). However, HIV-positive clients are unlikely to use their infection to intentionally harm another person. Instead, concerns relevant to AIDS revolve around the failure to protect others, principally by failing to disclose their HIV serostatus. In addition, most people at risk of exposure to HIV are not easily identified by clinicians

(Perry, 1989). Duty to protect only extends to people who can be identified and who could reasonably be harmed. Unlike *Tarasoff*, people at risk for HIV infection are probably already aware of the risks associated with their own behavior, given that high-risk practices are well known and everyone is advised to protect themselves (Perry, 1989). Nevertheless, mental-health treatment may require breaking confidentiality to warn a third party. For example, an HIV-infected client who states that he or she refuses to use condoms during sexual intercourse with his or her spouse involves a statement of intentional harm toward an identifiable third person who is known to be at risk. Psychologists who view potential risks to others as serious and imminent are likely to break confidentiality to protect third parties (McGuire, Nieri, Abbott, Sheridan, & Fisher, 1995). Thus, several professional associations have developed ethical policy statements regarding duty to warn in cases of AIDS.

The American Medical Association recommends that when physicians know that an HIV-seropositive patient is endangering a third party, the patient should be persuaded to stop engaging in risk behaviors. If the person fails to comply, the physician should notify public health authorities, and if the authorities do not act, the physician should notify the endangered party him- or herself (Kermani & Weiss, 1989). Similarly, the Canadian Medical Association states that physicians can ethically disclose a patient's HIV status to a spouse when the patient is unwilling to inform the spouse (I. Kleinman, 1991). Following these general parameters, the American Psychiatric Association (1992, 1993a) has proposed its own guidelines. A policy statement recommending that psychiatrists work with all patients to reduce their risk for HIV transmission, regardless of serostatus, and be competent in counseling about HIV testing (American Psychiatric Association, 1992) has been developed. In terms of protecting third parties, the policy statement reads

> In a situation where a psychiatrist received convincing clinical information that the patient is infected with HIV, the psychiatrist should advise and work with the patient either to obtain agreement to cease behaviors that places others at risk of infection or to notify individuals who may be at continuing risk of

exposure. If a patient refuses to agree to change behavior or to notify the person(s) at on-going risk or if the psychiatrist has good reason to believe that the patient has failed to or is unable to comply with this agreement, it is ethically permissible for the psychiatrist to notify identifiable persons who the psychiatrist believes to be in danger of contracting the virus, or to arrange for public health authorities to do so. (p. 721)

The American Psychiatric Association (1993a) also states that it is ethically permissible to notify public health authorities when a patient's behavior constitutes a risk to people who cannot be identified, as well as to past sexual or drug-injecting partners. Similar guidelines were established for professionals working with psychiatric inpatients (American Psychiatric Association, 1993b), as well for other professions, including social workers (Reamer, 1991).

When clinicians feel they must breach confidentiality to warn a third party, they are advised to proceed with caution (Melton, 1988). Protective actions can include interventions to eliminate risk behaviors and therefore remove potential harm. When clients are noncompliant, therapists may notify public health authorities of the danger rather than directly warning the third party. Partner notification falls within the professional role of public health workers rather than that of psychotherapists and counselors. Certain clients, such as those who are sexually impulsive, manic, psychotic, or antisocial, may require involuntary hospitalization, in effect isolating them from others (Knapp & VandeCreek, 1990; Winiarski, 1991). Hospitalization should, however, only be used to treat mental illness; decisions to quarantine again fall within professional roles of public health authorities and not mental health professionals (Melton, 1988). Finally, clients should be informed of the limits of confidentiality before they start treatment as a part of routine informed consent procedures. When clients are informed that information pertaining to potential harm to others must be reported to appropriate authorities, clinicians are less likely to encounter problems in releasing confidential information (Boyd, 1992; Kalichman, 1993).

CONCLUSION

The mental health professions are playing an increasingly important role in the AIDS epidemic. Unfortunately, many in the helping professions have little experience and often no training in treating HIV-seropositive clients (Campos, Brasfield, & Kelly, 1989; Kinderman, Matteo, & Morales, 1993). The many challenges that AIDS poses to people living with HIV are the same factors that require attention in counseling and therapy. Mental health providers are well positioned to aid in the care of people living with HIV infection. As medical treatments for HIV infection continue to advance, counselors and therapists must make an effort to keep up with the rapid pace of change in the epidemic. To remain optimally effective, providers must be informed about the progression of HIV infection and the progress of medical science in battling AIDS. The most recent of what will hopefully be many new treatments will bring new challenges to the psychological care of people living with HIV and AIDS.

References

Abid, S., Joseph, J., Ostrow, D., & James, S. (1991). Predictors of relapse in sexual practices among homosexual men. *AIDS Education and Prevention, 3,* 293–304.

Abrams, D. I. (1997). Alternative therapies for HIV. In M. A. Sande & P. A. Volberding (Eds.), *The medical management of AIDS* (pp. 143–158). Philadelphia: Saunders.

Adelman, M. (1989). Social support and AIDS. *AIDS and Public Policy Journal, 4,* 31–39.

Adjorolo-Johnson, E. G., DeCock, K., Ekpini, E., Vetter, K., Sibailly, T., Brattegaard, K., Yavo, D., Doorly, R., Whitaker, J., Kestens, L., Ou, C., George, J., & Gayle, H. (1994). Prospective comparison of mother-to-child transmission of HIV-1 and HIV-2 in Abidjan, Ivory Coast. *Journal of the American Medical Association, 272,* 462–466.

Adler, G., & Beckett, A. (1989). Psychotherapy of the patient with an HIV infection: Some ethical and therapeutic dilemmas. *Psychosomatics, 30,* 203–208.

Affleck, G., Tennen, H., Pfeiffer, C., & Fifield, J. (1987). Appraisals of control and predictability in adapting to a chronic disease. *Journal of Personality and Social Psychology, 53,* 273–279.

Agle, D., Gluck, H., & Pierce, G. F. (1987). The risk of AIDS: Psychologic impact on the hemophilic population. *General Hospital Psychiatry, 9,* 11–17.

Alfonso, C. A., Cohen, M. A. A., Aldajem, A. D., Morrison, F., Powell, D. R., Winters, R. A., & Orlowski, B. K. (1994). HIV seropositivity as a major risk factor for suicide in the general hospital. *Psychosomatics, 35,* 368–373.

Ambroziak, J. A., Blackbourn, D. J., Herndier, B. G., Glogau, R. G., Gullett, J. H., McDonald, A. R., Lennette, E. T., & Levy, J. A. (1995). Herpes-like sequences in HIV-infected and uninfected Kaposi's sarcoma patients. *Science, 268*, 582–583.

American Psychiatric Association. (1987). *Diagnostic and statistical manual cf mental disorders* (3rd ed., Rev.). Washington, DC: Author.

American Psychiatric Association. (1992). AIDS policy: Guidelines for outpatient psychiatric services. *American Journal of Psychiatry, 149*, 721.

American Psychiatric Association. (1993a). AIDS policy: Position statement on confidentiality, disclosure, and protection of others. *American Journal of Psychiatry, 150*, 852.

American Psychiatric Association. (1993b). AIDS policy: Guidelines for inpatient psychiatric services. *American Journal of Psychiatry, 150*, 853.

American Psychiatric Association. (1994). *Diagnostic and statistical manual of mental disorders* (4th ed.). Washington, DC: Author.

Anders, K. H., Guerra, W. F., Tomiyasu, U., Verity, M. A., & Vinters, H. V. (1986). The neuropathology of AIDS: UCLA experience and review. *American Journal of Pathology, 124*, 537–558.

Anderson, R. M., & May, R. M. (1992). Understanding the AIDS pandemic. *Scientific American, 266*, 58–66.

Andrulis, D. P., Weslowski, V. B., Hintz, E., & Spolarich, A. W. (1992). Comparisons of hospital care for patients with AIDS and other HIV-related conditions. *Journal of the American Medical Association, 267*, 2482–2486.

Antoni, M. H., Baggett, L., Ironson, G., LaPerriere, A., August, S., Klimas, N., Schneiderman, N., & Fletcher, M. A. (1991). Cognitive–behavioral stress management intervention buffers distress responses and immunologic changes following notification of HIV-1 seropositivity. *Journal of Consulting and Clinical Psychology, 59*, 906–915.

Aral, S. O., & Holmes, K. K. (1991). Sexually transmitted diseases in the AIDS era. *Scientific American, 264*, 62–69.

Aral, S. O., & Wasserheit, J. (1996). Interactions among HIV, other sexually transmitted diseases, socioeconomic status, and poverty in women. In A. O'Leary & L. S. Jemmott (Eds.), *Women at Risk* (pp. 13–42). New York: Plenum.

Armistead, L., & Forehand, R. (1995). For whom the bell tolls: Parenting decisions and challenges faced by mothers who are HIV seropositive. *Clinical Psychology: Science and Practice, 2*, 239–250.

Armistead, L., Klein, K., Forehand, R., & Wierson, M. (1997). Disclosure of parental HIV infection to children in the families of men with hemophilia: Description, outcomes, and the role of family process. *Journal of Family Psychology, 11*, 49–61.

Aronow, H. A., Brew, B. J., & Price, R. W. (1988). The management of the neurological complications of HIV infection and AIDS. *AIDS, 2*(Suppl. 1), S151–S159.

Athey, J. L. (1991). HIV infection and homeless adolescents. *Child Welfare, 70*, 517–528.

Atkinson, J. H., Grant, I., Kennedy, C. J., Richman, D. D., Spector, S. A., & McCutchan, J. A. (1988). Prevalence of psychiatric disorders among men infected with human immunodeficiency virus. *Archives of General Psychiatry, 45*, 859–864.

Aversa, S. L., & Kimberlin, C. (1996). Psychosocial aspects of antiretroviral medication use among HIV patients. *Patient Education and Counseling, 29*, 207–219.

Ayehunie, S., Groves, R. W., Bruzzese, A., Ruprecht, R. M., Kupper, T. S., & Langhoff, E. (1995). Acutely infected Langerhans cells are more efficient than T cells in disseminating HIV type 1 to activate T cells following a short cell-cell contact. *AIDS Research and Human Retroviruses, 11*, 877–884.

Baba, T. W., Sampson, J. E., Fratazzi, C., Greene, M. F., & Ruprecht, R. M. (1993). Maternal transmission of the human immunodeficiency virus: Can it be prevented? *Journal of Women's Health, 2*, 231–242.

Baba, T. W., Trichel, A. M., An, L., Liska, V., Martin, L. N., Murphey-Corb, M., & Ruprecht, R. M. (1996). Infection and AIDS in adult macaques after nontraumatic oral exposure to cell-free SIV. *Science, 272*, 1486–1489.

Bacchetti, P., Osmond, D., Chaisson, R. E., & Moss, A. R. (1988). Survival with AIDS in New York [Letter to the editor]. *New England Journal of Medicine, 318*, 1464.

Bacellar, H., Munoz, A., Miller, E. N., Cohen, B., Besley, D., Selnes, O., Becker, J., & McArthur, J. (1994). Temporal trends in the incidence of HIV-1-related neurologic diseases: Multicenter AIDS cohort study, 1985–1992. *Neurology, 44*, 1892–1900.

Bakal, D. A. (1992). *Psychology and health* (2nd ed.). New York: Springer.

Bandura, A. (1997). *Self-efficacy: The exercise of control.* New York: Freeman.

Bangsberg, D., Tulsky, J. P., Hecht, F. M., & Moss, A. R. (1997). Protease inhibitors in the homeless. *Journal of the American Medical Association, 278,* 63–65.

Barbour, R. S. (1994). The impact of working with people with HIV/AIDS: A review of the literature. *Social Science Medicine, 39,* 221–232.

Barrett, R. L. (1997). Countertransference issues in HIV-related psychotherapy. In M. G. Winiarski (Ed.), *HIV mental health for the 21st century.* New York: New York University Press.

Barsky, A. J., Cleary, P. D., Sarnie, M. K., & Klerman, G. L. (1993). The course of transient hypochondriasis. *American Journal of Psychiatry, 150,* 484–488.

Barsky, A. J., Wyshak, G., & Klerman, G. L. (1990). Transient hypochondriasis. *Archives of General Psychiatry, 47,* 746–752.

Bartholow, B. N., Doll, L. S., Joy, D., Douglas, J. M., Bolan, G., Harrison, J. S., Moss, P. M., & McKirnan, D. (1994). Emotional, behavioral, and HIV risks associated with sexual abuse among adult homosexual and bisexual men. *Child Abuse and Neglect, 18,* 747–761.

Bartlett, J. G. (1993a). *The Johns Hopkins Hospital guide to medical care of patients with HIV infection* (3rd ed.). Baltimore: Williams & Wilkins.

Bartlett, J. G. (1993b). Zidovudine now or later? *New England Journal of Medicine, 329,* 351–352.

Bartrop, R. W., Luckhurst, E., Lazarus, L., Kiloh, L., & Penny, R. (1977). Depressed lymphocyte function after bereavement. *The Lancet, 1,* 834–836.

Bayer, R. (1996). AIDS prevention—Sexual ethics and responsibility. *New England Journal of Medicine, 334,* 1540–1542.

Beck, A. T. (1976). *Cognitive therapy and emotional disorders.* Madison, CT: International Universities Press.

Beck, A. T., Kovacs, M., & Weissman, A. (1975). Hopelessness and suicidal behavior: An overview. *Journal of the American Medical Association, 234,* 1146–1149.

Beck, A. T., & Steer, R. A. (1993). *BDI: Beck Depression Inventory manual.* New York: Psychological Corporation.

Beck, E. J., Mandalia, S., Leonard, K., Griffith, R. J., Harris, J. R. W., & Miller, D. L. (1996). Case-control study of sexually transmitted diseases as cofactors for HIV-1 transmission. *International Journal of STD and AIDS, 7,* 34–38.

Beckett, A., & Rutan, J. S. (1990). Treating persons with ARC and AIDS in group psychotherapy. *International Journal of Group Psychotherapy, 40,* 19–29.

Bednarik, D. P., & Folks, T. M. (1992). Mechanisms of HIV-1 latency. *AIDS, 6,* 3–16.

Beevor, A. S., & Catalan, J. (1993). Women's experience of HIV testing: The views of HIV positive and HIV negative women. *AIDS Care, 5,* 177–186.

Belkin, G. S., Fleishman, J. A., Stein, M. D., Piette, J., & Mor, V. (1992). Physical symptoms and depressive symptoms among individuals with HIV infection. *Psychosomatics, 33,* 416–427.

Benight, C. C., Antoni, M. H., Kilbourn, K., Ironson, G., Kumar, M. A., Fletcher, M. A., Redwine, L., Baum, A., & Schneiderman, N. (1997). Coping self-efficacy buffers psychological and physiological disturbances in HIV-infected men following a natural disaster. *Health Psychology, 16,* 248–255.

Benjamin, A. E., & Preston, S. D. (1993, Spring). A comparative perspective on hospice care for persons with AIDS. *AIDS and Public Policy Journal, 36–* 43.

Bennett, L., & Kelaher, M. (1993). Variables contributing to experiences of grief in HIV/AIDS health care professionals. *Journal of Community Psychology, 21,* 210–217.

Bennett, L., Miller, D., & Ross, M. W. (1993). Review of the research to date on impact of HIV/AIDS on health workers. In L. Bennett, D. Miller, & M. Ross (Eds.), *Health workers and AIDS: Research, intervention and current issues in burnout and response* (pp. 15–34). New York: Hardwood Academic.

Beral, V., Bull, D., Darby, S., Weller, I., Carne, C., Beecham, M., & Jaffe, H. (1992). Risk of Kaposi's sarcoma and sexual practices associated with faecal contact in homosexual or bisexual men with AIDS. *The Lancet, 339,* 632–635.

Berenson, A. B., San Miguel, V., & Wilkinson, G. S. (1992). Violence and its relationship to substance use in adolescent pregnancy. *Journal of Adolescent Health, 13,* 470–474.

Berger, T. G. (1997). Dermatologic care in the AIDS patient. In M. A. Sande & P. A. Volberding (Eds.), *The medical management of AIDS* (5th ed., pp. 159–168). Philadelphia: Saunders.

Bergey, E., Cho, M., Blumberg, B., Hammarskjold, M. L., Rekosh, D., Epstein, L., & Levine, M. (1994). Interaction of HIV-1 and human salivary mucins. *Journal of Acquired Immune Deficiency Syndromes, 1*, 995–1002.

Besch, C. L. (1995). Compliance in clinical trials. *AIDS, 9*, 1–10.

Biggar, R. J., Pahwa, S., Minkoff, H., Mendes, H., Willoughby, A., Landesman, S., & Goedert, J. J. (1989). Immunosuppression in pregnant women infected with human immunodeficiency virus. *American Journal of Obstetrics and Gynecology, 161*, 1239–1244.

Billings, A. G., & Moos, R. H. (1981). The role of coping resources in attenuating the stress of life events. *Journal of Behavioral Medicine, 7*, 139–157.

Billings, A. G., & Moos, R. H. (1984). Coping, stress, and social resources among adults with unipolar depression. *Journal of Personality and Social Psychology, 46*, 877–891.

Billy, J. O. G., Tanfer, K., Grady, W., & Klepinger, D. H. (1993). The sexual behavior of men in the United States. *Family Planning Perspectives, 25*, 52–60.

Bliwise, N. G., Grade, M., Irish, T. M., & Ficarrotto, T. J. (1991). Measuring medical and nursing students' attitudes toward AIDS. *Health Psychology, 10*, 289–295.

Blumenfield, M., Smith, P. J., Milazzo, J., Seropian, S., & Wormser, G. P. (1987). Survey of attitudes of nurses working with AIDS patients. *General Hospital Psychiatry, 9*, 58–63.

Boivin, M. J., Green, S. D. R., Davies, A. G., Giordani, B., Mokili, J. K. L., Cutting, W. A. M. (1995). A preliminary evaluation of the cognitive and motor effects of pediatric HIV infection in Zairian children. *Health Psychology, 14*, 13–21.

Bolan, G. (1992). Management of syphilis in HIV-infected persons. In M. A. Sande & P. A. Volberding (Eds.), *The medical management of AIDS* (3rd ed., pp. 383–398). Philadelphia: Saunders.

Bollinger, R. C., & Siliciano, R. (1992). Immunodeficiency in HIV-1 infection. In G. P. Wormser (Ed.), *AIDS and other manifestations of HIV infection* (2nd ed., pp. 145–164). New York: Raven Press.

Bono, G., Mauri, M., Sinforiani, E., Barbarini, G., Minoli, L., & Fea, M. (1996). Longitudinal neuropsychological evaluation of HIV-infected intravenous drug users. *Addiction, 91*, 263–268.

Booth, R. E., Watters, J. K., & Chitwood, D. D. (1993). HIV risk-related sex behaviors among injection drug users, crack smokers, and injection drug users who smoke crack. *American Journal of Public Health, 83,* 1144–1148.

Booth, W. (1988). AIDS and drug abuse: No quick fix. *Science, 239,* 717–719.

Bor, R., Perry, L., & Miller, R. (1989). A systems approach to AIDS counseling. *Journal of Family Therapy, 11,* 77–86.

Bor, R., Prior, N., & Miller, R. (1990). Complementarity in relationships of couples affected by HIV. *Counseling Psychology Quarterly, 3,* 217–220.

Borden, W. (1989). Life review as a therapeutic frame in the treatment of young adults with AIDS. *Health and Social Work, 14,* 253–259.

Borden, W. (1991). Beneficial outcomes in adjustment to HIV seropositivity. *Social Service Review, 65,* 434–450.

Bornstein, R. A. (1993, April). *Neuropsychological function in the course of HIV infection.* Paper presented at the meeting of the Michigan Psychiatric Society, Detroit.

Bornstein, R. A., Nasrallah, H. A., Para, M. G., Whitacre, C. C., Rosenberger, P., Fass, R. J., & Rice, R. (1992). Neuropsychological performance in asymptomatic HIV infection. *Journal of Neuropsychiatry and Clinical Neurosciences, 4,* 386–394.

Bornstein, R. A., Pace, P., Rosenberger, P., Nasrallah, H., Para, M., Whitacre, C., & Fass, R. (1993). Depression and neuropsychological performance in asymptomatic HIV infection. *American Journal of Psychiatry, 150,* 922–927.

Bottomley, P. A., Hardy, C. J., Cousins, J. P., Armstrong, M., & Wagle, W. A. (1990). AIDS dementia complex: Brain high-energy phosphate metabolite deficits. *Radiology, 176,* 407–411.

Boyd, K. M. (1992). HIV infection and AIDS: The ethics of medical confidentiality. *Journal of Medical Ethics, 18,* 173–179.

Bozovich, A., Cianelli, L., Johnson, J., Wagner, L., Chrash, M., & Mallory, G. (1992). Assessing community resources for rural PWAs. *AIDS Patient Care, 6,* 229–231.

Bozzette, S. A., Finkelstein, D. M., Spector, S. A., Frame, P., Powderly, W. G., He, W., Phillips, L., Craven, D., van der Horst, C., & Feinberg, J. (1995). A randomized trial of three antipneumocystis agents in patients with advanced human immunodeficiency virus infection. *New England Journal of Medicine, 332,* 693–699.

Brennan, T. A. (1991). Transmission of the human immunodeficiency virus in the health care setting: Time for action. *New England Journal of Medicine, 324,* 1504–1509.

Brettle, R. P., & Leen, L. S. (1991). The natural history of HIV and AIDS in women. *AIDS, 5,* 1283–1292.

Broadhead, W. E., Kaplan, B. H., James, S. A., Wagner, E. H., Schoenbach, V. J., Grimson, R., Heyden, S., Tibblin, G., & Gehlbach, S. H. (1983). Reviews and commentary: The epidemiologic evidence for a relationship between social support and health. *American Journal of Epidemiology, 117,* 521–537.

Broder, S., Merigan, T. C., & Bolognesi, D. (1994). *Textbook of AIDS medicine.* Baltimore: Williams & Wilkins.

Brooner, R., Greenfield, L., Schmidt, C., & Bigelow, G. (1993). Antisocial personality disorder and HIV infection among intravenous drug abusers. *American Journal of Psychiatry, 150,* 53–58.

Brown, G., & Rundell, J. (1990). Prospective study of psychiatric morbidity in HIV-seropositive women without AIDS. *General Hospital Psychiatry, 12,* 30–35.

Brown, L. K., Kessel, S. M., Lourie, K. J., Ford, H. H., & Lipsitt, L. P. (1997). Influence of sexual abuse on HIV-related attitudes and behaviors in adolescent psychiatric inpatients. *Journal of the American Academy of Child Adolescent Psychiatry, 36,* 316–322.

Brown, W. A. (1996). Is interpersonal psychotherapy superior to supportive psychotherapy? *American Journal of Psychiatry, 153,* 1509–1510.

Buck, B. A. (1991, October). Support groups for hospitalized AIDS patients. *AIDS Patient Care,* pp. 255–258.

Buehler, J. W., & Ward, J. W. (1993). A new definition for AIDS surveillance. *Annals of Internal Medicine, 118,* 390–392.

Buiss, A. (1989). A peer counselling program for persons testing HIV antibody positive. *Canadian Journal of Counseling, 23,* 127–132.

Bumbalo, J. A., Patsdaughter, C. A., & McShane, R. E. (1993, January). Impact of AIDS on the family: Family functioning and symptoms among family members. *Wisconsin AIDS/HIV Update,* pp. 15–18.

Burish, T., Carey, M., Wallston, K., Stein, M., Jamison, P., & Lyles, J. (1984). Health locus of control and chronic disease: An external orientation may be advantageous. *Journal of Social and Clinical Psychology, 2*, 326–332.

Burns, B. H., & Howell, J. B. L. (1969). Disproportionately severe breathlessness in chronic bronchitis. *Quarterly Journal of Medicine, 38*, 277–294.

Burrack, J. H., Barrett, D. C., Stall, R., Chesney, M. A., Ekstrand, M. L., & Coates, T. J. (1993). Depressive symptoms and CD4 lymphocyte decline among HIV-infected men. *Journal of the American Medical Association, 270*, 2568–2573.

Butters, E., Higginson, I., George, R., & McCarthy, M. (1993). Palliative care for people with HIV/AIDS: Views of patients, caregivers and providers. *AIDS Care, 5*, 105–116.

Butters, N., Grant, I., Haxby, J., Judd, L. L., Martin, A., McClelland, J., Pequegnat, W., Schacter, D., & Stover, E. (1990). Assessment of AIDS-related cognitive changes: Recommendations of the NIMH workshop on neuropsychological assessment approaches. *Journal of Clinical and Experimental Neuropsychology, 12*, 963–978.

Cadwell, S. A. (1997). Transference and countertransference. In I. D. Yalom (Ed.), *Treating the psychological consequences of HIV* (pp. 1–32). San Francisco, CA: Jossey-Bass Publishers.

Calabrese, J., Kling, M., & Gold, P. (1987). Alterations in immunocompetence during stress, bereavement, and depression: Focus on neuroendocrine regulation. *American Journal of Psychiatry, 144*, 1123–1134.

Caldwell, J. C., & Caldwell, P. (1996). The African AIDS epidemic. *Scientific American, 274*, 62–63, 66–68.

Callen, M. (1990). *Surviving AIDS*. New York: HarperCollins.

Campbell, C. A. (1990). Prostitution and AIDS. In D. G. Ostrow (Ed.), *Behavioral aspects of AIDS* (pp. 121–137). New York: Plenum.

Campos, P. E., Brasfield, T. L., & Kelly, J. A. (1989). Psychology training related to AIDS: Survey of doctoral graduate programs and predoctoral internship programs. *Professional Psychology: Research and Practice, 20*, 214–220.

Camus, A. (1948). *The plague*. New York: Vintage.

Cao, Y., Qin, L., Zhang, L., Safrit, J., & Ho, D. (1995). Virologic and immunologic characterization of long-term survivors of human immunodeficiency virus type 1 infection. *New England Journal of Medicine, 332*, 201–208.

Capaldini, L. (1997). HIV disease: Psychosocial issues and psychiatric complications. In M. A. Sande & P. A. Volberding (Eds.), *The medical management
of AIDS* (5th ed., pp. 217–238). Philadelphia: Saunders.

Capitanio, J. (1994, January). *Variability in HIV disease: Toward an animal
model of psychosocial influences.* Paper presented at the NIMH Neuroscience Findings in AIDS Research, Rockville, MD.

Carey, M. A., Jenkins, R. A., Brown, G. R., Temoshok, L., & Pace, J. (1991,
June). *Gender differences in psychosocial functioning in early stage HIV pa-
tients.* Paper presented at the Seventh International Conference on AIDS,
Florence, Italy.

Carey, M. P., Carey, K., & Kalichman, S. C. (1997). Risk for human immunodeficiency virus (HIV) infection among persons with severe mental illnesses. *Clinical Psychology Review, 17,* 271–291.

Carey, M. P., Morrison-Beedy, D., & Johnson, B. T. (1997). The HIV-knowledge
questionnaire: Development and evaluation of a reliable, valid, and
practical self-administered questionnaire. *AIDS and Behavior, 1,* 61–
74.

Carey, M. P., Weinhardt, L. S., & Carey, K. B. (1995). Prevalence of infection
with HIV among the seriously mentally ill: Review of research and implications for practice. *Professional Psychology: Research and Practice, 26,*
262–268.

Carmen, E., & Brady, S. (1990). AIDS risk and prevention for the chronic
mentally ill. *Hospital and Community Psychiatry, 41,* 652–657.

Carpenter, C. C. J., Fischl, M. A., Hammer, S. M., Hirsch, M. S., Jacobsen,
D. M., Katzenstein, D. A., Montaner, J. S. G., Richman, D. D., Saag, M. S.,
Schooley, R. T., Thompson, M. A., Vella, S., Yeni, P. G., & Volberding,
P. A. (1997). Antiretroviral therapy for HIV infection in 1997. *Journal of
the American Medical Association, 277,* 1962–1969.

Carpenter, C. C. J., Mayer, K. H., Stein, M. D., Leibman, B. D., Fisher, A., &
Fiore, T. C. (1991). Human immunodeficiency virus infection in North
American women: Experience with 200 cases and a review of the literature.
Medicine, 70, 307–325.

Carr, A., & Cooper, D. A. (1997). Primary HIV infection. In M. A. Sande &
P. A. Volberding (Eds.), *The medical management of AIDS* (pp. 89–106).
Philadelphia: Saunders.

Carr, J. N. (1975). Drug patterns among drug-addicted mothers: Incidence, variance in use, and effects on children. *Pediatric Annals, 4,* 65–77.

Carson, V. (1990). Hope and spiritual well-being: Essentials for living with AIDS. *Perspectives in Psychiatric Care, 26,* 28–34.

Cassileth, B. R., Lusk, E. J., Strouse, T. B., Miller, D. S., Brown, L. L., Cross, P. A., & Tenaglia, A. N. (1984). Psychosocial status in chronic illness: A comparative analysis of six diagnostic groups. *New England Journal of Medicine, 311,* 506–511.

Cassileth, B. R., Lusk, E. J., Strouse, T. B., Miller, D. S., Brown, L. L., & Cross, P. A. (1985). A psychological analysis of cancer patients and their next-of-kin. *Cancer, 55,* 72–76.

Castro, K. G., Lieb, S., Jaffe, H. W., Narkunas, J. P., Calisher, C. H., Bush, T. J., & Witte, J. J. (1988). Transmission of HIV in Belle Glade, Florida: Lessons for other communities in the United States. *Science, 239,* 193–197.

Castro, K. G., Lifson, A. R., White, C. R., Bush, T. J., Chamberland, M. E., Lekatsas, A. M., & Jaffe, H. W. (1988). Investigations of AIDS patients with no previously identified risk factors. *Journal of the American Medical Association, 259,* 1338–1342.

Catalan, J. (1988). Invited review: Psychosocial and neuropsychiatric aspects of HIV infection: Review of their extent and implications for psychiatry. *Journal of Psychosomatic Research, 32,* 237–248.

Catalan, J., Beevor, A., Cassidy, L., Burgess, A. P., Meadows, J., Pergami, A., Gazzard, B., & Barton, S. (1996). Women and HIV infection: Investigation of its psychosocial consequences. *Journal of Psychosomatic Research, 41,* 39–47.

Catalan, J., & Burgess, A. (1991). Neuroscience of HIV infection: Basic and clinical frontiers. *AIDS Care, 3,* 467–471.

Catalan, J., & Thornton, S. (1993). Editorial review: Whatever happened to HIV dementia? *International Journal of STD and AIDS, 4,* 1–4.

Catania, J. A., Coates, T. J., Stall, R., Turner, H., Peterson, J., Hearst, N., Dolcini, M. M., Hudes, E., Gagnon, J., Wiley, J., & Groves, R. (1992). Prevalence of AIDS-related risk factors and condom use in the United States. *Science, 258,* 1101–1106.

Catania, J. A., Kegeles, S. M., & Coates, T. J. (1990). Towards an understanding of risk behavior: An AIDS risk reduction model (ARRM). *Health Education Quarterly, 17,* 53–72.

Catania, J. A., Turner, H. A., Choi, K., & Coates, T. J. (1992). Coping with death anxiety: Help-seeking and social support among gay men with various HIV diagnoses. *AIDS, 6,* 999–1005.

Catania, J. A., Turner, H., Kegeles, S. M., Stall, R., Pollack, L., & Coates, T. J. (1989). Older Americans and AIDS: Transmission risks and primary prevention research needs. *The Gerontologist, 29,* 373–381.

Ceballos-Capitaine, A., Szapocznik, J., Blaney, N., Morgan, R., Millon, C., & Eisdorfer, C. (1990). Ethnicity, emotional distress, stress-related disruption, and coping among HIV seropositive gay males. *Hispanic Journal of Behavioral Sciences, 12,* 135–152.

Cello, J. P. (1992). Gastrointestinal tract manifestations of AIDS. In M. A. Sande & P. A. Volberding (Eds.), *The medical management of AIDS* (3rd ed., pp. 176–192). Philadelphia: Saunders.

Centers for Disease Control and Prevention. (1987a). Antibody to human immunodeficiency virus in female prostitutes. *Morbidity and Mortality Weekly Report, 36,* 157–161.

Centers for Disease Control and Prevention. (1987b). Recommendations for prevention of HIV transmission in health-care settings. *Morbidity and Mortality Weekly Report, 36*(2S), 35S–18S.

Centers for Disease Control and Prevention. (1991a). Characteristics and risk behaviors of homeless Black men seeking services from the community homeless assistance plan—Dade County, Florida, August 1991. *Morbidity and Mortality Weekly Report, 40,* 865–868.

Centers for Disease Control and Prevention. (1991b). HIV/AIDS knowledge and awareness of testing and treatment—Behavioral risk factors surveillance system, 1990. *Morbidity and Mortality Weekly Report, 40,* 855–860.

Centers for Disease Control and Prevention. (1992a). Condom use among male injecting-drug users—New York City, 1987–1990. *Morbidity and Mortality Weekly Report, 41,* 617–620.

Centers for Disease Control and Prevention. (1992b). Heterosexual transmission of HIV—Puerto Rico, 1981–1991. *Morbidity and Mortality Weekly Report, 41,* 899–906.

Centers for Disease Control and Prevention. (1992c). HIV infection, syphilis, and tuberculosis screening among migrant farm workers—Florida, 1992. *Morbidity and Mortality Weekly Report, 41,* 723–725.

Centers for Disease Control and Prevention. (1992d). HIV seroprevalence among adults treated for cardiac arrest before reaching a medical facility —Seattle, Washington, 1989–1990. *Morbidity and Mortality Weekly Report, 41*, 381–383.

Centers for Disease Control and Prevention. (1992e). 1993 revised classification system for HIV infection and expanded surveillance case definition for AIDS among adolescents and adults. *Morbidity and Mortality Weekly Report, 41*(whole no. RR-17).

Centers for Disease Control and Prevention. (1992f). Patient exposures to HIV during nuclear medicine procedures. *Morbidity and Mortality Weekly Report, 41*, 575–578.

Centers for Disease Control and Prevention. (1992g). Selected behaviors that increase risk for HIV infection among high school students—United States, 1990. *Morbidity and Mortality Weekly Report, 41*, 231–240.

Centers for Disease Control and Prevention. (1992h). Selected behaviors that increase risk for HIV infection, other sexually transmitted diseases, and unintended pregnancy among high school students—United States, 1991. *Morbidity and Mortality Weekly Report, 41*, 945–950.

Centers for Disease Control and Prevention. (1992i). Surveillance for occupationally acquired HIV infection—United States, 1981–1992. *Morbidity and Mortality Weekly Report, 41*, 823–825.

Centers for Disease Control and Prevention. (1992j). Update: Investigations of patients who have been treated by HIV-infected health care workers. *Morbidity and Mortality Weekly Report, 41*, 344–346.

Centers for Disease Control and Prevention. (1993a). Recommendations on prophylaxis and therapy for disseminated mycobacterium avium complex for adults and adolescents infected with human immunodeficiency virus. *Morbidity and Mortality Weekly Report, 42*, 17–20.

Centers for Disease Control and Prevention. (1993b). Update: Barrier protection against HIV infection and other sexually transmitted diseases. *Morbidity and Mortality Weekly Report, 42*, 589–591, 597.

Centers for Disease Control and Prevention. (1993c). Update: Investigations of persons treated by HIV-infected health-care workers—United States. *Morbidity and Mortality Weekly Report, 42*, 329–331, 337.

Centers for Disease Control and Prevention. (1994a). Human immunodeficiency virus transmission in household settings—United States. *Morbidity and Mortality Weekly Report, 43*, 347–356.

Centers for Disease Control and Prevention. (1994b). Recommendations of the U.S. Public Health Service Task Force on the use of zidovudine to reduce perinatal transmission of human immunodeficiency virus. *Morbidity and Mortality Weekly Report, 43*(whole no. RR-11).

Centers for Disease Control and Prevention. (1997). *HIV/AIDS surveillance report*. Atlanta: Author.

Chaisson, R. E. (1992). Bacterial infections in HIV disease. In M. A. Sande & P. A. Volberding (Eds.), *The medical management of AIDS* (3rd ed., pp. 346–358). Philadelphia: Saunders.

Chaisson, R. E., Keruly, J. C., & Moore, R. D. (1995). Race, sex, drug use, and progression of human immunodeficiency virus disease. *New England Journal of Medicine, 333*, 751–756.

Chan, I. S. F., Neaton, J. D., Saravolatz, L. D., Crane, L. R., & Osterberger, J. (1995). Frequencies of opportunistic diseases prior to death among HIV-infected persons. *AIDS, 9*, 1145–1151.

Chang, S. W., Katz, M. H., & Hernandez, S. R. (1992). The new AIDS case definition: Implications for San Francisco. *Journal of the American Medical Association, 267*, 973–975.

Chang, Y., Cesarman, E., Pessin, M. S., Lee, F., Culpepper, J., Knowles, D. M., & Moore, P. S. (1994). Identification of herpesvirus-like DNA sequences in AIDS-associated Kaposi's sarcoma. *Science, 266*, 1865–1869.

Chesney, M. (November, 1997). Behavioral factors in HIV treatment adherence. Paper presented at *Adherence to New HIV Therapies: A Research Conference*, Washington, D.C.

Chesney, M., Folkman, S., & Chambers, D. (1996). Coping effectiveness training for men living with HIV: Preliminary findings. *International Journal of STD and AIDS, 7*(Suppl. 2), 75–82.

Chesney, M. A., Lurie, P., & Coates, T. J. (1995). Strategies for addressing the social and behavioral challenges of prophylactic HIV vaccine trials. *Journal of Acquired Deficiency Syndromes and Human Retrovirology, 9*, 30–35.

Chiasson, M. A., Stoneburner, R. L., Hildebrandt, D. S., Ewing, W. E., Telzak, E. E., & Jaffe, H. W. (1991). Heterosexual transmission of HIV-1 associated with the use of smokable freebase cocaine (crack). *AIDS, 5*, 1121–1126.

Chidwick, A., & Borrill, J. (1996). Dealing with a life-threatening diagnosis: The experience of people with the human immunodeficiency virus. *AIDS Care, 8,* 271–284.

Chitwood, D. D., McCoy, C. B., Inciardi, J. A., McBride, D. C., Comerford, M., Trapido, E., McCoy, V., Page, J. B., Griffin, J., Fletcher, M. A., & Ashman, M. A. (1990). HIV seropositivity of needles from shooting galleries in South Florida. *American Journal of Public Health, 80,* 150–152.

Chmiel, J. S., Detels, R., Kaslow, R. A., Van Raden, M., Kingsley, L. A., & Brookmeyer, R. (1987). Factors associated with prevalent human immunodeficiency virus (HIV) infection in the Multicenter AIDS Cohort Study. *American Journal of Epidemiology, 126,* 568–575.

Chochinov, H. M., Wilson, K. G., Enns, M., Mowchun, N., Lander, S., Levitt, M., & Clinch, J. J. (1995). Desire for death in the terminally ill. *American Journal of Psychiatry, 152,* 1185–1191.

Chorba, T. L., Holman, R. C., & Evatt, B. L. (1993). Heterosexual and mother-to-child transmission of AIDS in the hemophilia community. *Public Health Reports, 108,* 99–105.

Christ, G. H., & Wiener, L. S. (1985). Psychosocial issues in AIDS. In V. T. DeVita, S. Hellman, & S. A. Rosenberg (Eds.), *AIDS: Etiology, diagnosis, treatment and prevention* (pp. 275–297). Philadelphia: Lippincott.

Chu, S. Y., Buehler, J. W., & Berkelman, R. L. (1990). Impact of the human immunodeficiency virus epidemic on mortality in women of reproductive age, United States. *Journal of the American Medical Association, 264,* 225–229.

Chu, S. Y., Buehler, J. W., Fleming, P. L., & Berkelman, R. L. (1990). Epidemiology of reported cases of AIDS in lesbians. *American Journal of Public Health, 80,* 1380–1381.

Chu, S. Y., Conti, L., Schable, B., & Diaz, T. (1994). Female-to-female sexual contact and HIV transmission. *Journal of the American Medical Association, 272,* 443.

Chuang, H. T., Devins, G., Hunsley, J., & Gill, M. J. (1989). Psychosocial distress and well-being among gay and bisexual men with Human Immunodeficiency Virus infection. *American Journal of Psychiatry, 146,* 876–880.

Chuang, H. T., Jason, G., Pajurkova, E., & Gill, J. (1992). Psychiatric morbidity in patients with HIV infection. *Canadian Journal of Psychiatry, 37,* 109–115.

Chuck, S., & Rodvold, K. (in press). Pharmacokinetics of protease inhibitors and drug interactions with psychoactive drugs. In D. Ostrow & S. Kalichman (Eds.), *Behavioral and mental health impacts of new HIV therapies*. New York: Plenum Press.

Chun, T. W., Carruth, L., Finzi, D., Shen, X., DiGiuseppe, J. A., Taylor, H., Hermankova, M., Chadwick, K., Margolick, J., Quinn, T. C., Kuo, Y. H., Brookmeyer, R., Zeiger, M. A., Barditch-Crovo, P., & Siliciano, R. F. (1997). Quantification of latent tissue reservoirs and total body viral load in HIV-1 infection. *Nature, 387*, 183–188.

Cleary, P. D., Van Devanter, N., Rogers, T., Singer, E., Shipton-Levy, R., Steilen, M., Stuart, A., Avorn, J., & Pindyck, J. (1993). Depressive symptoms in blood donors notified of HIV infection. *American Journal of Public Health, 83*, 534–539.

Cleary, P. D., Van Devanter, N., Steilen, M., Stuart, A., Shipton-Levy, R., McMullen, W., Rogers, T., Singer, E., Avron, J., & Pindyck, J. (1995). A randomized trial of an education and support program for HIV-infected individuals. *AIDS, 9*, 1271–1278.

Clement, M., & Hollander, H. (1992). Natural history and management of the seropositive patient. In M. A. Sande & P. A. Volberding (Eds.), *The medical management of AIDS* (3rd ed., pp. 87–96). Philadelphia: Saunders.

Clifford, D. B., Jacoby, R. G., Miller, J. P., Seyfried, W. R., & Glicksman, M. (1990). Neuropsychometric performance of asymptomatic HIV-infected subjects. *AIDS, 4*, 767–774.

Clumeck, N., Taelman, H., Hermans, P., Piot, P., Schoumacher, M., & De Wit, S. (1989). A cluster of HIV infection among heterosexual people without apparent risk factors. *New England Journal of Medicine, 321*, 1460–1462.

Coates, T., McKusick, L., Kuno, R., & Stites, D. (1989). Stress reduction training changed number of sexual partners but not immune function in men with HIV. *American Journal of Public Health, 79*, 885–886.

Coates, T. J., Temoshok, L., & Mandel, J. (1984). Psychosocial research is essential to understanding and treating AIDS. *American Psychologist, 39*, 1309–1314.

Cobb, S. (1976). Social support as a moderator of life stress. *Psychosomatic Medicine, 38*, 300–314.

Cochran, S. D., & Mays, V. M. (1994). Depressive distress among homosexually active African American men and women. *American Journal of Psychiatry, 151,* 524–529.

Cockerell, C. J. (1992). Cutaneous and histologic signs of HIV infection other than Kaposi's sarcoma. In G. P. Wormser (Ed.), *AIDS and other manifestations of HIV infection* (2nd ed., pp. 463–476). New York: Raven Press.

Cohen, F. L., & Nehring, W. M. (1994). Foster care of HIV-positive children in the United States. *Public Health Reports, 109,* 60–67.

Cohen, H., Marmor, M., Wolfe, H., & Ribble, D. (1993). Risk assessment of HIV transmission among lesbians. *Journal of Acquired Immune Deficiency Syndromes and Human Retrovirology, 6,* 1173–1174.

Cohen, J. (1996a). SIV data raise concern on oral-sex risk. *Science, 272,* 1421–1422.

Cohen, J. (1996b). Chemokines share center stage with drug therapies. *Science, 273,* 302–303.

Cohen, J. (1997). Advances painted in shades of gray at a D.C. conference. *Science, 275,* 615–616.

Cohen, S. (1988). Psychosocial models of the role of social support in the etiology of physical disease. *Health Psychology, 7,* 269–297.

Cohen, S., & Willis, T. A. (1985). Stress, social support, and the buffering hypothesis. *Psychological Bulletin, 98,* 310–357.

Cohen, S., & Williamson, G. (1991). Stress and infectious disease in humans. *Psychological Bulletin, 109,* 5–24.

Cole, S. W., Kemeny, M. E., Taylor, S. E., & Visscher, B. R. (1996). Elevated physical health risk among gay men who conceal their homosexual identity. *Health Psychology, 15,* 243–251.

Cole, S. W., Kemeny, M. E., Taylor, S. E., Visscher, B. R., & Fahey, J. L. (1996). Accelerated course of human immunodeficiency virus infection in gay men who conceal their homosexual identity. *Psychosomatic Medicine, 58,* 219–231.

Coleman, V. E., & Harris, G. N. (1989). Clinical notes: A support group for individuals recently testing HIV positive—A psycho-educational group model. *Journal of Sex Research, 26,* 539–548.

Collier, A. C., Marra, C., Coombs, R. W., Claypoole, K., Cohen, W., Longstreth,

W. T., Townes, B. D., Maravilla, K. R., Critchlow, C., Murphy, V. L., & Handsfield, H. H. (1992). Central nervous system manifestations in human immunodeficiency virus infection without AIDS. *Journal of Acquired Immune Deficiency Syndromes and Human Retrovirology, 5,* 229–241.

Conant, M., Hardy, D., Sernatinger, J., Spicer, D., & Levy, J. A. (1986). Condoms prevent transmission of AIDS-associated retrovirus. *Journal of the American Medical Association, 255,* 1706.

Cooper, D. A. (1994). Early antiretroviral therapy. *AIDS, 8*(Suppl. 3), S9–S14.

Coreless, I. B., Fulton, R., Lamers, E. P., Bendiksen, R., Hysing-Dahl, B., MacElveen-Hoehn, P., O'Connor, P., Harvei, U., Schjolberg, T., & Stevenson, E. (1992). Assumptions and principles concerning care for persons affected by HIV disease. *AIDS and Public Policy Journal, 7,* 28–31.

Crandall, C. S. (1991). Multiple stigma and AIDS: Illness stigma and attitudes toward homosexuals and IV drug users in AIDS-related stigmatization. *Journal of Community and Applied Social Psychology, 1,* 165–172.

Crandall, C. S., & Coleman, R. (1992). AIDS-related stigmatization and the disruption of social relationships. *Journal of Social and Personal Relationships, 9,* 163–177.

Crawford, I., Humfleet, G., Ribordy, S. C., Ho, F. C., & Vickers, V. L. (1991). Stigmatization of AIDS patients by mental health professionals. *Professional Psychology: Research and Practice, 5,* 357–361.

Crystal, S., & Jackson, M. M. (1989). Psychosocial adaptation and economic circumstances of persons with AIDS and ARC. *Family and Community Health, 12,* 77–88.

Cunningham, R. M., Stiffman, A. R., & Dore, P. (1994). The association of physical and sexual abuse with HIV risk behaviors in adolescence and young adulthood: Implications for public health. *Child Abuse and Neglect, 18,* 233–245.

Curtis, J. R., & Patrick, D. L. (1993). Race and survival time with AIDS: A synthesis of the literature. *American Journal of Public Health, 83,* 1425–1428.

Dannenberg, A. L., McNeil, J. G., Brundage, J. F., & Brookmeyer, R. (1996). Suicide and HIV infection. *Journal of the American Medical Association, 276,* 1743–1746.

Danner, S. A., Carr, A., Leonard, J. M., Lehman, L. M., Gudiol, F., Gonzales,

J., Raventos, A., Rubio, R., Bouza, E., Pintadio, V., Aguado, A. G., Lomas-de Garcia, J., Delgado, R., Borleffs, J. C., Hsu, A., Valdes, J. M., Boucher, C. A., & Cooper, D. A. (1995). A short-term study of the safety, pharmacokinetics, and efficacy of ritonavir, an inhibitor of HIV-1 protease. *New England Journal of Medicine, 333,* 1528–1533.

Darrow, W. W., Webster, R. D., Kurtz, S. P., Buckley, A. K., Patel, K. I., & Stempel, R. R. (in press). Impact of HIV counseling and testing on HIV-infected men who have sex with men: The South Beach health survey. *AIDS and Behavior.*

Davis, K. A., Cameron, B., & Stapleton, J. T. (1992). The impact of HIV patient migration to rural areas. *AIDS Patient Care, 6,* 225–228.

Dawson, J. M., Fitzpatrick, R. M., Reeves, G., Boulton, M., McLean, J., Hart, G. J., & Brookes, M. (1994). Awareness of sexual partners' HIV status as an influence upon high-risk sexual behaviour among gay men. *AIDS, 8,* 837–841.

Dax, E. M., Adler, W. H., Nagel, J. E., Lange, W. R., & Jaffe, J. H. (1991). Amyl nitrite alters human in vitro immune function. *Immunopharmacology and Immunotoxicology, 13,* 577–587.

Dean, L., & Meyer, I. (1995). HIV prevalence and sexual behavior in a cohort of New York City gay men (aged 18–24). *Journal of Acquired Immune Deficiency Syndromes and Human Retrovirology, 8,* 208–211.

Decker, C. F., & Masur, H. (1997). Pneumocystis and other protozoa. In V. T. DeVita, S. Hellman, & S. A. Rosenberg (Eds.), *AIDS: Biology, diagnosis, treatment, and prevention* (4th ed., pp. 215–229). Philadelphia: Lippincott-Raven.

Deeks, S. G. (1997, December). *Failure of HIV-1 protease inhibitors to fully suppress viral replication: Implications for salvage therapy.* Paper presented at the meeting of Clinical Care of the AIDS Patients, San Francisco, California.

Deeks, S. G., Smith, M., Holodnly, M., & Kahn, J. (1997). HIV-1 protease inhibitors: A review for clinicians. *Journal of the American Medical Association, 277,* 145–153.

Derix, M. M. A., de Gans, J., Stam, J., & Portegies, P. (1990). Mental changes in patients with AIDS. *Clinical Neurology and Neurosurgery, 92,* 215–222.

Derogatis, L. R., Abeloff, M. D., & Melisaratos, N. (1979). Psychological coping mechanisms and survival time in metastatic breast cancer. *Journal of the American Medical Association, 242*, 1504–1508.

Derogatis, L. R., Morrow, G. R., Fetting, J., Penman, D., Piasetsky, S., Schmale, A. M., Henrichs, M., & Carnicke, C. L. M. (1983). The prevalence of psychiatric disorders among cancer patients. *Journal of the American Medical Association, 249*, 751–757.

Des Jarlais, D. C., Friedman, S. R., & Casriel, C. (1990). Target groups for preventing AIDS among intravenous drug users: 2. The "hard" data studies. *Journal of Consulting and Clinical Psychology, 58*, 50–56.

Des Jarlais, D. C., Friedman, S. R., & Stoneburner, R. L. (1988). HIV infection and intravenous drug use: Critical issues in the transmission dynamics, infection outcomes, and prevention. *Reviews of Infectious Diseases, 10*, 151–158.

De Vincenzi, I. (1994). A longitudinal study of human immunodeficiency virus transmission by heterosexual partners. *New England Journal of Medicine, 331*, 341–346.

Dew, M. A., Ragni, M. V., & Nimorwicz, P. (1990). Infection with human immunodeficiency virus and vulnerability to psychiatric distress. *Archives of General Psychiatry, 47*, 737–744.

Dew, M. A., Ragni, M. V., & Nimorwicz, P. (1991). Correlates of psychiatric distress among wives of hemophilic men with and without HIV infection. *American Journal of Psychiatry, 148*, 1016–1022.

Dhooper, S. S., Royse, D. D., & Tran, T. V. (1987–1988). Social work practitioners' attitudes towards AIDS victims. *Journal of Applied Social Sciences, 12*, 109–123.

DiFranco, M. J., Sheppard, H. W., Hunter, D. J., Tosteson, T. D., & Ascher, M. S. (1996). The lack of associations of marijuana and other recreational drugs with progression to AIDS in the San Francisco Men's Health Study. *Annals of Epidemiology, 6*, 283–289.

Dilley, J., Ochitill, H., Perl, M., & Volberding, P. (1985). Findings in psychiatric consultations with patients with acquired immune deficiency syndrome. *American Journal of Psychiatry, 142*, 82–86.

Dilley, J. W., Shelp, E. E., & Batki, S. L. (1985). *Psychiatric and ethical issues in the care of patients with AIDS: An overview.* Paper presented at the annual meeting of American Academy of Psychosomatic Medicine, San Francisco.

Dilley, J. W., Woods, W. J., & McFarland, W. (1997). Are advances in treatment changing views about high-risk sex? [Letter to the editor]. *New England Journal of Medicine, 337,* 501–502.

Dingle, G. A., & Oei, T. P. S. (1997). Is alcohol a cofactor of HIV and AIDS? Evidence from immunological and behavioral studies. *Psychological Bulletin, 122,* 56–71.

DiPasquale, J. A. (1990). The psychological effects of support groups on individuals infected by the AIDS virus. *Cancer Nursing, 13,* 278–285.

Doll, L. S., Joy, D., Bartholow, B. N., Harrison, J. S., Bolan, G., Douglas, J. M., Saltzman, L. E., Moss, P. M., & Delgado, W. (1992). Self-reported childhood and adolescent sexual abuse among adult homosexual and bisexual men. *Child Abuse and Neglect, 16,* 855–864.

Donegan, E., Stuart, M., Niland, J. C., Sacks, H., Azen, S., Dietrich, S., Faucett, C., Fletcher, M. A., Kleinman, S., Operskalski, E., Perkins, H., Pindyck, J., Schiff, E., Stites, D., Tomasulo, P., Mosely, J., & the Transfusion Study Group. (1990). Infection with human immunodeficiency virus type-1 (HIV-I) among recipients of antibody-positive blood donations. *Annals of Internal Medicine, 113,* 733–739.

Donlou, J. N., Wolcott, D., Gottlieb, M., & Landsverk, J. (1985). Psychosocial aspects of AIDS and AIDS-related complex: A pilot study. *Journal of Psychosocial Oncology, 3,* 39–55.

Downs, A. M., & De Vincenzi, I. (1996). Probability of heterosexual transmission of HIV: Relationship to the number of unprotected sexual contacts. *Journal of Acquired Immune Deficiency Syndromes and Human Retrovirology, 11,* 388–395.

Drew, W. L., Buhles, W., & Erlich, K. S. (1992). Management of herpes virus infections (CMV, HSV, VZV). In M. A. Sande & P. A. Volberding (Eds.), *The medical management of AIDS* (3rd ed., pp. 359–382). Philadelphia: Saunders.

Drew, W. L., Stempien, M. J., & Erlich, K. S. (1997). Management of herpes virus infections (CMV, HSV, VZV). In M. A. Sande & P. A. Volberding (Eds.), *The medical management of AIDS* (5th ed., pp. 381–398). Philadelphia: Saunders.

Duesberg, P. (1988). HIV is not the cause of AIDS. *Science, 241,* 514, 517.

Duesberg, P. H. (1989). Human immunodeficiency virus and acquired immunodeficiency syndrome: Correlation but not causation. *Proceedings of the National Academy of Science, 86,* 755–764.

Dunkel-Schetter, C., Feinstein, L. G., Taylor, S. E., & Falke, R. L. (1992). Patterns of coping with cancer. *Health Psychology, 11,* 79–87.

Dwyer, J., Wood, C., McNamara, J., & Kinder, B. (1987). Transplantation of thymic tissue into patients with AIDS. *Archives of Internal Medicine, 147,* 513–517.

Edwards, S. K., & White, C. (1995). HIV seroconversion illness after orogenital contact with successful contact tracing. *International Journal of STD and AIDS, 6,* 50–51.

Egan, V. (1992). Neuropsychological aspects of HIV infection. *AIDS Care, 4,* 3–10.

Egan, V., Brettle, R. P., & Goodwin, G. M. (1992). The Edinburgh cohort of HIV-positive drug users: Pattern of cognitive impairment in relation to progression of disease. *British Journal of Psychiatry, 161,* 522–531.

Egan, V. G., Chiswick, A., Brettle, R. P., & Goodwin, G. M. (1993). The Edinburgh cohort of HIV-positive drug users: The relationship between auditory P3 latency, cognitive function and self-rated mood. *Psychological Medicine, 23,* 1–10.

Ekstrand, M., & Coates, T. J. (1990). Maintenance of safer sexual behaviors and predictors of risky sex: The San Francisco Men's Health Study. *American Journal of Public Health, 80,* 973–977.

Eldin, B., Irwin, K., Faraque, S., McCoy, C., Word, C., Serrano, Y., Inciardi, J., Bowser, B., Schilling, R., & Holmberg, S. (1994). Intersecting epidemic: Crack cocaine use and HIV infection among inner-city young adults. *New England Journal of Medicine, 331,* 422–427.

Elford, J., Bor, R., & Summers, P. (1991). Research into HIV and AIDS between 1981 and 1990: The epidemic curve. *AIDS, 5,* 1515–1519.

Eller, L. S. (1995). Effects of two cognitive-behavioral interventions on immunity and symptoms in persons with HIV. *Annals of Behavioral Medicine, 17,* 339–348.

Elliott, A. J., Uldall, K., Bergam, K., Russo, J., Claypoole, K., & Roy-Byrne, P. (1998). Randomized, placebo-controlled trial of paroxetine versus imipramine in depressed HIV-positive outpatients. *American Journal of Psychiatry, 155,* 367–372.

Ellis, A. (1962). *Reason and emotion in psychotherapy.* New York: Lyle Stuart.

Emmot, S. (1991, June). *Cognitive group therapy for coping with HIV infection.* Paper presented at the Seventh International Conference on AIDS, Florence, Italy.

Eng, T. T., & Butler, W. T. (1997). *The hidden epidemic: Confronting sexually transmitted diseases.* Washington, DC: National Academy Press.

Engel, G. L. (1980). The clinical application of the biopsychosocial model. *American Journal of Psychiatry, 137,* 535–544.

Enger, C., Graham, N., Peng, Y., Chmiel, J. S., Kingsley, L. A., Detels, R., & Munoz, A. (1996). Survival from early, intermediate, and late stages of HIV infection. *Journal of the American Medical Association, 275,* 1329–1334.

Ericksen, K. P., & Trocki, K. F. (1992). Behavioral risk factors for sexually transmitted diseases in American households. *Social Science Medicine, 34,* 843–853.

Essex, M. E. (1997). Origin of acquired immunodeficiency syndrome. In V. T. Devita, S. Hellman, & S. A. Rosenberg (Eds.), *AIDS: Etiology, diagnosis, treatment, and prevention* (4th ed., pp. 3–14). Philadelphia: Lippincott-Raven.

Esterling, B. A., Kiecolt-Glaser, J. K., Bodnar, J. C., & Glaser, R. (1994). Chronic stress, social support, and persistent alterations in the natural killer cell response to cytokines in older adults. *Health Psychology, 13,* 291–298.

Evans, D. L., Leserman, J., Perkins, D. O., Stern, R. A., Murphy, C., Zheng, B., Gettes, D., Longmate, J. A., Silva, S. G., van der Horst, C. M., Hall, C. D., Folds, J. D., Golden, R. N., & Petitto, J. M. (1997). Severe life stress as a predictor of early disease progression in HIV infection. *American Journal of Psychiatry, 154,* 630–634.

Eversole, T. (1997). Psychotherapy and counseling: Bending the frame. In M. G. Winiarski (Ed.), *HIV mental health for the 21st century* (pp. 23–38). New York: New York University Press.

Expert Group of the Joint United Nations Programme on HIV/AIDS. (1997). Implications of HIV variability for transmission: Scientific and policy issues. *AIDS, 11,* UNAIDS1–UNAIDS15.

Ezzell, C. (1996). Emergence of the protease inhibitors: A better class of AIDS drugs? *Journal of NIH Research, 8,* 41–45.

& Detels, R. (1984). Quantitative changes in T helper or T suppressor/cytotoxic lymphocyte subsets that distinguish acquired immune deficiency syndrome from other immune subset disorders. *American Journal of Medicine, 76,* 95–100.

Fatkenheurer, G., Theisen, A., Rockstroh, J., Grabow, T., Wicke, C., Becker, K., Wieland, U., Pfister, H., Reiser, M., Hegener, P., Franzen, C., Schwenk, A., & Salzberger, B. (1997). Virological treatment failure of protease inhibitor therapy in an unselected cohort of HIV-infected patients. *AIDS, 11,* F113–F116.

Fauci, A. S. (1986). Current issues in developing a strategy for dealing with the acquired immunodeficiency syndrome. *Proceedings of the National Academy of Sciences, 83,* 9278–9283.

Fauci, A. S. (1988). The human immunodeficiency virus: Infectivity and mechanisms of pathogenesis. *Science, 239,* 617–622.

Fauci, A., & Dale, D. (1975). Alternate-day prednisone therapy and human lymphocyte subpopulations. *Journal of Clinical Investigation, 55,* 22–32.

Fauci, A. S., Macher, A. M., Longo, D. L., Lane, H. C., Rook, A. H., Masur, H., & Gelmann, E. P. (1984). Acquired immunodeficiency syndrome: Epidemiologic, clinical, immunologic, and therapeutic considerations. *Annals of Internal Medicine, 100,* 92–106.

Faulstich, M. (1987). Psychiatric aspects of AIDS. *American Journal of Psychiatry, 144,* 551–555.

Feifel, H., Strack, S., & Nagy, V. T. (1987). Coping strategies and associated features of medically ill patients. *Psychosomatic Medicine, 49,* 616–625.

Feldblum, P. J., & Fortney, J. A. (1988). Condoms, spermicides and the transmission of human immunodeficiency virus. *American Journal of Public Health, 78,* 52–54.

Felton, B. J., & Revenson, T. A. (1984). Coping with chronic illness: A study of illness controllability and the influence of coping strategies on psychological adjustment. *Journal of Consulting and Clinical Psychology, 52,* 343–353.

Finkelhor, D. (1986). *A sourcebook on child sexual abuse.* Newbury Park, CA: Sage.

Finley, J. L., Joshi, V. V., & Neill, J. S. A. (1992). General pathology of HIV infection. In G. P. Wormser (Ed.), *AIDS and other manifestations of HIV infection* (2nd ed., pp. 499–542). New York: Raven Press.

Fischl, M. A. (1992). Treatment of HIV infection. In M. A. Sande & P. A. Volberding (Eds.), *The medical management of AIDS* (3rd ed., pp. 97–110). Philadelphia: Saunders.

Fisher, J. D., & Fisher, W. A. (1992). Changing AIDS-risk behavior. *Psychological Bulletin, 111,* 455–474.

Fisher, J. D., Kimble, D., Misovich, S., & Weinstein, B. (in press). Dynamics of sexual risk behavior in HIV infected men who have sex with men. *AIDS and Behavior.*

Fleishman, J. A., & Fogel, B. (1994). Coping and depressive symptoms among people with AIDS. *Health Psychology, 13,* 156–169.

Fleming, P. L., Ciesielski, C. A., Byers, R. H., Castro, K. G., & Berkelman, R. L. (1993). Gender differences in reported AIDS-indicative diagnoses. *Journal of Infectious Diseases, 168,* 61–67.

Fliszar, G. M., & Clopton, J. R. (1995). Attitudes of psychologists in training toward persons with AIDS. *Professional Psychology: Research and Practice, 26,* 274–277.

Flood, M. F., Hansen, D. J., & Kalichman, S. C. (in press). Ecological perspectives on maternal decisions regarding HIV-exposed infants. *Children's Services: Social Policy, Research, and Practice.*

Fogel, B. S., & Mor, V. (1993). Depressed mood and care preferences in patients with AIDS. *General Hospital Psychiatry, 15,* 203–207.

Folkman, S. (September, 1994). *The San Francisco AIDS Bereavement and Coping Project update.* Paper presented at the meeting of NIMH Prevention Centers, New York.

Folkman, S. (1997). Positive psychological states and coping with severe stress. *Social Science Medicine, 45,* 1207–1221.

Folkman, S., Chesney, M., Collette, L., Boccellari, A., & Cooke, M. (1996). Postbereavement depressive mood and its prebereavement predictors in HIV+ and HIV− gay men. *Journal of Personality and Social Psychology, 70,* 336–348.

Folkman, S., Chesney, M., Pollack, L., & Phillips, C. (1992). Stress, coping, and high-risk sexual behavior. *Health Psychology, 11,* 218–222.

Folkman, S., Chesney, M. A., Cooke, M., Boccellari, A., & Collette, L. (1994). Caregiver burden in HIV-positive and HIV-negative partners of men with AIDS. *Journal of Consulting and Clinical Psychology, 62,* 746–756.

Folkman, S., Lazarus, R., Dunkel-Schetter, C., DeLongis, A., & Gruen, R. (1986). Dynamics of a stressful encounter: Cognitive appraisal, coping, and encounter outcomes. *Journal of Personality and Social Psychology, 50,* 571–579.

Forehand, R., Steele, R., Armistead, L., Morse, E., Simon, P., & Clark, L. (in press). The Family Health Project: Psychosocial adjustment of children whose mothers are HIV-infected. *Journal of Consulting and Clinical Psychology.*

Foster, G. (1996). Orphans. *AIDS Care, 9,* 82–87.

Foster, G., Makufa, C., Drew, R., Mashumba, S., & Kambeu, S. (1997). Perceptions of children and community members concerning the circumstances of orphans in rural Zimbabwe. *AIDS Care, 9,* 391–405.

Fox, P., Wolff, A., Yeh, C., Atkinson, J., & Baum, B. (1989). Salivary inhibition of HIV-1 infectivity: Functional properties and distribution in men, women, and children. *Journal of the American Dental Association, 118,* 709–711.

Frankl, V. E. (1963). *Man's search for meaning.* New York: Pocket Books.

Friedland, G. H., Saltzman, B. R., Rogers, M. F., Kahl, P. A., Lesser, M. L., Mayers, M. M., & Klein, R. S. (1986). Lack of transmission of HTLV-III/LAV infection to household contacts of patients with AIDS or AIDS-related complex with oral candidasis. *New England Journal of Medicine, 314,* 344–349.

Friedman, S. R., Neaigus, A., Jose, B., Curtis, R., Goldstein, M., Ildefonso, G., Rothenberg, R. B., & Des Jarlais, D. C. (1997). Sociometric risk networks and risk for HIV infection. *American Journal of Public Health, 87,* 1289–1296.

Friedman, Y., Franklin, C., Freels, S., & Weil, M. H. (1991). Long-term survival of patients with AIDS, *Pneumocystis carinii* pneumonia, and respiratory failure. *Journal of the American Medical Association, 266,* 89–92.

Frierson, R. L., & Lippmann, S. B. (1987). Psychologic implications of AIDS. *American Family Physician, 35,* 109–116.

Frierson, R. L., & Lippmann, S. B. (1988). Suicide and AIDS. *Psychosomatics, 29,* 226–231.

Frierson, R. L., Lippmann, S. B., & Johnson, J. (1987). AIDS: Psychological stresses on the family. *Psychosomatics, 28,* 65–68.

Frost, J. C., Makadon, H. J., Judd, D., Lee, S., O'Neill, S. F., & Paulsen, R. (1991). Care for caregivers: A support group for staff caring for AIDS patients in hospital-based primary care practice. *General Internal Medicine, 6,* 162–167.

Gallo, R. C. (1986). The first human retrovirus. *Scientific American, 255,* 88–98.

Gallo, R. C. (1987). The AIDS virus. *Scientific American, 256,* 46–56.

Gallo, R. C. (1988). HIV: The cause of AIDS—An overview on its biology, mechanisms of disease induction, and our attempts to control it. *Journal of Acquired Immune Deficiency Syndromes and Human Retrovirology, 1,* 521–535.

Gallo, R. C. (1991). *Virus hunting AIDS, cancer, and the human retrovirus: A story of scientific discovery.* New York: Basic Books.

Gallo, R. C., & Montagnier, L. (1988). AIDS in 1988. *Scientific American, 259,* 41–48.

Gallop, R. M., Lancee, W. J., Taerk, G., Coates, R. A., & Fanning, M. (1992). Fear of contagion and AIDS: Nurses' perception of risk. *AIDS Care, 4,* 103–109.

Gallop, R. M., Lancee, W. J., Taerk, G., Coates, R. A., Fanning, M., & Keatings, M. (1991). The knowledge, attitudes and concerns of hospital staff about AIDS. *Canadian Journal of Public Health, 82,* 409–412.

Gallop, R. M., Taerk, G., Lancee, W. J., Coates, R. A., & Fanning, M. (1992). A randomized trial of group interventions for hospital staff caring for persons with AIDS. *AIDS Care, 4,* 177–185.

Gamble, R., & Getzel, G. S. (1989). Group work with gay men with AIDS. *Social Casework: The Journal of Contemporary Social Work, 70,* 172–179.

Garber, G. E., Cameron, D. W., Hawley-Foss, N., Greenway, D., & Shannon, M. E. (1991). The use of ozone-treated blood in the therapy of HIV infection and immune disease: A pilot study of safety and efficacy. *AIDS, 5,* 981–984.

Garrett, L. (1994). *The coming plague: Newly emerging diseases in a world out of balance.* New York: Farrar, Straus & Giroux.

Gayle, H. D., & D'Angelo, L. J. (1991). Epidemiology of acquired immunodeficiency syndrome and human immunodeficiency virus infection in adolescents. *Pediatric Infectious Disease Journal, 10,* 322–328.

Gelman, D. (1993, November 29). A resistance to reason. *Newsweek*, p. 79.

George, J. M., Reed, T., Ballard, K., Colin, J., & Fielding, J. (1993). Contact with AIDS patients as a source of work-related distress: Effects of organizational and social support. *Academy of Management Journal, 36,* 157–171.

Gerberding, J. L. (1992). HIV transmission to providers and their patients. In M. A. Sande & P. A. Volberding (Eds.), *The medical management of AIDS* (3rd ed., pp. 54–64). Philadelphia: Saunders.

Gerberding, J. L. (1997). Limiting the risks of health care workers. In M. A. Sande & P. A. Volberding (Eds.), *The medical management of AIDS* (5th ed., pp. 75–84). Philadelphia: Saunders.

Gerberding, J. L., Littell, C., Brown, A., & Schecter, W. P. (1990). Risk of exposure of surgical personnel to patients' blood during surgery at San Francisco General Hospital. *Journal of the American Medical Association, 322,* 1788–1793.

Gerbert, B., Maguire, B. T., & Coates, T. J. (1990). Are patients talking to their physicians about AIDS? *American Journal of Public Health, 80,* 467–469.

Gerbert, B., Maguire, B. T., Bleecker, T., Coates, T. J., & McPhee, S. J. (1991). Primary care physicians and AIDS: Attitudinal and structural barriers to care. *Journal of the American Medical Association, 266,* 2837–2842.

Geronimus, A. T., Bound, J., Waidmann, T. A., Hillemeier, M. M., & Burns, P. B. (1996). Excess mortality among blacks and whites in the United States. *New England Journal of Medicine, 335,* 1552–1558.

Gillies, P., Tolley, K., & Wolstenholme, J. (1996). Is AIDS a disease of poverty? *AIDS Care, 8,* 351–363.

Ginsburg, K. R., Slap, G. B., Cnaan, A., Forke, C. M., Balsley, C. M., & Rouselle, D. M. (1995). Adolescents' perceptions of factors affecting their decisions to seek health care. *Journal of the American Medical Association, 273,* 1913–1918.

Ginzburg, H. M., & Gostin, L. (1986). Legal and ethical issues associated with HTLV-III diseases. *Psychiatric Annals, 16,* 180–185.

Giulian, D., Vaca, K., & Noonan, C. A. (1990). Secretion of neurotoxins by mononuclear phagocytes infected with HIV-1. *Science, 250,* 1593–1596.

Glaser, J. B., Strange, T. J., & Rosati, D. (1989). Heterosexual human immunodeficiency virus transmission among the middle class. *Archives of Internal Medicine, 149,* 645–649.

Glaser, R., Kiecolt-Glaser, J., Speicher, C., & Holliday, J. (1985). Stress, loneliness, and changes in herpes virus latency. *Journal of Behavioral Medicine, 8,* 249–260.

Glasner, P. D., & Kaslow, R. A. (1990). The epidemiology of human immunodeficiency virus infection. *Journal of Consulting and Clinical Psychology, 58,* 13–21.

Glass, R. M. (1988). Editorial: AIDS and suicide. *Journal of the American Medical Association, 259,* 1369–1370.

Gochros, H. L. (1992). The sexuality of gay men with HIV infection. *Social Work, 37,* 105–109.

Goffman, E. (1963). *Stigma: Notes on the management of spoiled identity.* Englewood Cliffs, NJ: Prentice Hall.

Goggin, K., Engelson, E. S., Rabkin, J. G., & Kotler, D. P. (1997). *The relationship of mood, endocrine and sexual disorders in HIV+ women: An exploratory study.* Manuscript submitted for publication.

Goggin, K. J., Zisook, S., Heaton, R. K., Atkinson, J. H., Marshall, S., McCutchan, J. A., Chandler, J. L., & Grant, I. (1996). *Neuropsychological performance of HIV+ men with major depression.* Manuscript submitted for publication.

Gold, R. S., Skinner, M. J., & Ross, M. W. (1994). Unprotected anal intercourse in HIV-infected and non-HIV-infected gay men. *Journal of Sex Research, 31,* 69–77.

Golden, W. L., Gersh, W. D., & Robbins, D. M. (1992). *Psychological treatment of cancer patients: A cognitive-behavioral approach.* Needham Heights, MA: Allyn & Bacon.

Golombok, S., Sketchley, J., & Rust, J. (1989). Condom failure among homosexual men. *Journal of Acquired Immune Deficiency Syndromes and Human Retrovirology, 2,* 404–409.

Goodkin, K., Blaney, N. T., Feaster, D., Fletcher, M. A., Baum, M. K., Atienza, E. M., Klimas, N. G., Millon, C., Szapocznik, J., & Eisdorfer, C. (1992). Active coping style is associated with natural killer cell cytotoxicity in asymptomatic HIV-1 seropositive homosexual men. *Journal of Psychosomatic Research, 36,* 635–650.

Gordin, F. M., Nelson, E. T., Matts, J. P., Cohn, D. L., Ernst, J., Benator, D., Besch, C. L., Crane, L. R., Sampson, J. H., Bragg, P. S., El-Sadr, W., & the Terry Beirn Community Programs for Clinical Research on AIDS. (1996). The impact of human immunodeficiency virus infection on drug-resistant tuberculosis. *American Journal of Respiratory and Critical Care Medicine, 154*, 1478–1483.

Gordon, J. H., Ulrich, C., Feeley, M., & Pollack, S. (1993). Staff distress among hemophilia nurses. *AIDS Care, 5*, 359–367.

Gorman, J., Kertzner, R., Cooper, T., Goetz, R., Lagomasino, I., Novacenko, H., Williams, J., Stern, Y., Mayeux, R., & Ehrhardt, A. (1991). Glucocorticoid level and neuropsychiatric symptoms in homosexual men with HIV infection. *American Journal of Psychiatry, 148*, 41–45.

Gostin, L. O. (1989). Public health strategies for confronting AIDS: Legislative and regulatory policy in the United States. *Journal of the American Medical Association, 261*, 1621–1630.

Goudsmit, J. (1997). *Viral sex: The nature of AIDS.* New York: Oxford University Press.

Grady, W. R., Klepinger, D. H., Billy, J. O., & Tanfer, K. (1993). Condom characteristics: The perspectives and preferences of men in the United States. *Family Planning Perspectives, 25*, 67–73.

Graham, N., Zeger, S., Park, L., Vermund, S., Detels, R., Rinaldo, C., & Phair, J. (1992). The effects on survival of early treatment of human immunodeficiency virus infection. *New England Journal of Medicine, 326*, 1037–1042.

Grant, D., & Anns, M. (1988). Counseling AIDS antibody-positive clients: Reactions and treatment. *American Psychologist, 18*, 72–74.

Grant, I., and Heaton, R. K. (1990). Human immunodeficiency virus-type 1 (HIV-1) and the brain. *Journal of Consulting and Clinical Psychology, 58*, 22–30.

Grant, I., Olshen, R. A., Atkinson, H., Heaton, R. K., Nelson, J., McCutchan, J. A., & Weinrich, J. D. (1993). Depressed mood does not explain neuropsychological deficits in HIV-infected persons. *Neuropsychology, 7*, 53–61.

Grant, L. M., & Ostrow, D. G. (1995). Perceptions of social support and psychological adaptation to sexually acquired HIV among White and African American men. *Social Work, 40*, 215–224.

Green, G. (1993). Editorial review: Social support and HIV. *AIDS Care, 5*, 87–104.

Greenberg, A. E., Thomas, P., Landesman, S., Mildvan, D., Seidlin, M., Friedland, G., Holzman, R., Starrett, B., Braun, J., & Bryan, E. (1992). The spectrum of HIV-1-related disease among outpatients in New York City. *AIDS, 6*, 849–859.

Greenberg, J. B., Johnson, W. D., & Fichtner, R. R. (1996). A community support group for HIV-seropositive drug users: Is attendance associated with reductions in risk behaviour? *AIDS Care, 8*, 529–540.

Greenblatt, R. M., Hollander, H., McMaster, J. R., & Henke, C. J. (1991). Polypharmacy among patients attending an AIDS clinic: Utilization of prescribed, unorthodox, and investigational treatments. *Journal of Acquired Immune Deficiency Syndromes and Human Retrovirology, 4*, 136–143.

Greenspan, J. S., & Greenspan, D. (1992). Oral lesions associated with HIV infection. In G. P. Wormser (Ed.), *AIDS and other manifestations of HIV infection* (2nd ed., pp. 489–498). New York: Raven Press.

Greenspan, J. S., Greenspan, D., & Winkler, J. (1992). Oral complications of HIV infection. In M. A. Sande & P. A. Volberding (Eds.), *The medical management of AIDS* (3rd ed., pp. 161–175). Philadelphia: Saunders.

Greenwood, D. U. (1991). Neuropsychological aspects of AIDS dementia complex: What clinicians need to know. *Professional Psychology: Research and Practice, 22*, 407–409.

Greer, S., Morris, T., & Pettingale, K. W. (1979). Psychological responses to breast cancer: Effect on outcome. *The Lancet, 2*(8146), 785–787.

Gresenguet, G., Kreiss, J., Chapko, M., Hillier, S., & Weiss, N. (1997). HIV infection and vaginal douching in Central Africa. *AIDS, 11*, 101–106.

Griffiths, K., & Wilkins, E. G. L. (July, 1993). *Patterns of coping with an HIV+ diagnosis: Psychological responses, threat appraisal, and stress mediation.* Paper presented at the Ninth International AIDS Conference, Berlin, Germany.

Grossman, A. H. (1991). Gay men and HIV/AIDS: Understanding the double stigma. *Journal of the Association of Nurses in AIDS Care, 2*, 28–32.

Grossman, A. H., & Silverstein, C. (1993). Facilitating support groups for professionals working with people with AIDS. *Social Work, 38*, 144–151.

Guccione, B. (1993, September). Interview with professor Peter Duesberg. *Spin*, pp. 95–108.

Gulick, R. M., Mellors, J. W., Havlir, D., Eron, J. J., Gonzalez, C., McMahon, D., Richman, D. D., Valentine, F. T., Jonas, L., Meibohm, A., Emini, E. A., & Chodakewitz, J. A. (1997). Treatment with indinavir, zidovudine, and lamivudine in adults with human immunodeficiency virus infection and prior antiretroviral therapy. *New England Journal of Medicine, 337*, 734–739.

Gwinn, M., Pappaioanou, M., George, R., Hannon, H., Wasser, S. C., Redus, M. A., Hoff, R., Grady, G. F., Willoughby, A., Novello, A. C., Petersen, L. R., Dondero, T. J., & Curran, J. W. (1991). Prevalence of HIV infection in childbearing women in the United States. *Journal of the American Medical Association, 265*, 1704–1708.

Haas, J. S., Weissman, J. S., Cleary, P. D., Goldberg, J., Gatsonis, C., Seage, G. R., Fowler, F. J., Massagli, M. P., Makadon, H. J., & Epstein, A. M. (1993). Discussion of preferences for life-sustaining care by persons with AIDS. *Archives of Internal Medicine, 153*, 1241–1248.

Haburchak, D. R., Harrison, S. M., Miles, F. W., & Hannon, R. N. (1989). Resolving patient feelings of guilt: A need for physician-chaplain liaison. *AIDS Patient Care, 3*, 42–43.

Hackl, K., Kalichman, S. C., & Somlai, A. (1995, February). *Women with HIV/AIDS: The dual challenges of patient and primary caregiver.* Paper presented at the HIV Infection in Women Conference, Washington, DC.

Hackl, K. L., Somlai, A., Kelly, J. A., & Kalichman, S. C. (1997). Women living with HIV/AIDS: The dual challenges of being a medical patient and a primary family caregiver. *Health and Social Work, 22*, 53–62.

Halstead, S., Riccio, M., Harlow, P., Oretti, R., & Thompson, C. (1988). Psychosis associated with HIV infection. *British Journal of Psychiatry, 153*, 618–623.

Hamburg, M. A., Koenig, S., & Fauci, A. S. (1990). Immunology of AIDS and HIV infection. In G. L. Mandell, R. G. Douglas, & J. E. Bennett (Eds.), *Principles and practice of infectious diseases* (pp. 1046–1059). New York: Churchill Livingstone.

Hammer, S. M., Katzenstein, D., Hughes, M., Gundacker, H., Schooley, R., Haubrich, R., Henry, K., Lederman, M., Phair, J., Niu, M., Hirsch, M., & Merigan, T. (1996). A trial comparing nucleoside monotherapy with combination therapy in HIV-infected adults with CD4 cell counts from 200 to 500 per cubic millimeter. *New England Journal of Medicine, 335,* 1081–1090.

Hammer, S. M., Squires, K. E., Hughes, M. D., Grimes, J. M., Demeter, L. M., Currier, J. S., Eron, J. J., Feinberg, J. E., Balfour, H. H., Deyton, L. R., Chodakewitz, J. A., & Fischl, M. A. (1997). A controlled trial of two nucleoside analogues plus indinavir in persons with human immunodeficiency virus infection and CD4 cell counts of 200 per cubic millimeter or less. *New England Journal of Medicine, 337,* 725–733.

Hankins, C., Gendron, S., Tran, T., Lamping, N., & LaPointe, J. (1997). Sexuality in Montreal women living with HIV. *AIDS Care, 9,* 261–272.

Hanson, M., Kramer, T. H., Gross, W., Quintana, J., Li, P. W., & Asher, R. (1992). AIDS awareness and risk behaviors among dually disordered adults. *AIDS Education and Prevention, 4,* 1–51.

Hardy, A. (1991). Long-term survivor collaborative study group: Characterization of long-term survivors of AIDS. *Journal of Acquired Immune Deficiency Syndromes and Human Retrovirology, 4,* 386–391.

Hart, G., Fitzpatrick, R., McLean, J., Dawson, J., & Boulton, M. (1990). Gay men, social support and HIV disease: A study of social integration in the gay community. *AIDS Care, 2,* 163–170.

Hatcher, R. A., Guest, F., Stewart, F., Stewart, G. K., Trussell, J., Bowen, S. C., & Cates, W. (1988). *Contraceptive technology 1988–1989* (14th ed., Rev.). New York: Irvington.

Haverkos, H. W., & Battjes, R. J. (1992). Female-to-male transmission of HIV. *Journal of the American Medical Association, 268,* 1855–1856.

Haverkos, H. W., & Quinn, T. C. (1995). The third wave: HIV infection among heterosexuals in the United States and Europe. *International Journal of STD and AIDS, 6,* 227–232.

Haynes, B. F., Pantaleo, G., & Fauci, A. S. (1996). Toward an understanding of the correlates of protective immunity to HIV infection. *Science, 271,* 324–328.

Hays, R. B., Catania, J. A., McKusick, L., & Coates, T. J. (1990). Help-seeking for AIDS-related concerns: A comparison of gay men with various HIV diagnoses. *American Journal of Community Psychology, 18,* 743–755.

Hays, R. B., Chauncey, S., & Tobey, L. A. (1990). The social support networks of gay men with AIDS. *Journal of Community Psychology, 18,* 374–385.

Hays, R. B., Magee, R. H., & Chauncey, S. (1994). Identifying helpful and unhelpful behaviours of loved ones: The PWA's perspective. *AIDS Care, 6,* 379–392.

Hays, R. B., Turner, H., & Coates, T. J. (1992). Social support, AIDS-related symptoms, and depression among gay men. *Journal of Consulting and Clinical Psychology, 60,* 463–469.

Hays, R. D., Cunningham, W. E., Ettl, M. K., Beck, C. K., & Shapiro, M. F. (1995). Health-related quality of life in HIV disease. *Assessment, 2,* 363–380.

Hays, R. D., Wells, K., Sherbourne, C., Rogers, W., & Spitzer, K. (1995). Functioning and well-being outcomes of patients with depression compared with chronic general medical illnesses. *Archives of General Psychiatry, 52,* 11–19.

Hecht, F. M. (1997, December). *Adherence to HIV treatment.* Paper presented at the meeting of Clinical Care of the AIDS Patients, San Francisco, California.

Heckman, T. G., Kelly, J. A., & Somlai, A. M. (in press). Predictors of continued high-risk sexual behavior in a community sample of persons living with HIV/AIDS. *AIDS and Behavior.*

Heckman, T. G., Somlai, A. M., Kalichman, S. C., Franzoi, S. L., & Kelly, J. A. (in press). Psychosocial differences between urban and rural persons living with HIV/AIDS. *Journal of Rural Health.*

Heckman, T. G., Somlai, A. M., Otto-Salau, L., & Davantes, B. R. (in press). Health-related quality of life among people living with HIV disease in small communities and rural areas. *Psychology and Health.*

Heckman, T. G., Somlai, A. M., Sikkema, K. J., Kelly, J. A., & Franzoi, S. L. (1997). Psychosocial predictors of life satisfaction among persons living with HIV infection and AIDS. *Journal of the Association of Nurses in AIDS Care, 8,* 21–30.

Hedge, B., & Glover, L. F. (1990). Group intervention with HIV seropositive patients and their partners. *AIDS Care, 2,* 147–154.

Hein, K. (1990). Lessons from New York City on HIV/AIDS in adolescents. *New York State Journal of Medicine, 90,* 143–145.

Hellinger, F. (1990). Updated forecasts of the costs of medical care for persons with AIDS, 1989–93. *Public Health Reports, 105,* 1–12.

Hellinger, F. J. (1993). The lifetime cost of treating a person with HIV. *Journal of the American Medical Association, 270,* 474–478.

Henderson, D. K., Saah, A. J., Zak, B. J., Kaslow, R. A., Lane, H. C., Folks, T., Blackwelder, W. C., Schmitt, J., LaCamera, D. J., Masur, H., & Fauci, A. S. (1986). Risk of nosocomial infection with human T-cell lymphocyte virus type-III/lymphadenopathy-associated virus in a large cohort of intensively exposed health care workers. *Annals of Internal Medicine, 104,* 644–647.

Henrad, D. R., Phillips, J. F., Muenz, L. R., Blattner, W. A., Wiesner, D., Eyster, M. E., & Goedert, J. J. (1995). Natural history of HIV-1 cell-free viremia. *Journal of the American Medical Association, 274,* 554–558.

Herbert, T. B., & Cohen, S. (1993). Depression and immunity: A meta-analytic review. *Psychological Bulletin, 113,* 472–486.

Herek, G. (1990). Illness, stigma, and AIDS. In G. M. Herek, S. M. Levy, S. Maddi, S. Taylor, & D. Wertlieb (Eds.), *Psychological aspects of chronic illness: Chronic conditions, fatal diseases, and clinical care* (pp. 7–60). Washington, DC: American Psychological Association.

Herek, G. M., & Capitanio, J. P. (1993). Public reactions to AIDS in the United States: A second decade of stigma. *American Journal of Public Health, 83,* 574–577.

Herek, G. M., & Glunt, E. K. (1988). An epidemic of stigma: Public reactions to AIDS. *American Psychologist, 43,* 886–891.

Herndier, B. G., Kaplan, L. D., & McGrath, M. S. (1994). Pathogenesis of AIDS lymphomas. *AIDS, 8,* 1025–1049.

Higgins, D. L., Galavotti, C., O'Reilly, K. R., Schnell, D. J., Moore, M., Rugg, D. L., & Johnson, R. (1991). Evidence for the effects of HIV antibody counseling and testing on risk behavior. *Journal of the American Medical Association, 266,* 2419–2429.

Hinkin, C. H., van Gorp, W. G., Satz, P., Weisman, J. D., Thommes, J., & Buckingham, S. (1992). Depressed mood and its relationship to neuropsychological test performance in HIV-1 seropositive individuals. *Journal of Clinical and Experimental Neuropsychology, 14,* 289–297.

Hintz, S., Kuck, J., Peterkin, J. J., Volk, D. M., & Zisook, S. (1990). Depression in the context of human immunodeficiency virus infection: Implications for treatment. *Journal of Clinical Psychiatry, 51,* 497–501.

Hirsch, M., Schooley, R., Ho, D., & Kaplan, J. (1984). Possible viral interactions in the acquired immunodeficiency syndrome (AIDS). *Reviews of Infectious Diseases, 6,* 726–731.

Hirsch, M. S., Wormser, G. P., Schooley, R. T., Ho, D. D., Felsenstein, D., Hopkins, C. C., Joline, C., Duncanson, F., Sarngadharan, M. G., Saxinger, C., & Gallo, R. C. (1985). Risk of nosocomial infection with human T-cell lymphotropic virus III (HTLV-III). *New England Journal of Medicine, 312,* 1–4.

Hirschtick, R. E., Glassroth, J., Jordan, M. C., Wilcosky, T. C., Wallace, J. M., Kvale, P. A., Markowitz, N., Rosen, M. J., Mangura, B. T., & Hopewell, P. C. (1995). Bacterial pneumonia in persons infected with the human immunodeficiency virus. *New England Journal of Medicine, 333,* 845–851.

Ho, D. D. (1995). Time to hit HIV, early and hard. *New England Journal of Medicine, 333,* 450–451.

Ho, D. D. (1996). Therapy of HIV infections: Problems and prospects. *Bulletin of the New York Academy of Medicine, 73,* 37–45.

Ho, D. D., Bredesen, D. E., Vinters, H. V., & Daar, E. S. (1989). The acquired immunodeficiency syndrome (AIDS) dementia complex. *Annals of Internal Medicine, 111,* 400–410.

Hogg, R. S., Heath, K. V., Yip, B., Craib, K. J., O'Shaughnessy, M. V., Schechter, M. T., & Montaner, J. S. G. (1998). Improved survival among HIV-infected individuals following initiation of antiretroviral therapy. *Journal of the American Medical Association, 279,* 450–454.

Hogg, R. S., Strathdee, S. A., Craib, K. J., O'Shaughnessy, M. V., Montaner, J. S., & Schechter, M. T. (1994). Lower socioeconomic status and shorter survival following HIV infection. *The Lancet, 344,* 1120–1124.

Holland, H. K., Saral, R., Rossi, J., Donnenberg, A., Burns, W., Beschorner, W., Farzadegan, H., Jones, R., Quinnan, G., Vogelsang, G., Vriesendorp, H., Wingard, J., Zaia, J., & Santos, G. (1989). Allogeneic bone marrow transplantation, zidovudine, and human immunodeficiency virus type 1 (HIV-1) infection. *Annals of Internal Medicine, 111,* 973–981.

Holland, J. (1982). Psychological aspects of cancer. In J. Holland & E. Frei

(Eds.), *Cancer medicine* (2nd ed., pp. 1175–1203). Philadelphia: Lea & Febiger.

Hoover, D. R., Saah, A. J., Bagellar, H., Phair, J., Detels, R., Anderson, R., & Kaslow, R. A. (1993). Clinical manifestations of AIDS in the era of pneumocystis prophylaxis. *New England Journal of Medicine, 329,* 1922–1926.

Hopewell, P. C. (1992). *Pneumocystis carinii* pneumonia: Current concepts. In M. A. Sande & P. A. Volberding (Eds.), *The medical management of AIDS* (3rd ed., pp. 261–283). Philadelphia: Saunders.

Hopewell, P. C. (1997). Tuberculosis in persons with human immunodeficiency virus infection. In M. A. Sande & P. A. Volberding (Eds.), *The medical management of AIDS* (5th ed., pp. 311–326). Philadelphia: Saunders.

Horsburgh, C. R. (1991). *Mycobacterium avium* complex infection in the acquired immunodeficiency syndrome. *New England Journal of Medicine, 324,* 1332–1338.

Horstman, W. R., & McKusick, L. (1986). The impact of AIDS on the physician. In L. McKusick (Ed.), *What to do about AIDS: Physicians and mental health professionals discuss the issues* (pp. 63–74). Berkeley: University of California Press.

House, J. S., Landis, K. R., & Umberson, D. (1988). Social relationships and health. *Science, 241,* 540–545.

Huggins, J., Elman, N., Baker, C., Forrester, R., & Lyter, D. (1991). Affective and behavioral responses of gay and bisexual men to HIV antibody testing. *Social Work, 36,* 61–66.

Humphry, D. (1991). *Final exit: The practicalities of self-deliverance and assisted suicide for dying patients.* Secaucus, NJ: Carol.

Huston, D. P. (1997). The biology of the immune system. *Journal of the American Medical Association, 278,* 1804–1814.

Hutchinson, C. M., Wilson, C., Reichart, C. A., Marsiglia, V. C., Zenilman, J. M., & Hook, E. W. (1991). CD4 lymphocyte concentrations in patients with newly identified HIV infection attending STD clinics: Potential impact on policy funded health care resources. *Journal of the American Medical Association, 266,* 253–256.

Ickovics, J. R., & Meisler, A. W. (in press). Adherence in AIDS clinical trials: A framework for clinical research and clinical care. *Journal of Clinical Epidemiology.*

Ickovics, J. R., & Rodin, J. (1992). Women and AIDS in the United States: Epidemiology, natural history, and mediating mechanisms. *Health Psychology, 11,* 1–16.

Imagawa, D. T., Lee, M., Wolinsky, S., Sano, K., Morales, F., & Kwok, S. (1989). Human immunodeficiency virus type 1 infection in homosexual men who remain seronegative for prolonged periods. *New England Journal of Medicine, 320,* 1458–1462.

Imperato, P. J., Feldman, J. G., Nayeri, K., & DeHovitz, J. A. (1988). Medical students' attitudes towards caring for patients with AIDS in a high incidence area. *New York State Journal of Medicine, 88,* 223–227.

Inciardi, J. A. (1994). HIV/AIDS risks among male, heterosexual noninjecting drug users who exchange crack for sex. In R. Battjes, Z. Sloboda, & F. W. Grace (Eds.), *The context of HIV risk among drug users and their sexual partners: NIDA Research Monograph* (Vol. 143). Washington, DC: NIDA.

Ironson, G., LaPerriere, A., Antoni, M., O'Hearn, P., Schneiderman, N., Klimas, N., & Fletcher, M. (1990). Changes in immune and psychological measures as a function of anticipation and reaction to news of HIV-1 antibody status. *Psychosomatic Medicine, 52,* 247–270.

Israelski, D. M., & Remington, J. S. (1992). AIDS-associated toxoplasmosis. In M. A. Sande & P. A. Volberding (Eds.), *The medical management of AIDS* (3rd ed., pp. 319–345). Philadelphia: Saunders.

Jackson, G., Perkins, J., Rubenis, M., Paul, D., Knigge, M., Despotes, J., & Spencer, P. (1988). Passive immunoneutralisation of human immunodeficiency virus in patients with advanced AIDS. *The Lancet, 1,* 647–652.

Jacobsberg, L., Frances, A., & Perry, S. (1995). Axis II diagnoses among volunteers for HIV testing and counseling. *American Journal of Psychiatry, 152,* 1222–1224.

Jacobsen, P., Perry, S., & Hirsch, D. A. (1990). Behavioral and psychological responses to HIV antibody testing. *Journal of Consulting and Clinical Psychology, 58,* 31–37.

Jacobson, M. (1992). Mycobacterial diseases: Tuberculosis and disseminated

Mycobacterial avium complex infection. In M. A. Sande & P. A. Volberding (Eds.), *The medical management of AIDS* (3rd ed., pp. 284–296). Philadelphia: Saunders.

Jacobson, M. A. (1997). Disseminated *Mycobacterium avium* complex and other bacterial infections. In M. A. Sande & P. A. Volberding (Eds.), *The medical management of AIDS* (5th ed., pp. 301–310). Philadelphia: Saunders.

Jacobson, M. A., Bacchetti, P., Kolokathis, A., Chaisson, R. E., Szabo, S., Polsky, B., Valainis, G. T., Mildvan, D., Abrams, D., Wilber, J., Winger, E., Sacks, H. S., Hendricksen, C., & Moss, A. (1991). Surrogate markers for survival in patients with AIDS and AIDS related complex treated with zidovudine. *British Journal of Medicine, 302,* 73–78.

Janssen, R. S., Cornblath, D. R., Epstein, L. G., Foa, R. P., McArthur, J. C., & Price, R. W. (1991). Nomenclature and research case definitions for neurologic manifestations of human immunodeficiency virus-type 1 (HIV-1) infection. *Neurology, 41,* 778–785.

Jemmott, J., & Locke, S. (1984). Psychosocial factors, immunologic mediation, and human susceptibility to infectious diseases: How much do we know? *Psychological Bulletin, 95,* 78–108.

Jenike, M. A., & Pato, C. (1986). Case report: Disabling fear of AIDS responsive to imipramine. *Psychosomatics, 27,* 143–144.

Jillson-Boostrom, I. (1992). The impact of HIV on minority populations. In P. I. Ahmed & N. Ahmed (Eds.), *Living and dying with AIDS* (pp. 235–254). New York: Plenum.

Johnston, D., Stall, R., & Smith, K. (1995). Reliance by gay men and intravenous drug users on friends and family for AIDS-related care. *AIDS Care, 7,* 307–319.

Jones, M., Klimes, I., & Catalan, J. (1994). Psychosexual problems in people with HIV infection: Controlled study of gay men and men with haemophilia. *AIDS Care, 6,* 587–593.

Joseph, J., Montgomery, S., Emmons, C., Kirscht, J., Kessler, R., Ostrow, D., Wortman, C., O'Brien, K., Eller, M., & Eshleman, S. (1987). Perceived risk of AIDS: Assessing the behavioral and psychosocial consequences in a cohort of gay men. *Journal of the American Medical Association, 322,* 1788–1793.

Judd, F. K., Mijch, A. M., & Cockram, A. (1995). Fluoxetine treatment of depressed patients with HIV infection. *Australian and New Zealand Journal of Psychiatry, 29*, 433–436.

Kain, C. (1996). *HIV affirmative counseling*. Alexandria, VA: American Counseling Association.

Kalichman, S. C. (1993). *Mandated reporting of suspected child abuse: Ethics, law, and policy*. Washington, DC: American Psychological Association.

Kalichman, S. C. (1995). *Understanding AIDS: A Guide for Mental Health Professionals*. Washington, DC: American Psychological Association.

Kalichman, S. C. (in press). Post-exposure prophylaxis for HIV infection in gay and bisexual men: Implications for the future of HIV prevention. *American Journal of Preventive Medicine*.

Kalichman, S. C., & Behavioral Intervention Research Branch, CDC. (1996). Continued sexual risk behavior among HIV seropositive, drug-using men—Atlanta, Washington, DC, and San Juan, Puerto Rico, 1993. *Morbidity and Mortality Weekly Report, 45*, 150–152.

Kalichman, S. C., Belcher, L., Cherry, C., Williams, E. A., Sanders, M., & Allers, C. (1998). Risk for human immunodeficiency virus (HIV) infection and use of cocaine among indigent African American men. *American Journal of Health Behavior, 22*, 141–150.

Kalichman, S. C., Carey, M. P., & Carey, K. B. (1996). Human immunodeficiency virus (HIV) risk among the seriously mentally ill. *Clinical Psychology: Science and Practice, 3*, 130–143.

Kalichman, S. C., Cherry, C., Williams, E., Nachimson, D., Abush-Kirsh, T., Schaper, P., Belcher, L., & Smith, S. (1997). Oral sex anxiety and its relationship to oral sexual behavior and perceptions of risk among gay and bisexual men. *Journal of the Gay and Lesbian Medical Association, 1*, 157–164.

Kalichman, S. C., Greenberg, J., & Abel, G. G. (1997). Sexual compulsivity among HIV positive men who engage in high-risk sexual behavior with multiple partners: An exploratory study. *AIDS Care, 9*, 443–452.

Kalichman, S. C., Hunter, T. L., & Kelly, J. A. (1992). Perceptions of AIDS risk susceptibility among minority and nonminority women at risk for HIV infection. *Journal of Consulting and Clinical Psychology, 60*, 725–732.

Kalichman, S. C., Kelly, J. A., Johnson, J., & Bulton, M. (1994). Factors associated with risk for human immunodeficiency virus (HIV) infection among chronic mentally ill adults. *American Journal of Psychiatry, 151,* 221–227.

Kalichman, S. C., Kelly, J. A., & Rompa, D. (1997). Continued high-risk sex among HIV seropositive men. *Health Psychology, 16,* 369–373.

Kalichman, S. C., & Nachimson, D. (1998). *Psychological and social factors associated with high-risk sexual behavior among people living with HIV– AIDS.* Manuscript submitted for publication.

Kalichman, S. C., Nachimson, D., Cherry, C., & Williams, E. (in press). *AIDS treatment advances and behavioral prevention set-backs: Preliminary assessment of reduced threat perceptions. Health Psychology.*

Kalichman, S. C., Roffman, R., & Picciano, J. (1997). Sexual relationships and sexual risk behaviors among human immunodeficiency virus (HIV) seropositive gay and bisexual men seeking risk reduction services. *Professional Psychology: Research and Practice, 28,* 355–360.

Kalichman, S. C., Roffman, R., Picciano, J., & Balan, M. (in press). Risk of human immunodeficiency virus (HIV) infection among gay and bisexual men seeking HIV-prevention services and risks posed to their female partners. *Health Psychology.*

Kalichman, S. C., Sikkema, K., & Somlai, A. (1995). Assessing persons with human immunodeficiency virus (HIV) infection using the Beck Depression Inventory: Disease processes and other potential confounds. *Journal of Personality Assessment, 64,* 86–100.

Kalichman, S. C., Sikkema, K. J., & Somlai, A. (1996). People living with HIV infection who attend and do not attend support groups: A pilot study of needs, characteristics and experiences. *AIDS Care, 8,* 589–599.

Kalichman, S. C., Somlai, A., Adair, V., & Weir, S. (1996). Psychological and social factors associated with HIV testing among sexually transmitted disease clinic patients. *Psychology and Health, 11,* 593–604.

Kalish, R. A. (1985). *Death, grief, and caring relationships* (2nd ed.). Monterey, CA: Brooks/Cole.

Kandel, E. R., Schwartz, J. H., & Jessell, T. M. (1991). *Principles of neural science* (3rd ed.). Norwalk, CT: Appleton & Lange.

Kaplan, L. D., & Northfelt, D. W. (1992). Malignancies associated with

AIDS. In M. A. Sande & P. A. Volberding (Eds.), *The medical management of AIDS* (3rd ed., pp. 399–429). Philadelphia: Saunders.

Kaplan, L. D. & Northfelt, D. W. (1997). Malignancies associated with AIDS. In M. A. Sande & P. A. Volberding (Eds.), *The medical management of AIDS* (5th ed., pp. 413–442). Philadelphia: Saunders.

Karasu, T. B., Docherty, J. P., Gelenberg, A., Kupfer, D. J., Merriam, A. E., & Shadoan, R. (1993). Practice guideline for major depressive disorder in adults. *American Journal of Psychiatry, 150*(Suppl.), 4–26.

Karon, J. M., Dondero, T. J., & Curran, J. W. (1988). The projected incidence of AIDS and estimated prevalence of HIV infection in the United States. *Journal of Acquired Immune Deficiency Syndromes and Human Retrovirology, 1*, 542–550.

Kaslow, R. A., Phair, J. P., Friedman, H. B., Lyter, D., Solomon, R. E., Dudley, J., Polk, F., & Blackwelder, W. (1987). Infection with the human immunodeficiency virus: Clinical manifestations and their relationship to immune deficiency. *Annals of Internal Medicine, 107*, 474–480.

Kassler, W. J. (1997). Advances in HIV testing technology and their potential impact on prevention. *AIDS Education and Prevention, 9*, 27–40.

Katz, M. H., Douglas, J. M., Bolan, G. A., Marx, R., Sweat, M., Park, M.-S., & Buchbinder, S. P. (1996). Depression and use of mental health services among HIV-infected men. *AIDS Care, 8*, 433–442.

Katz, M., & Gerberding, J. L. (1997). Postexposure treatment of people exposed to the human immunodeficiency virus through sexual contact or injection drug use. *New England Journal of Medicine, 336*, 1097–1100.

Katzenstein, D. A., Hammer, S. H., Hughes, M. D., Gundacker, H., Jackson, J. B., Fiscus, S., Rasheed, S., Elbeik, T., Reichman, R., Japour, A., Merigan, T. C., & Hirsch, M. S. (1996). The relation of virologic and immunologic to clinical outcomes after nucleoside therapy in HIV-infected adults with 200–500 CD4 cells per cubic millimeter. *New England Journal of Medicine, 335*(15), 1091–1098.

Kedes, D. H., Ganem, D., Ameli, N., Bacchetti, P., & Greenblatt, R. (1997). The prevalence of serum antibody to human herpesvirus 8 (Kaposi sarcoma-associated herpesvirus) among HIV-seropositive and high-risk HIV-seronegative women. *Journal of the American Medical Association, 277*, 478–481.

Keet, I. P. M., van Lent, N. A., Sandfort, T. G. M., Coutinho, R. A., & van Griensven, J. P. (1992). Orogenital sex and transmission of HIV among homosexual men. *AIDS, 6,* 223–226.

Kegeles, S. M., Coates, T. J., Christopher, T. A., & Lazarus, J. L. (1989). Perceptions of AIDS: The continuing saga of AIDS-related stigma. *AIDS, 3*(Suppl.), S253–S258.

Kegeles, S. M., Coates, T. J., Lo, B., & Catania, J. A. (1989). Mandatory reporting of HIV testing would deter men from being tested. *Journal of the American Medical Association, 261,* 1275–1276.

Kelly, J. A. (1991). Changing the behavior of an HIV-seropositive man who practices unsafe sex. *Hospital and Community Psychiatry, 42,* 239–240, 264.

Kelly, J. A. (1996). *Changing HIV risk behavior.* New York: Guilford Press.

Kelly, J. A., Heckman, T. G., Helfrich, S. E., Mence, R., Adair, V., & Broyles, L. (1995). HIV risk factors and behaviors in a Milwaukee homeless shelter. *American Journal of Public Health, 85,* 1585.

Kelly, J. A., & Kalichman, S. C. (1997). Increased attention to human sexuality can improve HIV/AIDS prevention efforts: Key research issues and directions. *Journal of Consulting and Clinical Psychology, 63,* 907–918.

Kelly, J. A., Kalichman, S. C., Kauth, M., Kilgore, H., Hood, H., Campos, P., Rao, S., et al. (1991). Situational factors associated with AIDS risk behavior lapses and coping strategies used by gay men who successfully avoid lapses. *American Journal of Public Health, 81,* 1335–1338.

Kelly, J. A., Murphy, D. A., Bahr, G. R., Kalichman, S. C., Morgan, M. G., Stevenson, L. Y., Koob, J. J., Brasfield, T. L., & Bernstein, B. M. (1993). Outcome of cognitive-behavioral and support group brief therapies for depressed persons diagnosed with HIV infection. *American Journal of Psychiatry, 150,* 1679–1680.

Kelly, J. A., Murphy, D. A., Bahr, G. R., Koob, J., Morgan, M., Kalichman, S. C., Stevenson, L. Y., Brasfield, T. L., Bernstein, B., & St. Lawrence, J. (1993). Factors associated with severity of depression and high-risk sexual behavior among persons diagnosed with human immunodeficiency virus (HIV) infection. *Health Psychology, 12,* 215–219.

Kelly, J. A., Murphy, D. A., Roffman, R. A., Solomon, L. J., Winnett, R. A., Stevenson, L. Y., Koob, J., Ayotte, D., Flynn, B., Desiderato, L., Hauth, A., Lemke, A., Lombard, D., Morgan, M., Norman, A., Sikkema, K., Steiner,

S., & Yaffe, D. (1992). Acquired immunodeficiency syndrome/human immunodeficiency virus risk behavior among gay men in small cities. *Archives of Internal Medicine, 152,* 2293–2297.

Kelly, J. A., St. Lawrence, J. S., Smith, S., Hood, H. V., & Cook, D. J. (1987a). Medical students' attitudes toward AIDS and homosexual patients. *Journal of Medical Education, 62,* 549–556.

Kelly, J. A., St. Lawrence, J. S., Smith, S., Hood, H. V., & Cook, D. J. (1987b). Stigmatization of AIDS patients by physicians. *American Journal of Public Health, 77,* 789–791.

Kelly, J., & Sykes, P. (1989). Helping the helpers: A support group for family members of persons with AIDS. *Social Work, 34,* 239–242.

Kemeny, M. E. (1991). Psychological factors, immune processes, and the course of herpes simplex and human immunodeficiency virus infection. In N. Plotnikoff, A. Murgo, R. Faith, & J. Wybran (Eds.), *Stress and immunity* (pp. 199–210). Boca Raton, FL: CRC Press.

Kemeny, M. E., Cohen, F., Zegans, L. S., & Conant, M. A. (1989). Psychological and immunological predictors of genital herpes recurrence. *Psychosomatic Medicine, 51,* 195–208.

Kemeny, M. E., Weiner, H., Taylor, S. E., Schneider, S., Visscher, B., & Fahey, J. L. (1994). Repeated bereavement, depressed mood, and immune parameters in HIV seropositive and seronegative gay men. *Health Psychology, 13,* 14–24.

Kennedy, C. A., Skurnick, J., Wan, J., Quattrone, G., Sheffet, A., Quinones, M., Wang, W., & Louria, D. (1993). Psychological distress, drug and alcohol use as correlates of condom use in HIV-serodiscordant heterosexual couples. *AIDS, 7,* 1493–1499.

Kennedy, M., Scarlett, M. I., Duerr, A., & Chu, S. (1995). Assessing HIV risk among women who have sex with women: Scientific and communication issues. *Journal of the Medical Women's Association, 50,* 103–107.

Keogh, P., Allen, S., Almedal, C., & Temahagili, B. (1994). The social impact of HIV infection on women in Kigali, Rwanda: A prospective study. *Social Science in Medicine, 38,* 1047–1053.

Kermani, E. J., & Weiss, B. A. (1989). AIDS and confidentiality: Legal concept and its application in psychotherapy. *American Journal of Psychotherapy, 43,* 25–31.

Kertzner, R. M., Goetz, R., Todak, G., Cooper, T., Lin, S., Reddy, M., Novacenko, H., Williams, J., Ehrhardt, A., & Gorman, J. (1993). Cortisol levels, immune status and mood in homosexual men with and without HIV infection. *American Journal of Psychiatry, 150,* 1674–1678.

Kessler, R. C., Foster, C., Joseph, J., Ostrow, D., Wortman, C., Phair, J., & Chmiel, J. (1991). Stressful life events and symptom onset in HIV infection. *American Journal of Psychiatry, 148,* 733–738.

Kessler, R. C., O'Brien, K., Joseph, J. G., Ostrow, D. G., Phair, J. P., Chmiel, J. S., Wortman, C. B., & Emmons, C. A. (1988). Effects of HIV infection, perceived health and clinical status on a cohort at risk for AIDS. *Society of Science and Medicine, 27,* 569–578.

Kiecolt-Glaser, J., & Glaser, R. (1988a). Major life changes, chronic stress, and immunity. In T. P. Bridge, A. F. Mirsky, & F. K. Goodwin (Eds.), *Psychological, neuropsychiatric, and substance abuse aspects of AIDS* (pp. 217–224). New York: Raven Press.

Kiecolt-Glaser, J., & Glaser, R. (1988b). Psychological influences on immunity. *American Psychologist, 43,* 892–898.

Kiecolt-Glaser, J., Fisher, L., Ogrocki, P., Stout, J., Speicher, C., & Glaser, R. (1987). Marital quality, marital disruption, and immune function. *Psychosomatic Medicine, 49,* 13–34.

Kiecolt-Glaser, J., Garner, W., Speicher, C., Penn, G., Holliday, J., & Glaser, R. (1984). Psychosocial modifiers of immunocompetence in medical students. *Psychosomatic Medicine, 46,* 7–14.

Kiecolt-Glaser, J., Kennedy, S., Malkoff, S., Fisher, L., Speicher, C., & Glaser, R. (1988). Marital discord and immunity in males. *Psychosomatic Medicine, 50,* 213–229.

Killeen, M. E. (1993). Getting through our grief: For caregivers of persons with AIDS. *American Journal of Hospice and Palliative Care, 10,* 18–24.

Kinderman, S. S., Matteo, T. M., & Morales, E. (1993). HIV training and perceived competence among doctoral students in psychology. *Professional Psychology: Research and Practice, 24,* 224–227.

King, G., Delaronde, S. R., Dinoi, R., & Forsberg, A. D. (1996). Substance use, coping, and safer sex practices among adolescents with hemophilia and human immunodeficiency virus. *Journal of Adolescent Health, 18,* 435–441.

Kingsley, L. A., Detels, R., Kaslow, R., Polk, B. F., Rinaldo, C. R., & Chmiel, J. (1987). Risk factors for seroconversion to human immunodeficiency virus among male homosexuals. *The Lancet, 1*(8529), 345–349.

Kinloch-de Loes, S., Hirschel, B. J., Hoen, B., Cooper, D. A., Tindall, B., Carr, A., Saurat, J.-H., Clumeck, N., Lazzarin, A., Mathiesen, L., Raffi, F., Antunes, F., von Overbeck, J., Luthy, R., Glauser, M., Hawkins, D., Baumberger, C., Yerly, S., Perneger, T. V., & Perrin, L. (1995). A controlled trial of zidovudine in primary human immunodeficiency virus infection. *New England Journal of Medicine, 333*, 408–413.

Kippax, S., Crawford, J., Davis, M., Rodden, P., & Dowsett, G. (1993). Sustaining safe sex: A longitudinal sample of homosexual men. *AIDS, 7*, 257–263.

Kishlansky, M., Geary, P., & O'Brien, P. (1991). *Civilization in the West.* New York: HarperCollins.

Kitahata, M. M., Koepsell, T. D., Deyo, R. A., Maxwell, C. L., Dodge, W. T., & Wagner, E. H. (1996). Physician's experience with the acquired immunodeficiency syndrome as a factor in patients' survival. *New England Journal of Medicine, 334*, 701–706.

Kleck, R. E. (1968). Self-disclosure patterns of the nonobviously stigmatized. *Psychological Reports, 23*, 1239–1248.

Kleiber, D., Enzman, D., & Guzy, B. (1993). Stress and burnout among health care personnel in the field of AIDS: Causes and prevalence. In H. Van Dis & E. Van Dongen (Eds.), *Burnout in HIV/AIDS health care and support: Impact on professionals and volunteers* (pp. 23–40). Amsterdam: University of Amsterdam Press.

Kleinman, A. (1988). *The illness narratives: Suffering, healing and the human condition.* New York: Basic Books.

Kleinman, I. (1991). HIV transmission: Ethical and legal considerations in psychotherapy. *Cancer Journal of Psychiatry, 36*, 121–123.

Kloser, P., & Craig, J. (1994). *The woman's HIV sourcebook: A guide to better health and well-being.* Dallas, TX: Taylor.

Knapp, S., & VandeCreek, L. (1990). Application of the duty to protect HIV-positive patients. *Professional Psychology: Research and Practice, 21*, 161–166.

Knox, M. D., & Dow, M. G. (1989). Staff discomfort in working with

HIV spectrum patients [Abstract]. *International Conference on AIDS, 5,* 720.

Koblin, B. A.. Hessol, N. A., Zauber, A. G., Taylor, P. E., Buchbinder, S. P., Katz, M. H., & Stevens, C. E. (1996). Increased incidence of cancer among homosexual men, New York City and San Francisco, 1978–1990. *American Journal of Epidemiology, 144,* 916–923.

Koenig, H. G., Meador, K. G., Cohen, H., & Blazer, D. (1988). Depression in elderly hospitalized patients with medical illness. *Archives of Internal Medicine, 148,* 1929–1936.

Kokkevi, A., Hatzakis, G., Maillis, A., Pittadaki, J., Zalonis, J., Samartzis, D., Touloumi, G., Mandalaki, T., & Stefanis, C. (1991). Neuropsychological assessment of HIV-seropositive haemophiliacs. *AIDS, 5,* 1223–1229.

Koppel, B. S. (1992). Neurological complications of AIDS and HIV infection. In G. P. Wormser (Ed.), *AIDS and other manifestations of HIV infection* (2nd ed., pp. 315–348). New York: Raven Press.

Kotchick, B. A., Forehand, R., Brody, G., Armistead, L., Morse, E., Simon, P., & Clark, L. (in press). The impact of maternal HIV infection on parenting in inner-city African American families. *Journal of Clinical and Consulting Psychology.*

Kourtis, A. P., Ibegbu, C., Nahmias, A. J., Lee, F. K., Clark, W. S., Sawyer, M. K., & Neshiem, S. (1996). Early progression of disease in HIV-infected infants with thymus dysfunction. *New England Journal of Medicine, 335,* 1431–1436.

Kovacs, J. A. (1995). Toxoplasmosis in AIDS: Keeping the lid on. *Annals of Internal Medicine, 123,* 230–231.

Krikorian, R., & Worbel, A. J. (1991). Cognitive impairment in HIV infection. *AIDS, 5,* 1501–1507.

Krupp, L., Belman, A., & Schneidman, P. (1992). Progressive multifocal leukoencephalopathy and HIV-1 infection. In G. P. Wormser (Ed.), *AIDS and other manifestations of HIV infection* (2nd ed., pp. 409–418). New York: Raven Press.

Kübler-Ross, E. (1969). *On death and dying.* New York: Macmillan.

Kübler-Ross, E. (1975). *Death: The final stage of growth.* Englewood Cliffs, NJ: Prentice Hall.

Kübler-Ross, E. (1981). *Living with death and dying.* New York: Macmillan.

Kurdek, L. A. (1988). Perceived social support in gays and lesbians in cohabitating relationships. *Journal of Personality and Social Psychology, 54,* 504–509.

Kurdek, L. A., & Siesky, G. (1990). The nature and correlates of psychological adjustment in gay men with AIDS-related conditions. *Journal of Applied Social Psychology, 20,* 846–860.

Kuritzkes, D. R. (1996). Clinical significance of drug resistance in HIV-1 infection. *AIDS, 10*(Suppl. 5), S27–S31.

Kwitkowski, C. F., & Booth, R. E. (in press). HIV-seropositive drug users and unprotected sex. *AIDS and Behavior.*

Lackritz, E., Satten, G., Aberle-Grasse, J., Dodd, R., Raimondi, V., Janssen, R., Lewis, F., Notari, E., & Petersen, L. (1995). Estimated risk of transmission of the human immunodeficiency virus by screened blood in the United States. *New England Journal of Medicine, 333,* 1721–1725.

Lagakos, S., Fischl, M. A., Stein, D. S., Lim, L., & Volberding, P. (1991). Effects of zidovudine therapy in minority and other subpopulations with early HIV infection. *Journal of the American Medical Association, 266,* 2709–2712.

Lakey, B., & Cassady, P. B. (1990). Cognitive processes in perceived social support. *Journal of Personality and Social Psychology, 59,* 337–343.

Lamping, D. L., Abrahamowicz, M., Gilmore, N., Edgar, L., Grover, S. A., Tsoukas, C., Falutz, J., Lalonde, R., Hamel, M., & Darsigny, R. (1993, June). *A randomized, controlled trial to evaluate a psychosocial intervention to improve quality of life in HIV infection.* Paper presented at the Ninth International Conference on AIDS, Berlin, Germany.

Land, H., & Harangody, G. (1990). A support group for partners of persons with AIDS. *Families in Society: The Journal of Contemporary Human Services, 71,* 471–481.

Landau-Stanton, J., Clements, C. D., & Stanton, M. D. (1993). Psychotherapeutic intervention: From individual through group to extended network. In J. Landau-Stanton & C. D. Clements (Eds.), *AIDS, health, and mental health: A primary sourcebook* (pp. 214–266). New York: Brunner/Mazel.

LaPerriere, A., Schneiderman, N., Antoni, M., & Fletcher, M. (1990). Aerobic exercise and psychoneuroimmunology in AIDS research. In L. Temoshok & A. Baum (Eds.), *Psychological perspectives on AIDS: Etiology, prevention, and treatment* (pp. 259–286). Hillsdale, NJ: Erlbaum.

LaPerriere, A. R., Antoni, M. H., Schneiderman, N., Ironson, G., Klimas, N., Caralis, P., & Fletcher, M. A. (1990). Exercise intervention attenuates emotional distress and natural killer cell decrements following notification of positive serologic status for HIV-1. *Biofeedback and Self-Regulation, 15,* 229–242.

Laumann, E., Masi, C., & Zuckerman, E. (1997). Circumcision in the United States: Prevalence, prophylactic effects, and sexual practice. *Journal of the American Medical Association, 277,* 1052–1057.

Laurence, J. (1992). Viral cofactors in the pathogenesis of HIV disease. In G. P. Wormser (Ed.), *AIDS and other manifestations of HIV infection* (2nd ed., pp. 77–84). New York: Raven Press.

Lazarus, R. S., & Folkman, S. (1984). *Stress, appraisal, and coping.* New York: Springer.

Lee, B. L. (1997). Drug interactions and toxicities in patients with AIDS. In M. A. Sande & P. A. Volberding (Eds.), *The medical management of AIDS* (5th ed., pp. 125–142). Philadelphia: Saunders.

Leigh, J. P., Lubeck, D. P., Farnham, P. G., & Fries, J. F. (1995). Hours at work and employment status among HIV-infected patients. *AIDS, 9,* 81–88.

Lemp, G. F., Hirozawa, A. M., Givertz, D., Nieri, G. N., Anderson, L., Lindergren, M. L., & Janssen, R. S. (1994). Seroprevalence of HIV and risk behaviors among young homosexual and bisexual men. *Journal of the American Medical Association, 272,* 449–454.

Lemp, G. F., Payne, S. F., Neal, D., Temelso, T., & Rutherford, G. W. (1990). Survival trends for patients with AIDS. *Journal of the American Medical Association, 263,* 402–406.

Lennon, M. C., Martin, J. L., & Dean, L. (1990). The influence of social support on AIDS-related grief reaction among gay men. *Social Science and Medicine, 31,* 477–484.

Leonard, A. S. (1985). Employment discrimination against persons with AIDS. *University of Dayton Law Review, 10,* 681–703.

Leserman, J., Perkins, D., & Evans, D. (1992). Coping with the threat of AIDS: The role of social support. *American Journal of Psychiatry, 149,* 1514–1520.

Levine, A., Gill, P., & Salahuddin, S. (1992). Neoplastic complications of HIV infection. In G. P. Wormser (Ed.), *AIDS and other manifestations of HIV infection* (2nd ed., pp. 443–454). New York: Raven Press.

Levine, S. H., Bystritsky, A., Baron, D., & Jones, L. D. (1991). Group psychotherapy for HIV-seropositive patients with major depression. *American Journal of Psychotherapy, 45,* 413–424.

Levy, J. A. (1992). Viral and immunologic factors in HIV infection. In M. A. Sande & P. A. Volberding (Eds.), *The medical management of AIDS* (3rd ed., pp. 18–32). Philadelphia: Saunders.

Levy, J. A. (1996). Infection by human immunodeficiency virus-CD4 is not enough. *New England Journal of Medicine, 335,* 1528–1530.

Levy, J. A., Kaminsky, L. S., Morrow, W. J., Steimer, K., Luciw, P., Dina, D., Hoxie, J., & Oshiro, L. (1985). Infection by the retrovirus associated with the acquired immunodeficiency syndrome: Clinical, biological, and molecular features. *Annals of Internal Medicine, 103,* 689–699.

Levy, J. A., Kaminsky, R. M., & Bredesen, D. E. (1988). Central nervous system dysfunction in acquired immunodeficiency syndrome. *Journal of Acquired Immune Deficiency Syndromes and Human Retrovirology, 1,* 41–64.

Levy, J. A., Shimabukuro, J., Hollander, H., Mills, J., & Kaminsky, L. (1985). Isolation of AIDS-associated retroviruses from cerebrospinal fluid and brain of patients with neurological symptoms. *The Lancet, 2,* 586–588.

Lifson, A. R. (1988). Do alternative modes of transmission of human immunodeficiency virus exist? *Journal of the American Medical Association, 259,* 1353–1356.

Lifson, A. R., Hessol, N. A., Buchbinder, S., & Holmberg, S. (1991). The association of clinical conditions and serological tests with CD4+ lymphocyte counts in HIV-infected subjects without AIDS. *AIDS, 5,* 1209–1215.

Lifson, A. R., O'Malley, P., Hessol, N. A., Buchbinder, S. P., Cannon, L., & Rutherford, G. (1990). HIV seroconversion in two homosexual men after receptive oral intercourse with ejaculation: Implications for counseling concerning safe sex. *American Journal of Public Health, 81,* 1509–1511.

Lindsay, M. K., Peterson, H. B., Boring, J., Gramling, J., Willis, S., & Klein, L. (1992). Crack cocaine: A risk factor for human immunodeficiency virus infection type 1 among inner-city patients. *Obstetrics and Gynecology, 80,* 981–984.

Linn, J. G., Lewis, F. M., Cain, V. A., & Kimbrough, G. A. (1993). HIV-illness, social support, sense of coherence, and psychosocial well-being in a sample of help-seeking adults. *AIDS Education and Prevention, 5,* 254–262.

Lipowski, Z. J. (1988). Somatization: The concept and its clinical application. *American Journal of Psychiatry, 145,* 1358–1368.

Lipsitz, J. D., Williams, J., Rabkin, J., Remien, R., Bradbury, M., Sadr, W., Goetz, R., Sorrell, S., & Gorman, J. (1994). Psychopathology in male and female intravenous drug users with and without HIV infection. *American Journal of Psychiatry, 151,* 1662–1668.

Lipsky, J. J. (1996). Antiretroviral drugs for AIDS. *The Lancet, 348,* 800–803.

Lipton, S. A., & Gendelman, H. E. (1995). Dementia associated with the acquired immunodeficiency syndrome. *New England Journal of Medicine, 332,* 934–940.

Lodico, M. A., & DiClemente, R. J. (1994). The association between childhood sexual abuse and prevalence of HIV-related risk behaviors. *Clinical Practices, 33,* 498–502.

Longo, M., Spross, J., & Locke, A. (1990). Identifying major concerns of persons with acquired immunodeficiency syndrome: A replication. *Clinical Nurse Specialist, 4,* 21–26.

Lui, K. J., Darrow, W. W., & Rutherford, G. W. (1988). A model-based estimate of the mean incubation period for AIDS in homosexual men. *Science, 240,* 1333–1335.

Lundgren, J. D., Phillips, A. N., Pedersen, C., Clumeck, N., Gatell, J. M., Johnson, A. M., Ledergerber, B., Vella, S., Nielsen, J. O., & the AIDS in Europe Study Group. (1994). Comparison of long-term prognosis of patients with AIDS treated and not treated with zidovudine. *Journal of the American Medical Association, 271,* 1088–1092.

Luo, L., Law, M., Kaldor, J. M., McDonald, A. M., & Cooper, D. A. (1995). The role of initial AIDS-defining illness in survival following AIDS. *AIDS, 9,* 57–63.

Lutgendorf, S. K., Antoni, M. H., Ironson, G., Klimas, N., Kumar, M., Starr, K., McCabe, P., Cleven, K., Fletcher, M. A., & Schneiderman, N. (1997). Cognitive–behavioral stress management decreases dysphoric mood and herpes simplex virus-type 2 antibody titers in symptomatic HIV-seropositive gay men. *Journal of Consulting and Clinical Psychology, 65,* 31–43.

Lyketsos, C. G., Hoover, D. R., Guccione, M., Dew, M. A., Wesch, J. E., Bing,

E. G., & Treisman, G. J. (1996). Changes in depressive symptoms as AIDS develops. *American Journal of Psychiatry, 153*, 1430–1437.

Lyketsos, C. G., Hoover, D., Guccione, M., Senterfitt, W., Dew, A., Wesch, J., VanRaden, M., Treisman, G., & Morgenstern, H. (1993). Depressive symptoms as predictors of medical outcomes in HIV infection. *Journal of the American Medical Association, 270*, 2563–2567.

Lyketsos, C., Hanson, A., Fishman, M., Rosenblatt, A., McHugh, P., & Treisman, G. (1993). Manic syndrome early and late in the course of HIV. *American Journal of Psychiatry, 150*, 326–327.

Lyman, A. (1997). Prescribing protease inhibitors for the homeless. *Journal of the American Medical Association, 278*, 1235–1236.

Lyter, D., Valdiserri, R., Kingsley, L., Amoroso, W., & Rinaldo, C. (1987). The HIV antibody test: Why gay and bisexual men want or do not want to know their results. *Public Health Reports, 102*, 468–474.

Maddox, J. (1993). Where the AIDS virus hides away. *Nature, 362*, 287.

Magura, S., Grossman, J. I., Lipton, D. S., Siddiqi, Q., Shapiro, J., Marion, I., & Amann, K. R. (1989). Determinants of needle sharing among intravenous drug users. *American Journal of Public Health, 79*, 459–462.

Maj, M. (1990). Psychiatric aspects of HIV-1 infection and AIDS. *Psychological Medicine, 20*, 547–563.

Manly, J. J., Patterson, T. L., Heaton, R. K., Semple, S. J., White, D. A., Velin, R. A., Atkinson, J. H., McCutchan, J. A., Chandler, J. L., & Grant, I. (1997). The relationship between neuropsychological functioning and coping activity among HIV-positive men. *AIDS and Behavior, 1*, 81–91.

Mann, J., & Tarantola, D. J. (1996). *AIDS in the world: II.* New York: Oxford University Press.

Mansfield, S., Barter, G., & Singh, S. (1992). Editorial review: AIDS and palliative care. *International Journal of STD and AIDS, 3*, 248–250.

Mapou, R. L., & Law, W. A. (1994). Neurobehavioral aspects of HIV disease and AIDS: An update. *Professional Psychology: Research and Practice, 25*, 132–140.

Marcus, R., & CDC Cooperative Needlestick Surveillance Group. (1988). Surveillance of health care workers exposed to blood from patients infected with the human immunodeficiency virus. *New England Journal of Medicine, 319,* 1118–1123.

Mariuz, P. R., & Luft, B. J. (1992). Toxoplasmic encephalitis. *AIDS Clinical Review,* 105–130.

Markham, P., Salahuddin, S. Z., Veren, K., Orndorff, S., & Gallo, R. (1986). Hydrocortisone and some other hormones enhance the expression of HTLV-III. *International Journal of Cancer, 37,* 67–72.

Markowitz, J. C., Klerman, G. L., Clougherty, K. F., Spielman, L. A., Jacobsberg, L. B., Fishman, B., Frances, A. J., Kocsis, J. H., & Perry, S. W. (1995). Individual psychotherapies for depressed HIV-positive patients. *American Journal of Psychiatry, 152,* 1504–1509.

Markowitz, J. C., Klerman, G. L., & Perry, S. W. (1992). Interpersonal psychotherapy of depressed HIV-positive outpatients. *Hospital and Community Psychiatry, 43,* 885–890.

Markowitz, J. C., Klerman, G. L., & Perry, S. W. (1993). An interpersonal psychotherapeutic approach to depressed HIV-seropositive patients. In W. H. Sledge & A. Tasman (Eds.), *Clinical challenges in psychiatry* (pp. 37–59). Washington, DC: American Psychiatric Press.

Markowitz, J. C., Klerman, G. L., Perry, S. W., Clougherty, K. F., & Josephs, L. S. (1993). Interpersonal psychotherapy for depressed HIV-seropositive patients. In G. L. Klerman & M. M. Weissman (Eds.), *New applications of interpersonal psychotherapy* (pp. 199–224). Washington, DC: American Psychiatric Press.

Markowitz, J. C., & Perry, S. W. (1992). Effects of human immunodeficiency virus on the central nervous system. In S. C. Yudofsky & R. E. Hales (Eds.), *The American Psychiatric Press textbook of neuropsychiatry* (pp. 499–518). Washington, DC: American Psychiatric Press.

Markowitz, J. C., Rabkin, J., & Perry, S. (1994). Treating depression in HIV-positive patients. *AIDS, 8,* 403–412.

Marks, G., Bundek, N., Richardson, J., Ruiz, M., Malonado, N., & Mason, H. (1992). Self-disclosure of HIV infection: Preliminary results from a sample of Hispanic men. *Health Psychology, 11,* 300–306.

Marks, G., Mason, H. R. C., & Simoni, J. M. (1995). The prevalence of patient disclosure of HIV infection to doctors [Letter to the editor]. *American Journal of Public Health, 85,* 1018–1019.

Marks, G., Richardson, J. L., & Maldonado, N. (1991). Self-disclosure of HIV infection to sexual partners. *American Journal of Public Health, 81*, 1321–1323.

Marks, G., Richardson, J., Ruiz, M., & Maldonado, N. (1992). HIV-infected men's practices in notifying past sexual partners of infection risk. *Public Health Reports, 107*, 100–105.

Marlatt, G. A., & Gordon, J. R. (1985). *Relapse prevention: Maintenance strategies in the treatment of addictive behaviors.* New York: Guilford Press.

Marmor, M., Weiss, L. R., Lynden, M., Weiss, S. H., Saxinger, W. C., Spira, T. J., & Feorino, P. M. (1986). Possible female-to-female transmission of human immunodeficiency virus. *Annals of Internal Medicine, 105*, 969.

Martin, D. (1993). Coping with AIDS and AIDS-risk reduction efforts among gay men. *AIDS Education and Prevention, 5*, 104–120.

Martin, D. J. (1992). Inappropriate lubricant use with condoms by homosexual men. *Public Health Reports, 107*, 468–473.

Martin, E. M., Robertson, L. C., Edelstein, H. E., Jagust, W. J., Sorensen, D. J., Giovanni, D. S., & Chirurgi, V. A. (1992). Performance of patients with early HIV-1 infection on the Stroop task. *Journal of Clinical and Experimental Neuropsychology, 14*, 857–868.

Martin, E. M., Robertson, L. C., Sorensen, D. J., Jagust, W. J., Mallon, K. N. F., & Chirurgi, V. A. (1993). Speed of memory scanning is not affected in early HIV-1 infection. *Journal of Clinical and Experimental Neuropsychology, 15*, 311–320.

Martin, E. M., Sorensen, D. J., Edelstein, H. E., & Robertson, L. C. (1992). Decision-making speed in HIV-1 infection: A preliminary report. *AIDS, 6*, 109–113.

Martin, E. M., Sorensen, D. J., Robertson, L. C., Edelstein, H. E., & Chirurgi, V. A. (1992). Spatial attention in HIV-1 infection: A preliminary report. *Journal of Neuropsychiatry and Clinical Neurosciences, 4*, 288–293.

Martin, J. L. (1988). Psychological consequences of AIDS-related bereavement among gay men. *Journal of Consulting and Clinical Psychology, 56*, 856–862.

Martin, J. L., & Dean, L. (1992). Effects of AIDS-related bereavement and HIV-related illness on psychological distress among gay men: A 7-year longitudinal study, 1985–1991. *Journal of Consulting and Clinical Psychology, 61*, 94–103.

Martin, J. L., & Dean, L. (1993). Bereavement following death from AIDS: Unique problems, reactions, and special needs. In M. Stroebe, W. Stroebe, & R. Hannson (Eds.), *Handbook of bereavement* (pp. 317–330). Cambridge, England: Cambridge University Press.

Marzuk, P. M., Tardiff, K., Leon, A., Hirsch, C., Hartwell, N., Portera, L., & Iqbal, M. (1997). HIV seroprevalence among suicide victims in New York City, 1991–1993. *American Journal of Psychiatry, 154*, 1720–1725.

Marzuk, P. M., Tierney, H., Gross, E. M., Morgan, E., Hsu, M., & Mann, J. (1988). Increased risk of suicide in persons with AIDS. *Journal of the American Medical Association, 259*, 1333–1337.

Masci, J. R., Poon, M., Wormser, G. P., & Bottone, E. J. (1992). *Cryptococcus neoformans* infections in the era of AIDS. In G. P. Wormser (Ed.), *AIDS and other manifestations of HIV infection* (2nd ed., pp. 393–408). New York: Raven Press.

Maslach, C., & Goldberg, J. (1998). Prevention of burnout: New perspectives. *Applied and Preventive Psychology, 7*, 63–74.

Mason, H., Marks, G., Simoni, J., Ruiz, M., & Richardson, J. (1995). Culturally sanctioned secrets? Latino men's nondisclosure of HIV infection to family, friends, and lovers. *Health Psychology, 14*, 6–12.

Masur, H., Ognibene, F., Yarchoan, R., Shelhamer, J. H., Baird, B. F., Travis, W., Suffredini, A. F., Deyton, L., Kovacs, J. A., & Fallon, J. (1989). CD4 counts as predictors of opportunistic pneumonias in human immunodeficiency virus (HIV) infection. *Annals of Internal Medicine, 111*, 223–231.

Mathews, B., & Bowes, J. (1989). A training model of group therapy with an HIV-seropositive population. *AIDS and Public Policy Journal, 4*, 51–55.

May, R. M. (1988). HIV infection in heterosexuals. *Nature, 331*, 655–666.

Mayer, K. H. (in press). The rationale for combination antiretroviral chemotherapy: An evolving process. In D. Ostrow & S. C. Kalichman (Eds.), *Behavioral and mental health aspects of new HIV treatments*. New York: Plenum Press.

McArthur, J. C., Cohen, B. A., Farzadegan, H., Cornblath, D. R., Selnes, O. A., Ostrow, D., Johnson, R. T., Phair, J., & Polk, B. F. (1988). Cerebrospinal fluid abnormalities in homosexual men with and without neuropsychiatric findings. *Annals of Neurology, 23*(Suppl.), S34–S37.

McCann, K., & Wadsworth, E. (1991). The experience of having a positive HIV antibody test. *AIDS Care, 3,* 43–53.

McCorkle, R., & Quint-Benoliel, J. (1983). Symptom distress, current concerns and mood disturbance after diagnosis of life-threatening disease. *Society of Science and Medicine, 17,* 431–438.

McCrae, R. R., & Costa, P. T. (1986). Personality, coping, and coping effectiveness in an adult sample. *Journal of Personality, 54,* 385–405.

McCusker, J., Stoddard, A., Mayer, K., Zapka, J., Morrison, C., & Saltzman, S. (1988). Effects of HIV antibody test knowledge on subsequent sexual behaviors in a cohort of homosexually active men. *American Journal of Public Health, 78,* 462–467.

McCutchan, J. A. (1990). Virology, immunology, and clinical course of HIV infection. *Journal of Consulting and Clinical Psychology, 58,* 5–12.

McDonell, J. R. (1993). Judgments of personal responsibility for HIV infection: An attributional analysis. *Social Work, 38,* 403–410.

McGuff, J., & Popovsky, M. A. (1989). Needlestick injuries in blood collection staff. *Transfusion, 29,* 693–695.

McGuire, J., Nieri, D., Abbott, D., Sheridan, K., & Fisher, M. (1995). Do Tarasoff principles apply in AIDS-related psychotherapy? Ethical decision making and the role of therapist homophobia and perceived client as dangerous. *Professional Psychology Research and Practice, 26,* 608–611.

McIntosh, J., Santos, J., Hubbard, R., & Overholser, J. (1994). *Elder suicide: Research, theory, and treatment.* Washington, DC: American Psychological Association.

McKegney, F. P., & O'Dowd, M. A. (1992). Suicidality and HIV status. *American Journal of Psychiatry, 149,* 396–398.

McKegney, F. P., O'Dowd, M. A., Feiner, C., Selwyn, P., Drucker, E., & Friedland, G. H. (1990). A prospective comparison of neuropsychologic function in HIV-seropositive and seronegative methadone-maintained patients. *AIDS, 4,* 565–569.

McNeely, T., Dealy, M., Dripps, D., Orenstein, J., Eisenberg, S., & Wahl, S. (1995). Secretory leukocyte protease inhibitor: A human saliva protein exhibiting anti-human immunodeficiency virus-1 activity in vitro. *Journal of Clinical Investigation, 96,* 456–464.

McShane, R. E., Bumbalo, J. A., & Patsdaughter, C. A. (1994). Psychological distress in family members living with human immunodeficiency virus/ acquired immune deficiency syndrome. *Archives of Psychiatric Nursing, 8,* 53–61.

Mebatsion, T., Finke, S., Weiland, F., & Conzelmann, K. (1997). A CXCR4/CD4 pseudotype rhabdovirus that selectively infects HIV-1 envelope protein-expressing cells. *Cell, 90,* 841–847.

Mehta, S., Moore, R. D., & Graham, N. M. H. (1997). Potential factors affecting adherence with HIV therapy. *AIDS, 11,* 1665–1670.

Meichenbaum, D. (1977). *Cognitive behavior modification.* New York: Plenum.

Melnick, S. L., Sherer, R., Louis, T. A., Hillman, D., Rodriguez, E. M., Lackman, C., Capps, L., Brown, L. S., Carlyn, M., Korvick, J. A., & Deyton, L. (1994). Survival and disease progression according to gender of patients with HIV infection. *Journal of the American Medical Association, 272,* 1915–1921.

Melton, G. B. (1988). Ethical and legal issues and AIDS-related practice. *American Psychologist, 43,* 941–947.

Merson, M. (June, 1991). *Opening address of the Director, Global Programme on AIDS, WHO.* Ninth International Conference on AIDS, Florence, Italy.

Messeri, P., Bartelli, D., Howard, J., Roegner, G., Sahar, M., & Kiperman, G. (1994). *Peer groups for HIV risk reduction and social support: Description of HIV peer group activities and assessment of outcomes.* New York: New York State Department of Health, AIDS Institute.

Metsch, L. R., McCoy, C. B., Lai, S., & Miles, C. (in press). Continuing risk behaviors among HIV seropositive chronic drug users in Miami, Florida. *AIDS and Behavior.*

Meyer-Bahlburg, H. F., Nostlinger, C., Exner, T. M., Ehrhardt, A. A., Gruen, R. S., Lorenz, G., Gorman, J. M., El-Sadr, W., & Sorrell, S. L. (1993). Sexual functioning in HIV+ and HIV− injected drug-using women. *Journal of Sex and Marital Therapy, 19,* 56–68.

Michaels, D., & Levine, C. (1992). Estimates of the number of motherless youth orphaned by AIDS in the United States. *Journal of the American Medical Association, 268,* 3456–3461.

Miller, D. (1990). Diagnosis and treatment of acute psychological problems related to HIV infection and disease. In D. Ostrow (Ed.), *Behavioral aspects of AIDS* (pp. 187–206). New York: Plenum.

Miller, D., & Pinching, A. (1989). HIV tests and counseling: Current issues. *AIDS, 3*(Suppl.), S187–S193.

Miller, D., & Riccio, M. (1990). Editorial review: Non-organic psychiatric and psychosocial syndromes associated with HIV-1 infection and disease. *AIDS, 4,* 381–388.

Miller, E. N., Selnes, O. A., McArthur, J. C., Satz, P., Becker, J. T., Cohen, B. A., Sheridan, K., Machado, A. M., van Gorp, W. G., & Visscher, B. (1990). Neuropsychological performance in HIV-1-infected homosexual men: The Multicenter AIDS Cohort Study (MACS). *Neurology, 40,* 197–203.

Miller, R. L., Holmes, J. M., & Auerbach, M. I. (1992, August). *Volunteer experiences of providing AIDS-related educational services.* Paper presented at the 100th Annual Convention of the American Psychological Association, Washington, DC.

Minkoff, H. L., & DeHovitz, J. A. (1991). Care of women infected with the human immunodeficiency virus. *Journal of the American Medical Association, 266,* 2253–2258.

Mondragon, D., Kirkman-Liff, B., & Schneller, E. S. (1991). Hostility to people with AIDS: Risk perception and demographic factors. *Society of Science and Medicine, 32,* 1137–1142.

Monzon, O. T., & Capellan, J. M. B. (1987). Female-to-female transmission of HIV. *The Lancet, 2,* 40–41.

Moore, R., Hidalgo, J., Sugland, B., & Chaisson, R. (1991). Zidovudine and the natural history of the acquired immunodeficiency syndrome. *New England Journal of Medicine, 324,* 1412–1416.

Moos, R. H., & Tsu, V. D. (1977). The crisis of physical illness: An overview. In R. H. Moos (Ed.), *Coping with physical illness.* New York: Plenum.

Morin, S. F., & Batchelor, W. F. (1984). Responding to the psychological crisis of AIDS. *Public Health Reports, 99,* 4–9.

Morrey, J., Bourn, S., Bunch, T., Jackson, K., Sidwell, R., Barrows, L., Daynes, R., & Rosen, C. (1991). In vivo activation of human immunodeficiency virus type 1 long terminal repeat by UV type A (UV-A) light plus psoralen and UV-B light in the skin of transgenic mice. *Journal of Virology, 65,* 5045–5051.

Morrow, R. H., Colebunders, R. L., & Chin, J. (1989). Interactions of HIV infection with endemic tropical diseases. *AIDS, 3*(Suppl.), S79–S87.

Morse, E. V., Simon, P. M., Coburn, M., Hyslop, N., Greenspan, D., & Balson, P. M. (1991). Determinants of subject compliance with an experimental anti-HIV drug protocol. *Social Science Medicine, 32,* 1161–1167.

Moses, S., Plummer, F. A., Bradley, J. E., Ndinya-Achola, J. O., Nagelkerke, J. D., & Ronald, A. R. (1994). The association between lack of male circumcision and risk for HIV infection: A review of the epidemiological data. *Sexually Transmitted Diseases, 21,* 201–210.

Moss, A. (1991). Surrogate markers for survival in patients with AIDS and AIDS related couples treated with zidovudine. *British Medical Journal, 302,* 73–78.

Moss, A. R., & Bacchetti, P. (1989). Natural history of HIV infection. *AIDS, 3*(Suppl.), S55–S61.

Moss, V. (1990). Palliative care in advanced HIV disease: Presentation, problems and palliation. *AIDS, 4*(Suppl. 1), S235–S242.

Moulton, J. M., Sweet, D. M., Temoshok, L., & Mandel, J. S. (1987). Attributions of blame and responsibility in relation to distress and health behavior change in people with AIDS and AIDS-related complex. *Journal of Applied Social Psychology, 17,* 493–506.

Mulder, C., & Antoni, M. (1992). Psychosocial correlates of immune status and disease progression in HIV-1 infected homosexual men: Review of preliminary findings and commentary. *Psychology and Health, 6,* 175–192.

Mulder, C. L., Emmelkamp, P. M. G., Mulder, J. W., Antoni, M. H., Sandfort, T., & Vries, M. J. (1992, July). *The immunological and psychosocial effects of group intervention for asymptomatic HIV infected homosexual men: The effects of cognitive-behavioral vs. experiential therapy.* Paper presented at the Eighth International AIDS Conference, Amsterdam.

Muram, D., Hostetler, B. R., Jones, C. E., & Speck, P. M. (1995). Adolescent victims of sexual assault. *Journal of Adolescent Health, 17,* 372–375.

Murrain, M. (1993). Differences in opportunistic infection rates in women with AIDS. *Journal of Women's Health, 2,* 243–248.

Myers, S. A., Prose, N. S., & Bartlett, J. A. (1993). Progress in the understanding of HIV infection: An overview. *Journal of the American Academy of Dermatology, 29,* 1–21.

Naficy, A. B., & Soave, R. (1992). Cryptosporidiosis, isosporiasis, and microsporidiosis in AIDS. In G. P. Wormser (Ed.), *AIDS and other manifestations of HIV infection* (2nd ed., pp. 433–442). New York: Raven Press.

Namir, S., Alumbaugh, M. J., Fawzy, F. I., & Wolcott, D. L. (1989). The relationship of social support to physical and psychological aspects of AIDS. *Psychology and Health, 3,* 77–86.

Namir, S., Wolcott, D., Fawzy, F. I., & Alumbaugh, M. J. (1987). Coping with AIDS: Psychological and health implications. *Journal of Applied Social Psychology, 17,* 309–328.

Namir, S., Wolcott, D., Fawzy, F., & Alumbaugh, M. (1990). Implications of different strategies for coping with AIDS. In L. Temoshok & A. Baum (Eds.), *Psychological perspectives on AIDS: Etiology, prevention, and treatment* (pp. 173–190). Hillsdale, NJ: Erlbaum.

National Institutes of Health. (1997). *National Institutes of Health consensus development statement on interventions to prevent HIV risk behaviors* (Vol. 15, No. 2). Bethesda, MD: Author.

Navia, B. A., Jordan, B. D., & Price, R. W. (1986). The AIDS dementia complex: I. Clinical features. *Annals of Neurology, 19,* 517–524.

Neugebauer, R., Rabkin, J., Williams, J., Remien, R., Goetz, R., & Gorman, J. (1992). Bereavement reactions among homosexual men experiencing multiple losses in the AIDS epidemic. *American Journal of Psychiatry, 149,* 1374–1379.

Newman, S. P., Lunn, S., & Harrison, M. J. G. (1995). Do asymptomatic HIV-seropositive individuals show cognitive deficit? *AIDS, 9,* 1211–1220.

Nichols, S. E. (1985). Psychosocial reactions of persons with the acquired immunodeficiency syndrome. *Annals of Internal Medicine, 103,* 765–767.

Nicholson, W. D., & Long, B. (1990). Self-esteem, social support, internalized homophobia, and coping strategies of HIV+ gay men. *Journal of Consulting and Clinical Psychology, 58,* 873–876.

Nicolosi, A., Musicco, M., Saracco, A., Lazzarin, A., & the Italian Study Group on HIV Heterosexual Transmission. (1994). Risk factors for woman-to-man sexual transmission of the human immunodeficiency virus. *Journal of Acquired Immune Deficiency Syndromes and Human Retrovirology, 7,* 296–300.

Noh, S., Chandarana, P., Field, V., & Posthuma, B. (1990). AIDS epidemic, emotional strain, coping and psychological distress in homosexual men. *AIDS Education and Prevention, 2,* 272–283.

Nolan, G. (1997). Harnessing viral devices as pharmaceuticals: Fighting HIV-1's fire with fire. *Cell, 90,* 821–824.

Novick, L. F., Glebatis, D. M., Stricof, R. L., MacCubbin, P. A., Lessner, L., & Berns, D. S. (1991). Newborn seroprevalence study: Methods and results. *American Journal of Public Health, 81,* 15–21.

Nowak, M. A., & McMichael, A. J. (August, 1995). How HIV defeats the immune system. *Scientific American,* 58–65.

Nyamathi, A., Bennett, C., & Leake, B. (1993). AIDS-related knowledge, perceptions, and behaviors among impoverished minority women. *American Journal of Public Health, 83,* 65–71.

O'Brien, T. R., Shaffer, N., & Jaffe, H. W. (1992). Acquisition and transmission of HIV. In M. A. Sande & P. A. Volberding (Eds.), *The medical management of AIDS* (3rd ed., pp. 3–17). Philadelphia: Saunders.

O'Connor, P. G., & Samet, J. H. (1996). The substance-using human immunodeficiency virus patient: Approaches to outpatient management. *American Journal of Medicine, 101,* 435–444.

O'Dowd, M. A. (1988). Psychosocial issues in HIV infection. *AIDS, 2*(Suppl. 1), S201–S205.

O'Dowd, M. A., Biderman, D. J., & McKegney, F. P. (1993). Incidence of suicidality in AIDS and HIV-positive patients attending a psychiatry outpatient program. *Psychosomatics, 34,* 33–40.

O'Dowd, M. A., & McKegney, F. P. (1990). AIDS patients compared with others seen in psychiatric consultation. *General Hospital Psychiatry, 12,* 50–55.

O'Dowd, M. A., Natali, C., Orr, D., & McKegney, F. P. (1991). Characteristics of patients attending an HIV-related psychiatric clinic. *Hospital and Community Psychiatry, 42,* 615–619.

O'Leary, A. (1990). Stress, emotion, and human immune function. *Psychological Bulletin, 108,* 363–382.

Omoto, A. M., & Snyder, M. (1995). Sustained helping without obligation: Motivation, longevity of service, and perceived attitude change among AIDS volunteers. *Journal of Personality and Social Psychology, 68,* 671–686.

Osmond, D., Charlebois, E., Lang, W., Shiboski, S., & Moss, A. (1994). Changes in AIDS survival time in two San Francisco cohorts of homosexual men, 1983–1993. *Journal of the American Medical Association, 271,* 1083–1087.

Ostrow, D. (1988). Models for understanding the psychiatric consequences of AIDS. In T. P. Bridge, A. F. Mirsky, & F. K. Goodwin (Eds.), *Psychological, neuropsychiatric, and substance abuse aspects of AIDS* (pp. 85–94). New York: Raven Press.

Ostrow, D. G. (1989). Psychiatry and AIDS: An American view. *Royal Society of Medicine, 82,* 192–197.

Ostrow, D. G. (1990). *Psychiatric aspects of human immunodeficiency virus infection.* Kalamazoo, MI: Upjohn.

Ostrow, D. G. (1994). Substance abuse and HIV infection. *Psychiatric Manifestations of HIV Disease, 17,* 69–89.

Ostrow, D., DiFranceisco, W., Chmeil, J., Wagstaff, D., & Wesch, J. (1995). A case-control study of human immunodeficiency virus type-1 seroconversion and risk-related behaviors in the Chicago MACS/CCS cohort, 1984–1992. *American Journal of Epidemiology, 142,* 1–10.

Ostrow, D., Grant, I., & Atkinson, H. (1988). Assessment and management of the AIDS patient with neuropsychiatric disturbances. *Journal of Clinical Psychiatry, 49,* 14–22.

Ostrow, D., Joseph, J., Kessler, R., Soucy, J., Tal, M., Eller, M., Chmiel, J., & Phair, J. (1989). Disclosure of HIV antibody status: Behavioral and mental health correlates. *AIDS Education and Prevention, 1,* 1–11.

Ostrow, D. G., Joseph, J., Monjan, A., Kessler, R., Emmons, C., Phair, J., Fox, R., Kingsley, L., Dudley, J., Chmiel, J., & Van Raden, M. (1986). Psychosocial aspects of AIDS risk. *Psychopharmacology Bulletin, 22,* 678–683.

Ostrow, D. G., Monjan, A., Joseph, J., Van Raden, M., Fox, R., Kingsley, L., Dudley, J., & Phair, J. (1989). HIV-related symptoms and psychological functioning in a cohort of homosexual men. *American Journal of Psychiatry, 146,* 737–742.

Ostrow, D. G., Whitaker, R. E. D., Frasier, K., Cohen, C., Wan, J., Frank, C., &

Fisher, E. (1991). Racial differences in social support and mental health in men with HIV infection: A pilot study. *AIDS Care, 3,* 55–62.

Ozawa, M., Auslander, W., & Slonim-Nevo, V. (1993). Problems in financing the care of AIDS patients. *Social Work, 38,* 369–377.

Ozer, E. M., & Bandura, A. (1990). Mechanisms governing empowerment effects: A self-efficacy analysis. *Journal of Personality and Social Psychology, 58,* 472–486.

Pace, J., Brown, G. R., Rundell, J. R., Paolucci, S., Drexler, K., & McManis, S. (1990). Prevalence of psychiatric disorders in a mandatory screening program for infection with human immunodeficiency virus: A pilot study. *Military Medicine, 155,* 76–80.

Padian, N., Marquis, L., Francis, D. P., Anderson, R. E., Rutherford, G., O'Malley, P. M., & Winkelstein, W. (1987). Male-to-female transmission of human immunodeficiency virus. *Journal of the American Medical Association, 258,* 788–790.

Padian, N. S., Shiboski, S. C., & Jewell, N. P. (1991). Female-to-male transmission of human immunodeficiency virus. *Journal of the American Medical Association, 266,* 1664–1667.

Pakenham, K. I., Dadds, M. R., & Terry, D. J. (1994). Relationships between adjustment to HIV and both social support and coping. *Journal of Consulting and Clinical Psychology, 62,* 1194–1203.

Panel on Clinical Practices for Treatment of HIV Infection. (1997). *Report of the NIH panel to define principles of therapy in HIV infection.* Bethesda, MD: National Institutes of Health.

Pantaleo, G., Graziosi, C., & Fauci, A. S. (1993). The role of lymphoid organs in the immunopathogenesis of HIV infection. *AIDS, 7*(Suppl.), S19–S23.

Pantaleo, G., Menzo, S., Vaccarezza, M., Graziosi, C., Cohen, O. J., Demarest, J. F., Montefiori, D., Orenstein, J. M., Fox, C., Schrager, L. K., Margolick, J. B., Buchbinder, S., Giorgi, J. V., & Fauci, A. S. (1995). Studies in subjects with long-term nonprogressive human immunodeficiency virus infection. *New England Journal of Medicine, 332,* 209–216.

Pearlin, L. I., Mullan, J. T., Aneshensel, C. S., Wardlaw, L., & Harrington, C. (1994). The structure and functions of AIDS caregiving relationships. *Psychosocial Rehabilitation Journal, 17,* 51–67.

Pearlin, L. I., & Schooler, C. (1978). The structure of coping. *Journal of Health and Social Psychology, 19,* 2–21.

Perdices, M., & Cooper, D. A. (1990). Neuropsychological investigation of patients with AIDS and ARC. *Journal of Acquired Immune Deficiency Syndromes and Human Retrovirology, 3,* 555–564.

Pergami, A., Gala, C., Burgess, A., Durbano, F., Zanello, D., Riccio, M., Invernizzi, G., & Catalan, J. (1993). The psychosocial impact of HIV infection in women. *Journal of Psychosomatic Research, 37,* 687–696.

Perkins, D., Davidson, E., Leserman, J., Liao, D., & Evans, D. (1993). Personality disorder in patients infected with HIV: A controlled study with implications for clinical care. *American Journal of Psychiatry, 150,* 309–315.

Perkins, D. O., Stern, R. A., Golden, R. N., Murphy, C., Naftolowitz, D., & Evans, D. L. (1994). Mood disorders in HIV infection: Prevalence and risk factors in a nonepicenter of the AIDS epidemic. *American Journal of Psychiatry, 151,* 233–236.

Perry, S. (1989). Warning third parties at risk of AIDS: APA's policy is a barrier to treatment. *Hospital and Community Psychiatry, 40,* 158–161.

Perry, S., & Fishman, B. (1993). Depression and HIV: How does one affect the other? *Journal of the American Medical Association, 270,* 2509–2510.

Perry, S., Fishman, B., Jacobsberg, L., & Frances, A. (1992). Relationships over 1 year between lymphocyte subsets and psychosocial variables among adults with infection by human immunodeficiency virus. *Archives of General Psychiatry, 49,* 396–401.

Perry, S., Jacobsberg, L., Card, C. A., Ashman, T., Frances, A., & Fishman, B. (1993). Severity of psychiatric symptoms after HIV testing. *American Journal of Psychiatry, 150,* 775–779.

Perry, S., Jacobsberg, L., & Fishman, B. (1990). Suicidal ideation and HIV testing. *Journal of the American Medical Association, 263,* 679–682.

Perry, S., Jacobsberg, L., Fishman, B., Frances, A., Bobo, J., & Jacobsberg, B. K. (1990). Psychiatric diagnosis before serological testing for the human immunodeficiency virus. *American Journal of Psychiatry, 147,* 89–93.

Perry, S., Jacobsberg, L., Fishman, B., Weiler, P., Gold, J. W. M., & Frances, A. (1990). Psychological responses to serological testing for HIV. *AIDS, 4,* 145–152.

Perry, S. W., & Markowitz, J. (1986). Psychiatric interventions for AIDS-spectrum disorders. *Hospital and Community Psychiatry, 37,* 1001–1006.

Perry, S., & Markowitz, J. (1988). Counseling for HIV testing. *Hospital and Community Psychiatry, 39,* 731–739.

Perry, S., & Marotta, R. F. (1987). AIDS dementia: A review of the literature. *Alzheimer Disease and Associated Disorders, 1,* 221–235.

Perry, S., Ryan, J., Ashman, T., & Jacobsberg, L. (1992). Refusal of zidovudine by HIV-positive patients. *AIDS, 6,* 514–515.

Perry, S. W., Card, C. A., Moffatt, M., Ashman, T., Fishman, B., & Jacobsberg, L. B. (1994). Self-disclosure of HIV infection to sexual partners after repeated counseling. *AIDS Education and Prevention, 6,* 403–411.

Perry, S. W., & Tross, S. (1984). Psychiatric problems of AIDS inpatients at the New York Hospital: Preliminary report. *Public Health Reports, 99,* 200–205.

Petersen, L. R., Doll, L., White, C., Chu, S., & the HIV Blood Donor Study Group. (1992). No evidence for female-to-female HIV transmission among 960,000 female blood donors. *Journal of Acquired Immune Deficiency Syndromes and Human Retrovirology, 5,* 853–855.

Peterson, C., Seligman, M. E. P., & Vaillant, G. E. (1988). Pessimistic explanatory style is a risk factor for physical illness: A thirty-five-year longitudinal study. *Journal of Personality and Social Psychology, 55,* 23–27.

Peterson, J. L., Folkman, S., & Bakeman, R. (1996). Stress, coping, HIV status, psychosocial resources, and depressive mood in African American gay, bisexual, and heterosexual men. *American Journal of Community Psychology, 24,* 461–487.

Pfeiffer, N. (1992). Long-term survival and HIV disease: The role of exercise and CD4 response in HIV disease. *AIDS Patient Care, October,* 237–239.

Phair, J., Munoz, A., Detels, R., Kaslow, R., Rinaldo, C., Saah, A., & the Multicenter AIDS Cohort Study Group. (1990). The risk of *Pneumocystis carinii* pneumonia among men infected with human immunodeficiency virus type 1. *New England Journal of Medicine, 322,* 161–165.

Physicians' Desk Reference. (1998). *Physicians' Desk References.* Montvale, NJ: Medical Economics Company.

Pillard, R. (1988). Sexual orientation and mental disorders. *Psychiatric Annals, 18,* 52–56.

Pitchenik, A., & Fertel, D. (1992). Mycobacterial disease in patients with HIV infection. In G. P. Wormser (Ed.), *AIDS and other manifestations of HIV infection* (2nd ed., pp. 277–314). New York: Raven Press.

Pliskin, M., Farrell, K., Crandles, S., & DeHovitz, J. (1993). *Factors influencing HIV positive mothers' disclosure to their non-infected children.* Unpublished manuscript.

Polk, B. F., Fox, R., Brookmeyer, R., Kanchanaraksa, S., Kaslow, R., Visscher, B., Rinaldo, C., & Phair, J. (1987). Predictors of the acquired immuno-deficiency syndrome in a cohort of seropositive homosexual men. *New England Journal of Medicine, 316,* 61–66.

Poretsky, L., Can, S., & Zurnoff, B. (1995). Testicular dysfunction in human immunodeficiency virus-infected men. *Metabolism, 44,* 946–953.

Potts, M., Anderson, R., & Baily, M. C. (1991). Slowing the spread of human immunodeficiency virus in developing countries. *The Lancet, 338,* 608–613.

Powderly, W. G., Finkelstein, D. M., Feinberg, J., Frame, P., He, W., van der Horst, C., Koletar, S. L., Eyster, E., Carey, J., Waskin, H., Hooton, T. M., Hyslop, N., Spector, S. A., & Bozzette, S. A. (1995). A randomized trial comparing fluconazole with clotrimazole troches for the pre-vention of fungal infections in patients with advanced human immuno-deficiency virus infection. *New England Journal of Medicine, 332,* 700–705.

Power, C., Selnes, O., Grim, J., & McArthur, J. (1995). HIV Dementia Scale: A rapid screening test. *Journal of Acquired Immunodeficiency Syndromes and Human Retrovirology, 8,* 273–278.

Price, R. W. (1997). Management of the neurologic complications of HIV-1 infection and AIDS. In M. A. Sande & P. A. Volberding (Eds.), *The medical management of AIDS* (5th ed., pp. 197–216). Philadelphia: Saunders.

Price, R. W., & Brew, B. (1991, May/June). Management of the neurologic complications of HIV-1 infection and AIDS: I. Dementia and diffuse brain disease. *The AIDS Reader,* pp. 97–102.

Price, R. W., & Sidtis, J. J. (1992). The AIDS dementia complex. In G. P. Worm-ser (Ed.), *AIDS and other manifestations of HIV infection* (2nd ed., pp. 373–382). New York: Raven Press.

Price, V., & Hsu, M. L. (1992). Public opinion about AIDS policies: The role of misinformation and attitudes toward homosexuals. *Public Opinion Quarterly, 56*, 29–52.

Pryor, J. B., Reeder, G. D., Vinacco, R., & Kott, T. (1989). The instrumental and symbolic functions of attitudes toward persons with AIDS. *Journal of Applied Social Psychology, 19*, 377–404.

Quadrel, M. J., Fischhoff, B. & Davis W. (1993). Adolescent (In)vulnerability. *American Psychologist, 48*, 102–116.

Quinn, T. C., Glaser, D., Cannon, R. O., Matuszak, D. L., Dunning, R. W., & Kline, M. S. (1988). Human immunodeficiency virus infection among patients attending clinics for sexually transmitted diseases. *New England Journal of Medicine, 318*, 197–203.

Quinn, T. C., Groseclose, S. L., Spence, M., Provost, V., & Hook, E. (1992). Evolution of the human immunodeficiency virus epidemic among patients attending sexually transmitted disease clinics: A decade of experience. *Journal of Infectious Diseases, 165*, 541–544.

Rabeneck, L., & Wray, N. P. (1993). Predicting the outcomes of human immunodeficiency virus infection: How well are we doing? *Archives of Internal Medicine, 153*, 2749–2755.

Rabkin, J. G. (1994, January). *Mood and immune effects of pharmacotherapy in HIV illness.* Paper presented at the NIMH Neuroscience Findings in AIDS Research Conference, Rockville, MD.

Rabkin, J. G., & Chesney, M. (in press). Treatment adherence to HIV medications: The Achilles heel of the new therapeutics. In D. Ostrow & S. Kalichman (Eds.), *Behavioral and mental health impacts of new HIV therapies.* New York: Plenum Press.

Rabkin, J. G., & Ferrando, S. (1997). A "second life" agenda: Psychiatric research issues raised by protease inhibitor treatments for people with human immunodeficiency virus or the acquired immunodeficiency syndrome. *Archives of General Psychiatry, 54*, 1049–1053.

Rabkin, J. G., Goetz, R. R., Remien, R. H., Williams, J. B. W., Todak, G., & Gorman, J. M. (1997). Stability of mood despite HIV illness progression in a group of homosexual men. *American Journal of Psychiatry, 154*, 231–238.

Rabkin, J. G., & Harrison, W. M. (1990). Effect of imipramine on depression and immune status in a sample of men with HIV infection. *American Journal of Psychiatry, 147,* 495–497.

Rabkin, J. G., Johnson, J., Lin, S., Lipsitz, J. D., Remien, R. H., Williams, J. B. W., & Gorman, J. M. (1997). Psychopathology in male and female HIV-positive and negative injecting drug users: Longitudinal course over 3 years. *AIDS, 11,* 507–515.

Rabkin, J. G., Rabkin, R., Harrison, W., & Wagner, G. (1994). Effect of imipramine on mood and enumerative measures of immune status in depressed patients with HIV illness. *American Journal of Psychiatry, 151,* 516–523.

Rabkin, J. G., Rabkin, R., & Wagner, G. (1994). Effects of fluoxetine on mood and immune status in depressed patients with HIV illness. *Journal of Clinical Psychiatry, 55,* 92–97.

Rabkin, J. G., Rabkin, R., & Wagner, G. (1995). Testosterone replacement therapy in HIV illness. *General Hospital Psychiatry, 17,* 37–42.

Rabkin, J. G., Remien, R., Katoff, L., & Williams, J. (1993). Resiliency in adversity among long-term survivors of AIDS. *Hospital and Community Psychology, 44,* 162–167.

Rabkin, J. G., Wagner, G., & Rabkin, R. (1996). Treatment of depression in HIV+ men: Literature review and report of an ongoing study of testosterone replacement therapy. *Annals of Behavioral Medicine, 18,* 24–29.

Rabkin, J. G., Williams, J. B., Neugebauer, R., Remien, R., & Goetz, R. (1990). Maintenance of hope in HIV-spectrum homosexual men. *American Journal of Psychiatry, 147,* 1322–1326.

Rabkin, J. G., Williams, J. B., Remien, R. H., Goetz, R., Kertzner, R., & Gorman, J. M. (1991). Depression, distress, lymphocyte subsets, and human immunodeficiency virus symptoms on two occasions in HIV-positive homosexual men. *Archives of General Psychiatry, 48,* 111–119.

Rabkin, J. G., Wilson, C., & Kimpton, D. J. (1993, January). The end of the line. . . . When is enough enough? *PAACNOTES,* pp. 25–47.

Raviglione, M. C., Snider, D. E., & Kochi, A. (1995). Global epidemiology of tuberculosis: Morbidity and mortality of a worldwide epidemic. *Journal of the American Medical Association, 273,* 220–226.

Reamer, F. G. (1991). AIDS, social work, and the "duty to protect." *Social Work, 36,* 56–60.

Reed, G. M., Kemeny, M. E., Taylor, S. E., Wang, H.-Y. J., & Visscher, B. R. (1994). "Realistic acceptance" as a predictor of survival time in gay men with AIDS. *Health Psychology, 13,* 299–307.

Reed, G. M., Taylor, S. E., & Kemeny, M. E. (1993). Perceived control and psychological adjustment in gay men with AIDS. *Journal of Applied Social Psychology, 23,* 791–824.

Reed, P., Wise, T. N., & Mann, L. S. (1984). Nurses' attitudes regarding acquired immunodeficiency syndrome (AIDS). *Nursing Forum, 11,* 153–156.

Reidy, M., Taggart, M. E., & Asselin, L. (1991). Psychosocial needs expressed by the natural caregivers of HIV infected children. *AIDS Care, 3,* 331–343.

Remien, R. H., Carballo-Dieguez, A., & Wagner, G. (1995). Intimacy and sexual behavior in serodiscordant male couples. *AIDS Care, 7,* 429–438.

Remien, R. H., Rabkin, J., Williams, J., & Katoff, L. (1992). Coping strategies and health beliefs of AIDS long-term survivors. *Psychology and Health, 6,* 335–345.

Resnick, L., diMarzo-Veronese, F., Schupbach, J., Tourtellotte, W. W., Ho, D. D., Muller, F., Shapshak, P., Vogt, M., Groopman, J. E., & Markham, P. D. (1985). Intra-blood-brain-barrier synthesis of HTLV-III specific IgG in patients with neurologic symptoms associated with AIDS or AIDS-related complex. *New England Journal of Medicine, 313,* 1498–1504.

Rich, J. D., Buck, A., Tuomala, R. E., & Kazanjian, P. H. (1993). Transmission of human immunodeficiency virus infection presumed to have occurred via female homosexual contact. *Clinical Infectious Diseases, 17,* 1003–1005.

Richters, J., Donovan, B., & Gerofi, J. (1993). How often do condoms break or slip off in use? *International Journal of STD and AIDS, 4,* 90–94.

Riley, J. L., & Greene, R. R. (1993). Influence of education on self-perceived attitudes about HIV/AIDS among human services providers. *Social Work, 38,* 396–401.

Ritchie, E. C., & Radke, A. Q. (1992). Depression and support systems in male Army HIV+ patients. *Military Medicine, 157,* 345–349.

Robiner, W. N., Melroe, N. H., Campbell, S., Phame, F. S., Colon, E., Chung, J., & Reaney, S. (1993). Psychological effects of participation and nonparticipation in a placebo-controlled zidovudine clinical trial with asymptomatic human immunodeficiency virus-infected individuals. *Journal of Acquired Immune Deficiency Syndromes, 6,* 795–808.

Robins, A. G., Dew, M. A., Davidson, S., Penkower, L., Becker, J. T., & Kingsley, L. (1994). Psychosocial factors associated with risky sexual behavior among HIV-seropositive gay men. *AIDS Education and Prevention, 6,* 483–492.

Rodin, G., & Voshart, K. (1986). Depression in the medically ill: An overview. *American Journal of Psychiatry, 143,* 696–705.

Rogers, M. F., & Kilbourne, B. W. (1992). Epidemiology of pediatric HIV infection. In G. P. Wormser (Ed.), *AIDS and other manifestations of HIV infection* (2nd ed., pp. 17–24). New York: Raven Press.

Root-Bernstein, R. S. (1990). Do we know the cause(s) of AIDS? *Perspectives in Biological Medicine, 33,* 480–500.

Rosenberg, M. J., Holmes, K. K., & the World Health Organization Working Group on Virucides. (1993). Virucides in prevention of HIV infection: Research priorities. *Sexually Transmitted Diseases, 20,* 41–44.

Rosenberg, Z. F., & Fauci, A. S. (1991). Immunopathology and pathogenesis of human immunodeficiency virus infection. *Pediatric Infectious Disease Journal, 10,* 230–238.

Rosengard, C., & Folkman, S. (1997). Suicidal ideation, bereavement, HIV serostatus and psychosocial variables in partners of men with AIDS. *AIDS Care, 9,* 373–384.

Rosser, B. R., Metz, M. E., Bockting, W. O., & Buroker, T. (1997). Sexual difficulties, concerns, and satisfaction in homosexual men: An empirical study with implications for HIV prevention. *Journal of Sex and Marital Therapy, 23,* 61–73.

Rothenberg, R., Woelfel, M., Stoneburner, R., Milberg, J., Parker, R., & Truman, B. (1987). Survival with the acquired immunodeficiency syndrome: Experience with 5833 cases in New York City. *New England Journal of Medicine, 317,* 1297–1302.

Rotheram-Borus, M. J., & Koopman, C. (1991). Sexual risk behaviors, AIDS knowledge, and beliefs about AIDS among runaways. *American Journal of Public Health, 81,* 208–210.

Rotheram-Borus, M. J., Rossario, M., Van Rossem, R., Reid, H., & Gillis, J. (1995). Prevalence, course, and predictors of multiple problem behaviors among gay bisexual male adolescents. *Developmental Psychology, 31,* 75–85.

Royce, R. A., Sena, A., Cates, W., & Cohen, M. S. (1997). Sexual transmission of HIV. *New England Journal of Medicine, 336,* 1072–1078.

Royce, R. A., & Winkelstein, W. (1990). HIV infection, cigarette smoking and CD4+ T-lymphocyte counts: Preliminary results from the San Francisco men's health study. *AIDS, 4,* 327–333.

Rundell, J. R., Paolucci, S. L., Beatty, D. C., & Boswell, R. N. (1988). Psychiatric illness at all stages of human immunodeficiency virus infection. *American Journal of Psychiatry, 145,* 652–653.

Ryder, R. W., & Hassig, S. E. (1988). The epidemiology of perinatal transmission of HIV. *AIDS, 2*(Suppl. 1), S83–S89.

Saag, M. S. (1992). AIDS testing: Now and in the future. In M. A. Sande & P. A. Volberding (Eds.), *The medical management of AIDS* (3rd ed., pp. 33–35). Philadelphia: Saunders.

Saag, M. S. (1995). AIDS testing now and in the future. In M. A. Sande & P. A. Volberding (Eds.), *The medical management of AIDS* (4th ed., pp. 65–88). Philadelphia: Saunders.

Saag, M. S. (1997). Quantitation of HIV viral load: A tool for clinical practice? In M. A. Sande & P. A. Volberding (Eds.), *The medical management of AIDS* (5th ed., pp. 57–74). Philadelphia: Saunders.

Saah, A. J., Hoover, D. R., Peng, Y., Phair, J. P., Visscher, B., Kingsley, L. A., & Schrager, L. K. (1995). Predictors for failure of *Pneumocystis carinii* pneumonia prophylaxis. *Journal of the American Medical Association, 273,* 1197–1202.

Saah, A. J., Horn, T. D., Hoover, D. R., Chen, C., Whitmore, S. E., Flynn, C., Wesch, J., Detels, R., & Anderson, R. (1997). Solar ultraviolet radiation exposure does not appear to exacerbate HIV infection in homosexual men. *AIDS, 11,* 1773–1778.

Saahs, J. A., Goetz, R., Reddy, M., Rabkin, J. G., Williams, J. B. W., Kertzner, R., & Gorman, J. M. (1994). Psychological distress and natural killer cells in gay men with and without HIV infection. *American Journal of Psychiatry, 151,* 1479–1484.

Sadovsky, R. (1991). Psychosocial issues in symptomatic HIV infection. *American Family Physician, 44,* 2065–2072.

Sales, E. (1991). Psychosocial impact of the phase of cancer on the family: An updated review. *Journal of Psychosocial Oncology, 9,* 1–18.

Sales, E., Schulz, R., & Biegel, D. (1992). Predictors of strain in families of cancer patients: A review of the literature. *Journal of Psychosocial Oncology, 10,* 1–26.

Samet, J. H., Libman, H., Steger, K. A., Dhwan, R. K., Chen, J., Shevitz, A. H., Dewees-Dunk, R., Leveson, S., Kufe, D., & Caven, D. E. (1992). Compliance with zidovudine therapy in patients infected with HIV type 1: A cross sectional study in a municipal hospital clinic. *American Journal of Medicine, 92*(5), 495–502.

Samuel, M. C., Hessol, N., Shiboski, S., Eagel, R., Speed, T. P., & Winkelstein, W. (1993). Factors associated with human immunodeficiency virus seroconversion in homosexual men in three San Francisco cohort studies, 1984–1989. *Journal of AIDS, 6,* 303–312.

Sande, M. A., & Volberding, P. A. (Eds.). (1997). *The medical management of AIDS* (5th ed.). Philadelphia: Saunders.

Sarason, I., Sarason, B., Potter, E., & Antoni, M. (1985). Life events, social support, and illness. *Psychosomatic Medicine, 47,* 156–163.

Sarosi, G. A. (1992). Endemic mycoses in HIV infection. In M. A. Sande & P. A. Volberding (Eds.), *The medical management of AIDS* (3rd ed., pp. 311–318). Philadelphia: Saunders.

Saunders, L. D., Rutherford, G. W., Lemp, G. F., & Barnhart, J. L. (1990). Impact of AIDS on mortality in San Francisco, 1979–1986. *Journal of Acquired Immune Deficiency Syndromes and Human Retrovirology, 3,* 921–924.

Saykin, A. J., Janssen, R., Sprehn, G., Spira, T., Cannon, L., Kaplan, J., O'Connor, B., Watson, S., & Allen, R. (1989). Neuropsychological and psychosocial function in two cohorts of gay men: Relation to stage of HIV-1 infection [Abstract]. *International Conference on AIDS, 5,* 389.

Schacker, T., Collier, A., Hughes, J., Shea, T., & Corey, L. (1996). Clinical and epidemiological features of primary HIV infection. *Annals of Internal Medicine, 125,* 257–264.

Schaefer, S., & Coleman, E. (1992). Shifts in meaning, purpose, and values following a diagnosis of human immunodeficiency virus (HIV) infection among gay men. *Journal of Psychology and Human Sexuality, 5,* 13–29.

Schaeffer, M. A., & Baum, A. (1984). Adrenal cortical response to stress at Three Mile Island. *Psychosomatic Medicine, 46*, 227–237.

Schechter, M. T., Craib, K. J. P., Le, T. N., Montaner, J. S. G., Douglas, B., Sestak, P., Willoughby, B., & O'Shaughnessy, M. V. (1990). Susceptibility to AIDS progression appears early in HIV infection. *AIDS, 4*, 185–190.

Scheier, M. F., & Carver, C. S. (1987). Dispositional optimism and physical well-being: The influence of generalized outcome expectancies on health. *Journal of Personality, 55*, 169–210.

Scheier, M. F., Matthews, K. A., Owens, J. F., Magovern, G. J., Lefebvre, R. C., Abbott, R. A., & Carver, C. S. (1989). Dispositional optimism and recovery from coronary artery bypass surgery: The beneficial effects on physical and psychological well-being. *Journal of Personality and Social Psychology, 57*, 1024–1040.

Schielke, E., Tatsch, K., Pfister, H. W., Trenkwalder, C., Leinsinger, G., Kirsch, C. M., Matuschke, A., & Einhaupl, K. M. (1990). Reduced cerebral blood flow in early stages of human immunodeficiency virus infection. *Archives of Neurology, 47*, 1342–1345.

Schilling, R., El-Bassel, N., Ivanoff, A., Gilbert, L., Su, K. H., & Safyer, S. M. (1994). Sexual risk behavior of incarcerated, drug-using women, 1992. *Public Health Reports, 109*, 539–547.

Schleifer, S. J., Keller, S. E., Bond, R. N., Cohen, J., & Stein, M. (1989). Major depressive disorder and immunity: Role of age, sex, severity, and hospitalization. *Archives of General Psychiatry, 46*, 81–87.

Schleifer, S., Keller, S., Camerino, M., Thornton, J., & Stein, M. (1983). Suppression of lymphocyte stimulation following bereavement. *Journal of the American Medical Association, 250*, 374–377.

Schleifer, S. J., Keller, S. E., Siris, S. G., Davis, K. L., & Stein, M. (1985). Depression and immunity. *Archives of General Psychiatry, 42*, 129–133.

Schmaling, K. B., & DiClementi, J. D. (1991, October). Cognitive therapy with the HIV seropositive patient. *The Behavior Therapist*, pp. 221–224.

Schmidt, N. B., Lerew, D. R., & Trakowski, J. H. (1997). Body vigilance in panic disorder: Evaluating attention to bodily pertubations. *Journal of Consulting and Clinical Psychology, 65*, 214–220.

Schmitt, F. A., Bigley, J. W., McKinnis, R., Logue, P. E., Evans, R. W., Drucker, J. L., & the AZT Collaborative Working Group. (1988). Neuropsychological outcome of zidovudine (AZT) treatment of patients with AIDS and AIDS-related complex. *New England Journal of Medicine, 319,* 1573–1578.

Schneider, S. G., Taylor, S. E., Hammen, C., Kemeny, M., & Dudley, J. (1991). Factors influencing suicide intent in gay and bisexual suicide ideators: Differing models for men with and without human immunodeficiency virus. *Journal of Personality and Social Psychology, 61,* 776–788.

Schnell, D., Higgins, D., Wilson, R., Goldbaum, G., Cohn, D., & Wolitski, R. (1992). Men's disclosure of HIV test results to male primary sex partners. *American Journal of Public Health, 82,* 1675–1676.

Schnell, M. J., Johnson, J. E., Buonocore, L., & Rose, J. K. (1997). Construction of a novel virus that targets HIV-1-infected cells and controls HIV-1 infection. *Cell, 90,* 849–857.

Schoenbaum, E. E., Weber, M. P., Vermund, S., & Gayle, H. (1990). HIV antibody in persons screened for syphilis: Prevalence in a New York City emergency room and primary care clinics. *Sexually Transmitted Diseases, 17,* 190–193.

Schooley, R. (1992). Antiretroviral chemotherapy. In G. P. Wormser (Ed.), *AIDS and other manifestations of HIV infection* (2nd ed., pp. 609–624). New York: Raven Press.

Schoub, B. D. (1993). *AIDS and HIV in perspective.* Cambridge, England: Cambridge University Press.

Schroder, K., & Barton, S. E. (1994). Patients' attitudes to zidovudine: The influence of the Concorde trial and the media. *AIDS, 8,* 1354–1355.

Schwarcz, S. K., Kellogg, T., Kohn, R., Katz, M., Lemp, G., & Bolan, G. (1995). Temporal trends in human immunodeficiency virus seroprevalence and sexual behavior at the San Francisco Municipal Sexually Transmitted Disease Clinic, 1989–1992. *American Journal of Epidemiology, 142,* 314–322.

Schwartzberg, S. S. (1993). Struggling for meaning: HIV-positive gay men make sense of AIDS. *Professional Psychology: Research and Practice, 24,* 483–490.

Scrager, L. K. (1988). Bacterial infections in AIDS patients. *AIDS, 2*(Suppl. 1), S183–S189.

Seed, J., Allen, S., Mertens, T., Hudes, E., Serufilira, A., Carael, M., Karita, E., Van de Perre, P., & Nsengumuremyi, F. (1995). Male circumcision, sexually transmitted disease, and risk of HIV. *Journal of Acquired Immune Deficiency Syndromes and Human Retrovirology, 8,* 83–90.

Segerstrom, S. C, Taylor, S. E., Kemeny, M. E., Reed, G. M., & Visscher, B. R. (1996). Causal attributions predict rate of immune decline in HIV-seropositive gay men. *Health Psychology, 15*, 485–493.

Selik, R. M., Chu, S. Y., & Buehler, J. W. (1993). HIV infection as leading cause of death among young adults in US cities and states. *Journal of the American Medical Association, 269*, 2991–2994.

Selnes, O. A., & Miller, E. N. (1992). Cognitive impairment of HIV infection. *AIDS, 6*, 602–603.

Selnes, O. A., Miller, E., McArthur, J., Gordon, B., Munoz, A., Sheridan, K., Fox, R., Saah, A. J., & the Multicenter AIDS Cohort Study. (1990). HIV-1 infection: No evidence of cognitive decline during the asymptomatic stages. *Neurology, 40*, 204–208.

Seltzer, E., Schulman, K. A., Brennan, P. J., & Lynn, L. A. (1993). Patient attitudes toward rooming with persons with HIV infection. *Journal of Family Practice, 37*, 564–568.

Serraino, D., Franceschi, S., Dal Maso, L., & La Vecchia, C. (1995). HIV transmission and Kaposi's sarcoma among European women. *AIDS, 9*, 971–973.

Sewell, D. D., Jeste, D. V., Atkinson, J. H., Heaton, R. K., Hesselink, J. R., Wiley, C., Thal, L., Chandler, J. L., Grant, I., & the San Diego HIV Neurobehavioral Research Center Group. (1994). HIV-associated psychosis: A study of 20 cases. *American Journal of Psychiatry, 151*, 237–242.

Shader, R. I., von Moltke, L., Schmider, J., Harmatz, J., & Greenblatt, G. J. (1996). The clinician and drug interactions—An update. *Journal of Clinical Psychopharmacology.*

Sharer, L. R. (1992). Pathology of HIV-1 infection of the central nervous system. *Journal of Neuropathology and Experimental Neurology, 51*, 3–11.

Shaw, G. M., Harper, M. E., Hahn, B. H., Epstein, L. G., Gajdusek, D. C., Price, R. W., Navia, B. A., Petito, C. K., O'Hara, C. J., Groopman, J. E., Cho, E. S., Oleske, J. M., Staal, F. W., & Sherer, R. (1988). Physician use of the HIV antibody test: The need for consent, counseling, confidentiality, and caution. *Journal of the American Medical Association, 259*, 264–265.

Shinn, M., Lehmann, S., & Wong, N. W. (1984). Social interaction and social support. *Journal of Social Issues, 40*, 55–76.

Siegel, K. (1986). AIDS: The social dimension. *Psychiatric Annals, 16*, 168–172.

Siegel, K., Karus, D., & Raveis, V. H. (1997). Correlates of change in depressive symptomatology among gay men with AIDS. *Health Psychology, 16,* 230–238.

Siegel, K., & Krauss, B. (1991). Living with HIV infection: Adaptive tasks of seropositive gay men. *Journal of Health and Social Behavior, 32,* 17–32.

Siegel, K., Levine, M., Brooks, C., & Kern, R. (1989). The motives of gay men for taking or not taking the HIV antibody test. *Social Problems, 36,* 368–383.

Siegl, D., & Morse, J. M. (1994). Tolerating reality: The experience of parents of HIV positive sons. *Society of Science and Medicine, 38,* 959–971.

Sikkema, K. J., Kalichman, S. C., Kelly, J. A., & Koob, J. J. (1995). Group intervention to improve coping with AIDS-related bereavement: Model development and an illustrative clinical example. *AIDS Care, 7,* 463–475.

Sikkema, K., & Kelly, J. (1996). Behavioral medicine interventions can improve quality of life and health of persons with HIV disease. *Annals of Behavioral Medicine, 18,* 40–48.

Sikkema, K. J., Koob, J., Cargill, V., Kelly, J. A., Desiderato, L., & Roffman, R. (1995). Levels and predictors of HIV risk behavior among women living in low-income housing developments. *Public Health Reports, 6,* 707–713.

Silva, J. A, Leong, G. B., & Weinstock, R. (1989). An HIV-infected psychiatric patient: Some clinicolegal dilemmas. *Bulletin of the American Academy of Psychiatry and Law, 17,* 33–43.

Silverman, D. C. (1993). Psychosocial impact of HIV-related caregiving on health providers: A review and recommendations for the role of psychiatry. *American Journal of Psychiatry, 150,* 705–712.

Simberkoff, M. S., & Leaf, H. (1992). Bacterial infections in patients with HIV infection. In G. P. Wormser (Ed.), *AIDS and other manifestations of HIV infection* (2nd ed., pp. 269–276). New York: Raven Press.

Simonds, R. J., Lindergren, M. L., Thomas, P., Hanson, D., Caldwell, B., Scott, G., & Rogers, M. (1995). Prophylaxis against pneumocystis carinii pneumonia among children with perinatally acquired human immunodeficiency virus infection in the United States. *New England Journal of Medicine, 332,* 786–790.

Simoni, J. M., Mason, H. R. C., Marks, G., Ruiz, M. S., Reed, D., & Richardson, J. L. (1995). Women's self-disclosure of HIV infection: Rates, reasons, and reactions. *Journal of Consulting and Clinical Psychology, 63,* 474–478.

Sinforiani, E., Mauri, M., Bono, G., Muratori, S., Alessi, E., & Minoli, L. (1991). Cognitive abnormalities and disease progression in a selected population of asymptomatic HIV-positive subjects. *AIDS, 5,* 1117–1120.

Singh, B. K., Koman, J. J., Catan, V., Souply, K., Birkel, R., & Golaszewski, T. (1993). Sexual risk behavior among injection drug-using human immunodeficiency virus positive clients. *International Journal of the Addictions, 28,* 735–747.

Singh, N., Squier, C., Sivek, C., Wagener, M., Nguyen, M. H., & Yu, V. L. (1996). Determinants of compliance with antiretroviral therapy in patients with human immunodeficiency virus: Prospective assessment with implications for enhancing compliance. *AIDS Care, 8,* 261–269.

Slovic, P., Fischhoff, B., & Lichtenstein, S. (1982). Facts versus fears: Understanding perceived risk. In D. Kahneman, P. Slovic, & A. Tversky (Eds.), *Judgment under uncertainty: Heuristics and biases* (pp. 463–489). Cambridge, England: Cambridge University Press.

Slowinski, J. W. (1989, September). Psychological needs of HIV-positive and AIDS patients. *Medical Aspects of Human Sexuality,* pp. 52–54.

Smith, D. A, & Smith, L. (1989). The isolation of HIV-positive patients. *Journal of the American Medical Association, 262,* 208.

Smith, M. Y., & Rapkin, B. D. (1996). Social support and barriers to family involvement in care giving for persons with AIDS: Implications for patient education. *Patient Education and Counseling, 27,* 85–94.

Smith, P. F., Mikl, J., Hyde, S., & Morse, D. L. (1991). The AIDS epidemic in New York State. *American Journal of Public Health, 81,* 54–60.

Snyder, S., Reyner, A., Schmeidler, J., Bogursky, E., Gomez, H., & Strain, J. (1992). Prevalence of mental disorders in newly admitted medical inpatients with AIDS. *Psychosomatics, 33,* 166–170.

Solano, L., Costa, M., Salvati, S., Coda, R., Aiuti, F., Mezzaroma, I., & Bertini, M. (1993). Psychosocial factors and clinical evolution in HIV-1 infection: A longitudinal study. *Journal of Psychosomatic Research, 37,* 39–51.

Solomon, G. F., Kemeny, M., & Temoshok, L. (1991). Psychoneuroimmunologic aspects of human immunodeficiency virus infection. In R. Ader, D.

Felten, & L. Cohen (Eds.), *Psychoneuroimmunology II* (pp. 1082–1113). Orlando, FL: Academic Press.

Somerfield, M., & Curbow, B. (1992). Methodological issues and research strategies in the study of coping with cancer. *Social Science and Medicine, 34,* 1203–1216.

Somlai, A., & Kalichman, S. (1994, August). *The spiritual practices and needs of people living with HIV-AIDS.* Paper presented at the 102nd Annual Convention of the American Psychological Association, Los Angeles.

Somlai, A. M., Kelly, J. A., Kalichman, S. C., Mulry, G., Sikkema, K. J., McAuliffe, T., Multhauf, K., & Devantes, B. (1996). An empirical investigation of the relationship between spirituality, coping, and emotional distress in people living with HIV infection and AIDS. *The Journal of Pastoral Care, 50,* 181–191.

Soto-Ramirez, L., Renjifo, B., McLane, M., Marlink, R., O'Hara, C., Sutthent, R., Wasi, C., Vithayasai, P., Vithayasai, V., Apichartpiyakul, C., Auewarakul, P., Cruz, V., Chui, D., Osathanondh, R., Mayer, K., Lee, T., & Essex, M. (1996). HIV-1 Langerhans cell tropism associated with heterosexual transmission of HIV. *Science, 271,* 1291–1293.

Spector, I. C., & Conklin, R. (1987). Brief reports: AIDS group psychotherapy. *International Journal of Group Psychotherapy, 37,* 433–439.

Spijkerman, I. J. B., Langendam, M. W., Veugelers, P. J., van Ameijden, E. J. C., Keet, I. P. M., Geskus, R. B., van den Hoek, A., & Coutinho, R. A. (1996). Differences in progression to AIDS between injection drug users and homosexual men with documented dates of seroconversion. *Epidemiology, 7,* 571–577.

Srinivasan, A., York, D., & Bohan, C. (1987). Lack of HIV replication in arthropod cells. *The Lancet, 1*(8541), 1094–1095.

St. Lawrence, J., & Brasfield, T. (1995). HIV risk behavior among homeless adults. *AIDS Education and Prevention, 7,* 22–31.

St. Lawrence, J. S., Kelly, J. A., Owen, A. D., Hogan, I. G., & Wilson, R. A. (1990). Psychologists' attitudes toward AIDS. *Psychology and Health, 4,* 357–365.

Stahly, G. B. (1988). Psychosocial aspects of the stigma of cancer: An overview. *Journal of Psychosocial Oncology, 6,* 3–27.

Stall, R., Heurtin-Roberts, S., McKusick, L., Hoff, C., & Lang, S. W. (1990).

Sexual risk for HIV transmission among singles-bar patrons in San Francisco. *Medical Anthropology Quarterly, 4,* 115–128.

Stall, R., Hoff, C., Coates, T. J., Paul, J., Phillips, K. A., Estrand, M., Kegeles, S., Catania, J., Daigle, D., & Diaz, R. (1996). Decisions to get HIV tested and to accept antiretroviral therapies among gay/bisexual men: Implications for secondary prevention efforts. *Journal of Acquired Immune Deficiency Syndromes and Human Retrovirology, 11,* 151–160.

Stansell, J. D., & Huang, L. (1997). *Pneumocystis carinii* pneumonia. In M. A. Sande & P. A. Volberding (Eds.), *The medical management of AIDS* (5th ed., pp. 275–300). Philadelphia: Saunders.

Stansell, J. D., & Sande, M. A (1992). Cryptococcal infection in AIDS. In M. A. Sande & P. A. Volberding (Eds.), *The medical management of AIDS* (3rd ed., pp. 297–310). Philadelphia: Saunders.

Staprans, S. I., & Feinberg, M. (1997). Natural history and immunopathogenesis of HIV-1 disease. In M. A. Sande & P. A. Volberding (Eds.), *The medical management of AIDS* (5th ed., pp. 29–56). Philadelphia: Saunders.

Stein, M. D., Freedberg, K. A., Sullivan, L. M., Savetsky, J., Levenson, S. M., Hingson, R., & Samet, J. H. (1997). Sexual ethics: Disclosure of HIV positive status to partners. Manuscript submitted for publication.

Stein, M., Miller, A. H., & Trestman, R. L. (1991). Depression, the immune system, and health and illness. *Archives of General Psychiatry, 48,* 171–177.

Stewart, D. L., Zuckerman, C. J., & Ingle, J. M. (1994). HIV seroprevalence in a chronically mentally ill population. *Journal of the National Medical Association, 86,* 519–523.

Stoneburner, R. L., Chiasson, M. A., Weisfuse, I. B., & Thomas, P. A. (1990). The epidemic of AIDS and HIV-1 infection among heterosexuals in New York City. *AIDS, 4,* 99–106.

Storosom, J., Van den Boom, F., Van Beauzekom, M., & Sno, H. (1990). *Stress and coping in people with HIV infection.* Paper presented at the Ninth International Conference on AIDS, San Francisco.

Storosum, J. G., Sno, H. N., Schalken, H. F. A., Krol, L. J., Swinkels, J. A., Nahuijs, M., Meijer, E. P., & Danner, S. A. (1991). Attitudes of health-care workers towards AIDS at three Dutch hospitals. *AIDS, 5,* 55–60.

Stowe, A., Ross, M. W., Wodak, A., Thomas, G. V., & Larson, S. A (1993).

Significant relationships and social supports of injecting drug users and their implications for HIV/AIDS services. *AIDS Care, 5,* 23–33.

Stricof, R. L., Kennedy, J. T., Nattell, T. C., Weisfuse, I. B., & Novick, L. F. (1991). HIV seroprevalence in a facility for runaway and homeless adolescents. *American Journal of Public Health, 81,* 50–53.

Strunin, L., Culbert, A., & Crane, S. (1989). First year medical students' attitudes and knowledge about AIDS. *AIDS Care, 1,* 105–110.

Sweat, M. D., & Levin, M. (1995). HIV/AIDS knowledge among the US population. *AIDS Education and Prevention, 7,* 355–372.

Taerk, G., Gallop, R. M., Lancee, W. J., Coates, R. A., & Fanning, M. (1993). Recurrent themes of concern in groups for health care professionals. *AIDS Care, 5,* 215–222.

Takigiku, S. K., Brubaker, T. H., & Hennon, C. B. (1993). A contextual model of stress among parent caregivers of gay sons with AIDS. *AIDS Education and Prevention, 5,* 25–42.

Tanfer, K., Grady, W. R., Klepinger, D. H., & Billy, J. O. (1993). Condom use among U.S. men, 1991. *Family Planning Perspectives, 25,* 61–66.

Tarasoff v. Regents of the University of California, 131 Cal. Rptr. 14, 551 P.2d 334 (1976).

Taylor, M. G., Huo, J. M., & Detels, R. (1991). Is the incubation period of AIDS lengthening? *Journal of Acquired Immune Deficiency Syndromes and Human Retrovirology, 4,* 69–75.

Taylor, J. M., Schwartz, K., & Detels, R. (1986). The time from infection with human immunodeficiency virus (HIV) to the onset of AIDS. *Journal of Infectious Diseases, 154,* 694–697.

Taylor, S. E. (1983). Adjustment to threatening events: A theory of cognitive adaptation. *American Psychologist, 38,* 1161–1173.

Taylor, S. E., & Aspinwall, L. (1990). Psychosocial aspects of chronic illness. In G. M. Herek, S. M. Levy, S. Maddi, S. Taylor, & D. Wertlieb (Eds.), *Psychological aspects of chronic illness: Chronic conditions, fatal diseases, and clinical care* (pp. 7–60). Washington, DC: American Psychological Association.

Taylor, S. E., & Brown, J. D. (1988). Illusion and well-being: A social psychological perspective on mental health. *Psychological Bulletin, 103,* 193–210.

Taylor, S. E., Helgeson, V. S., Reed, G. M., & Skokan, L. A. (1991). Self-generated feelings of control and adjustment to physical illness. *Journal of Social Issues, 47,* 91–109.

Taylor, S. E., Kemeny, M. E., Aspinwall, L. G., Schneider, S. G., Rodriguez, R., & Herbert, M. (1992). Optimism, coping, psychological distress, and high-risk sexual behavior among men at risk for acquired immunodeficiency syndrome (AIDS). *Journal of Personality and Social Psychology, 63,* 460–473.

Taylor, S. E., Lichtman, R. R., & Wood, J. V. (1984). Attributions, beliefs about control, and adjustment to breast cancer. *Journal of Personality and Social Psychology, 46,* 489–502.

Telzak, E. E, Sepkowitz, K., Alpert, P., Manheimer, S., Medard, F., El-Sadr, W., Blum, S., Gagliardi, A., Salomon, N., & Turett, G. (1995). Multidrug-resistant tuberculosis in patients without HIV infection. *New England Journal of Medicine, 333,* 907–911.

Temin, H. M., & Bolognesi, D. P. (1993). Where has HIV been hiding? *Nature, 362,* 292–293.

Terl, A. H. (1992). *AIDS and the law: A basic guide for the nonlawyer.* New York: Taylor & Francis.

Thomas, S., & Quinn, S. C. (1991). Public health then and now: The Tuskegee syphilis study, 1932 to 1972—Implications for HIV education and AIDS risk education programs in the Black community. *American Journal of Public Health, 81,* 1498–1505.

Tindall, B., Carr, A., & Cooper, D. A. (1995). Primary HIV infection: Clinical, immunologic, and serologic aspects. In M. A. Sande & P. A. Volberding (Eds.), *The medical management of AIDS* (4th ed., pp. 105–129). Philadelphia: Saunders.

Tindall, B., Forde, S., Goldstein, D., Ross, M. W., & Cooper, D. A. (1994). Sexual dysfunction in advanced HIV disease. *AIDS Care, 6,* 105–107.

Tindall, B., Imrie, A., Donovan, B., Penny, R., & Cooper, D. A. (1992). Primary HIV infection. In M. A. Sande & P. A. Volberding (Eds.), *The medical management of AIDS* (3rd ed., pp. 67–86). Philadelphia: Saunders.

Tolstoy, L. (1981). *The death of Ivan Ilyich.* New York: Bantam Books. (Original work published 1886)

Torres, R. A., Mani, S., & Altholz, J. (1990). Human immunodeficiency virus infection among homeless men in a New York City shelter: Association with mycobacterium tuberculosis infection. *Journal of the American Medical Association, 50*, 2030–2036.

Travers, K., Mboup, S., Marlink, R., Gueye-Ndiaye, A., Siby, T., Thior, I., Traore, I., Dieng-Sarr, A., Sankale, J., Mullins, C., Ndoye, I., Hsieh, C., Essex, M., & Kanki, P. (1995). Natural protection against HIV-1 infection provided by HIV-2. *Science, 268*, 1612–1615.

Treiber, F. A., Shawn, D., & Malcolm, R. (1987). Acquired immune deficiency syndrome: Psychological impact on health personnel. *Journal of Nervous and Mental Disease, 175*, 496–499.

Treisman, G. J., Lyketsos, C. G., Fishman, M., & McHugh, P. R. (1993). A brief guide to the psychiatric care and evaluation of patients infected with HIV. (Available from Johns Hopkins AIDS Psychiatry Service, Meyer 4-119, 600 North Wolfe Street, Baltimore, MD 21205)

Triplet, R. G. (1992). Discriminatory biases in the perception of illness: The application of availability and representativeness heuristics to the AIDS crisis. *Basic and Applied Social Psychology, 13*, 303–322.

Troop, M., Easterbrook, P., Thornton, S., Flynn, R., Gazzard, B., & Catalan, J. (1997). Reasons given by patients for 'non-progression' in HIV infection. *AIDS Care, 9*, 133–142.

Tross, S, & Hirsch, D. (1988). Psychological distress and neuropsychological complications of HIV infection and AIDS. *American Psychologist, 43*, 929–934.

Turnbull, P. (1997). Prisons. *AIDS Care, 9*, 92–95.

Turner, D. C. (1995, October). HIV, body image, and sexuality. *AIDS Patient Care*, pp. 245–248.

Turner, H. A., Hays, R. B., & Coates, T. J. (1993). Determinants of social support among gay men: The context of AIDS. *Journal of Health and Social Behavior, 34*, 37–53.

Uldall, K. K., Koutsky, L. A, Bradshaw, D. H., Hopkins, S. G., Katon, W., & Lafferty, W. E. (1994). Psychiatric comorbidity and length of stay in hospitalized AIDS patients. *American Journal of Psychiatry, 151*, 1475–1478.

Upchurch, D. M., Ray, P., Reichart, C., Celentano, D. D., Quinn, T., & Hook, E. W. (1992). Prevalence and patterns of condom use among patients attending a sexually transmitted disease clinic. *Sexually Transmitted Diseases, 19*, 175–180.

Urassa, M., Todd, J., Boerma, T., Hayes, R., & Isingo, R. (1997). Male circumcision and susceptibility to HIV infection among men in Tanzania. *AIDS, 11,* 73–80.

Vakil, N. B., Schwartz, S. M., Buggy, B. P., Brummitt, C. F., Kherellah, M., Letzer, D. M., Gilson, I. H., & Jones, P. G. (1996). Biliary cryptosporidiosis in HIV-infected people after the waterborne outbreak of cryptosporidiosis in Milwaukee. *New England Journal of Medicine, 334,* 19–23.

Van Cleef, G. F., Fisher, E., & Polk, R. (1997). Drug interaction potential with inhibitors of HIV protease. *Pharmacology, 17,* 774–778.

van Gorp, W. G., Satz, P., Hinkin, C., Evans, G., & Miller, E. N. (1989). The neuropsychological aspects of HIV-1 spectrum disease. *Psychiatric Medicine, 7,* 59–78.

Vanhems, P., Toma, E., & Pineault, R. (1996). Quality of life assessment and HIV infection: a review. *European Journal of Epidemiology, 12,* 221–228.

Van Servellen, G. & Leake, B. (1993). Introduction: burnout in HIV and AIDS care. In H. Van Dis & E. van Dongen (Eds.) *Burnout in HIV/AIDS Health Care and Support: Impact for professionals and volunteers* (pp. 7–9). Amsterdam: University of Amsterdam Press.

Van Servellen, G. M., Lewis, C. E., & Leake, B. (1988). Nurses' responses to the AIDS crisis: Implications for continuing education programs. *Journal of Continuing Education in Nursing, 19,* 4–8.

Vedhara, K., & Nott, K. H. (1996). Psychological vulnerability to stress: A study of HIV-positive homosexual men. *Journal of Psychosomatic Research, 41,* 255–267.

Vella, S., Giuliano, M., Floriia, M., Chiesi, A., Tomino, C., Seeber, A., Barcherini, S., Bucciardini, R., & Mariotti, S. (1995). Effect of sex, age, and transmission category on the progression to AIDS and survival of zidovudine-treated symptomatic patients. *AIDS, 9,* 51–56.

Velentgas, P., Bynum, C., & Zierler, S. (1990). The buddy volunteer commitment in AIDS care. *American Journal of Public Health, 80,* 1378–1380.

Vernazza, P. L., Gilliam, B., Dyer, M., Fiscus, S., Eron, J., Frank, A., & Cohen, M. (1997). Quantification of HIV in semen: Correlation with antiretroviral treatment and immune status. *AIDS, 11,* 987–993.

Viney, L. L., Crooks, L., Walker, B. M., & Henry, R. (1991). Psychological frailness and strength in an AIDS-affected community: A study of seropositive gay men and voluntary caregivers. *American Journal of Community Psychology, 19,* 279–287.

Vitkovic, L., & Koslow, S. H. (1994). *Neuroimmunology and mental health: A report on neuroimmunology research.* Rockville, MD: National Institute of Mental Health.

Vlahov, D., Graham, N., Hoover, D., Flynn, C., Bartlett, J., Margolick, J., Lyles, C., Nelson, K., Smith, D., Holmberg, S., & Farzadegan, H. (1998). Prognostic indicators of AIDS and infectious disease death in HIV-infected injection drug users: Plasma viral load and CD4 cell count. *Journal of the American Medical Association, 279,* 35–40.

Vogel, J., Cepeda, M., Tschachler, E., Napolitano, K., & Jay, G. (1992). UV activation of human immunodeficiency virus gene expression in transgenic mice. *Journal of Virology, 66,* 1–5.

Volberding, P. A. (1997). Antiretroviral therapy. In M. A. Sande & P. A. Volberding (Eds.), *The medical management of AIDS* (5th ed., pp. 113–124). Philadelphia: Saunders.

von Moltke, L., Grassi, J., Granda, B., Fogelman, S., Daily, J., Harmatz, J., & Shader, R. (in press). Protease inhibitors as inhibitors of human cytochromes P450: High risk associated with ritonavir. *Journal of Clinical Psychopharmacology.*

von Overbeck, J., Egger, M., Smith, G. D., Schoep, M., Ledergerber, B., Furrer, H., & Malinverni, R. (1994). Survival of HIV infection: Do sex and category of transmission matter? *AIDS, 8,* 1307–1313.

Wachtel, T., Piette, J., Mor, V., Stein, M., Fleishman, J., & Carpenter, C. (1992). Quality of life in persons with human immunodeficiency virus infection: Measurement by the medical outcomes study instrument. *Annals of Internal Medicine, 116,* 129–137.

Wagner, G., Rabkin, J. G., & Rabkin, R. (1995). Illness stage, concurrent medications, and other correlates of low testosterone in men with HIV illness. *Journal of Acquired Immune Deficiency Syndrome and Human Retrovirology, 1,* 204–207.

Wagner, G. J., Rabkin, J. G., & Rabkin, R. (1996). A comparative analysis of standard and alternative antidepressants in the treatment of human immunodeficiency virus patients. *Comprehensive Psychiatry, 37,* 402–408.

Waldorf, D., & Lauderback, D. (1993). Condom failure among male sex workers in San Francisco. *AIDS and Public Policy Journal, 8,* 79–90.

Walker, B. S., & Spenger, P. (1995). Clinical judgement of major depression in AIDS patients: The effects of clinician complexity and stereotyping. *Professional Psychology: Research and Practice, 26,* 269–272.

Wallace, B., & Lasker, J. (1992). Awakenings: UV light and HIV gene activation. *Science, 257,* 1211–1212.

Wallack, J. J. (1989). AIDS anxiety among health care professionals. *Hospital and Community Psychiatry, 40,* 507–510.

Wara, D. W., & Dorenbaum, A. (1997). Pediatric AIDS: Perinatal transmission and early diagnosis. In M. A. Sande & P. A Volberding (Eds.), *The medical management of AIDS* (5th ed., pp. 469–474). Philadelphia: Saunders.

Warner-Robins, C. G, & Christiana, N. (1989). The spiritual needs of persons with AIDS. *Family and Community Health, 12,* 43–51.

Warwick, H. (1989). AIDS hypochondriasis. *British Journal of Psychiatry, 155,* 125–126.

Watson, M. (1983). Psychosocial intervention with cancer patients: A review. *Psychological Medicine, 13,* 839–846.

Weber, J., & Weiss, R. (1988). HIV infection: The cellular picture. *Scientific American, 259,* 101–109.

Weinberger, M., Conover, C. J., Samsa, G. P., & Greenberg, S. M. (1992). Physicians' attitudes and practices regarding treatment of HIV-infected patients. *Southern Medical Journal, 85,* 683–686.

Weinstock, H., Sidhu, J., Gwinn, M., Karon, J., & Petersen, L. (1995). Trends in HIV seroprevalence among persons attending sexually transmitted disease clinics in the United States, 1998–1992. *Journal of Acquired Immune Deficiency Syndromes and Human Retrovirology, 9,* 514–522.

Weir, S. S., Feldblum, P. J., Roddy, R. E., & Zekeng, L. (1994). Gonorrhea as a risk factor of HIV acquisition. *AIDS, 8,* 1605–1608.

Weiss, R., & Hardy, L. M. (1990). HIV infection and health policy. *Journal of Consulting and Clinical Psychology, 58,* 70–76.

Weissman, D. (1997). Macrophage-topic HIV and SIV envelope proteins induce a signal through the CCR% chemokine receptor. *Nature, 389,* 981–985.

Weitz, R. (1989). Uncertainty and the lives of persons with AIDS. *Journal of Health and Social Behavior, 30,* 270–281.

Wenger, N., Kusseling, F., Beck, K., & Shapiro, M. (1994). Sexual behavior of individuals infected with human immunodeficiency virus. *Archives of Internal Medicine, 154,* 1849–1854.

White, R. (1987). Testimony before the President's Commission on AIDS. Available from the Ryan White Foundation. Internet address www.ryanwhite.org.

Wight, R. G., LeBlanc, A. J., & Anseshensel, C. S. (1995). Support service use by persons with AIDS and their caregivers. *AIDS Care, 7,* 509–520.

Williams, J. B. W., Rabkin, J. G., Remien, R. H., Gorman, J. M., & Ehrhardt, A. A. (1991). Multidisciplinary baseline assessment of homosexual men with and without human immunodeficiency virus infection. *Archives of General Psychiatry, 48,* 124–130.

Williams, M. L. (1990). HIV seroprevalence among male IVDUs in Houston, Texas. *American Journal of Public Health, 80,* 1507–1508.

Wingood, G. A., & DiClemente, R. J. (1997a). The effects of an abusive primary partner on the condom use and sexual negotiation practices of African-American women. *American Journal of Public Health, 87,* 1016–1018.

Wingood, G. M., & DiClemente, R. J. (1997b). Child sexual abuse, HIV sexual risk, and gender relations of African-American women. *American Journal of Preventive Medicine, 13,* 380–384.

Winiarski, M. G. (1991). *AIDS-related psychotherapy.* Elmsford, NY: Pergamon Press.

Wofsy, C. (1992). Therapeutic issues in women with HIV disease. In M. A. Sande & P. A. Volberding (Eds.), *The medical management of AIDS* (3rd ed., pp. 465–476). Philadelphia: Saunders.

Wolcott, D. L., Namir, S., Fawzy, F., Gottlieb, M., & Mitsuyasu, R. (1986). Illness concerns, attitudes towards homosexuality, and social support in gay men with AIDS. *General Hospital Psychiatry, 8,* 395–403.

Wolf, T., Balson, P., Morse, E., Simon, P., Gaumer, R., Dralle, P., & Williams, M. (1991). Relationship of coping style to affective state and perceived social support in asymptomatic HIV-infected persons: Implications for clinical management. *Journal of Clinical Psychiatry, 52,* 171–173.

Wong, J. K., Hezareh, M., Gunthard, H. F., Havlir, D. V., Ignacio, C. C., Spina,

C. A., & Richman, D. D. (1997). Recovery of replication-competent HIV despite prolonged suppression of plasma viremia. *Science, 278*, 1291–1293.

Wong, S. Y., Israelski, D. M., & Remington, J. S. (1995). AIDS-associated toxoplasmosis. In M. A. Sande & P. A. Volberding (Eds.), *The medical management of AIDS* (4th ed., pp. 460–493). Philadelphia: Saunders.

Woo, S. (1992). *Ending the isolation: HIV and mental health in the second decade.* Ottawa, Ontario, Canada: Minister of Health and Welfare.

Wood, K. A., Nairn, R., Kraft, H., & Kiegel, A. (1997). Suicidality among HIV-positive psychiatric in-patients. *AIDS Care, 9*, 385–389.

Woodhouse, D. E., Muth, J. B., Potterat, J. J., & Riffe, L. D. (1993). Restricting personal behaviour: Case studies on legal measures to prevent the spread of HIV. *International Journal of STD and AIDS, 4*, 114–117.

Worley, J. M., & Price, R. W. (1992). Management of neurologic complications of HIV-1 infection and AIDS. In M. A. Sande & P. A. Volberding (Eds.), *The medical management of AIDS* (3rd ed., pp. 193–217). Philadelphia: Saunders.

Wormser, G. P. (Ed.). (1992). *AIDS and other manifestations of HIV infection* (2nd ed.). New York: Raven Press.

Wu, A. W., Rubin, H. R., Mathews, W. C., Ware, J. E., Brysk, L. T., Hardy, W. D., Bozzette, S. A., Spector, S. A, & Richman, D. D. (1991). A health status questionnaire using 30 items from the medical outcomes study: Preliminary validation in persons with early HIV infection. *Medical Care, 29*, 786–798.

Yarrish, R. L. (1992). Cytomegalovirus infections in AIDS. In G. P. Wormser (Ed.), *AIDS and other manifestations of HIV infection* (2nd ed., pp. 249–268). New York: Raven Press.

Yates, J. (1991). AIDS: A Christian view. *International Journal of STD and AIDS, 2*, 38–40.

Zakowski, S., McAllister, C., Deal, M., & Baum, A. (1992). Stress, reactivity, and immune function in healthy men. *Health Psychology, 11*, 223–232.

Zamperetti, M., Goldwurm, G. F., Abbate, E., Gris, T., Muratori, S., & Vigo, B. (1990, June). *Attempted suicide and HIV infection: Epidemiological aspects in a psychiatric ward.* Paper presented at the Sixth International Conference on AIDS, San Francisco.

Zich, J., & Temoshok, L. (1987). Perceptions of social support in men with

AIDS and ARC: Relationships with distress and hardiness. *Journal of Applied Social Psychology, 17,* 193–215.

Zich, J., & Temoshok, L. (1990). Perceptions of social support, distress, and hopelessness in men with AIDS and ARC: Clinical implications. In L. Temoshok & A. Baum (Eds.), *Psychosocial perspectives on AIDS* (pp. 201–227). Hillsdale, NJ: Erlbaum.

Ziegler, P. (1969). *The black death.* New York: John Day.

Zierler, S., Feingold, L., Laufer, D., Velentgas, P., Kantrowitz-Gordon, I., & Mayer, K. (1991). Adult survivors of childhood sexual abuse and subsequent risk of HIV infection. *American Journal of Public Health, 81,* 572–575.

Zigmond, A. S., & Snaith, R. P. (1983). The Hospital Anxiety and Depression Scale. *Acta Psychiatrica Scandinavia, 67,* 361–370.

Zonderman, A. B., Costa, P. T., & McCrae, R. R. (1989). Depression as a risk for cancer morbidity and mortality in a nationally representative sample. *Journal of the American Medical Association, 262,* 1191–1195.

Summary of U.S. Epidemiology

Table A.1

Total AIDS Cases Reported in U.S. States Through June 1997

State	Cumulative Total AIDS Cases
Alabama	4,504
Alaska	385
Arizona	5,258
Arkansas	2,270
California	101,569
Colorado	5,962
Connecticut	9,174
Delaware	1,922
District of Columbia	9,946
Florida	62,200
Georgia	17,985
Hawaii	2,028
Idaho	394
Illinois	19,319
Indiana	4,779
Iowa	1,028
Kansas	1,919

Table continues

Table A.1 (Continued)

State	Cumulative Total AIDS Cases
Kentucky	2,401
Louisiana	9,660
Maine	783
Maryland	16,223
Massachusetts	12,523
Michigan	8,770
Minnesota	3,095
Mississippi	3,050
Missouri	7,487
Montana	249
Nebraska	843
Nevada	3,300
New Hampshire	729
New Jersey	34,871
New Mexico	1,517
New York	113,549
North Carolina	7,742
North Dakota	85
Ohio	9,109
Oklahoma	2,886
Oregon	4,021
Pennsylvania	18,388
Rhode Island	1,668

Table continues

Table A.1 (Continued)

State	Cumulative Total AIDS Cases
South Carolina	6,661
South Dakota	122
Tennessee	5,974
Texas	42,185
Utah	1,449
Vermont	316
Virginia	9,699
Washington	7,930
West Virginia	801
Wisconsin	2,916
Wyoming	153
Puerto Rico	19,583
Total	611,358

Table A.2

Estimated Total Persons Living With AIDS in U.S. States Through June 1997

State	People Living With AIDS
Alabama	1,977
Alaska	184
Arizona	1,812
Arkansas	1,094
California	34,832

Table continues

Table A.2 (Continued)

State	People Living with AIDS
Colorado	2,359
Connecticut	4,424
Delaware	857
District of Columbia	4,193
Florida	25,900
Georgia	7,739
Hawaii	686
Idaho	160
Illinois	6,597
Indiana	2,045
Iowa	439
Kansas	715
Kentucky	975
Louisiana	4,040
Maine	345
Maryland	6,803
Massachusetts	4,202
Michigan	3,487
Minnesota	1,217
Mississippi	1,253
Missouri	3,227
Montana	116
Nebraska	331
Nevada	1,525
New Hampshire	382

Table continues

Table A.2 (*Continued*)

State	People Living with AIDS
New Jersey	12,165
New Mexico	601
New York	37,091
North Carolina	2,847
North Dakota	33
Ohio	3,091
Oklahoma	1,209
Oregon	1,557
Pennsylvania	7,287
Rhode Island	689
South Carolina	2,985
South Dakota	45
Tennessee	2,740
Texas	17,133
Utah	605
Vermont	137
Virginia	3,813
Washington	3,129
West Virginia	333
Wisconsin	1,237
Wyoming	60
Puerto Rico	6,912
Total	229,616

Table A.3

U.S. AIDS Cases for HIV Exposure Categories Reported Through June 1997

Exposure Category	Males		Females	
	Number	%	Number	%
Men who have sex with men	289,699	58	—	
Injecting drug use	113,635	22	41,029	44
Men who have sex with men and inject drugs	38,923	8	—	
Hemophilia	4,378	1	189	0
Heterosexual contact	18,811	4	35,760	39
With injection drug user	6,906		15,984	
With bisexual man	—		2,768	
With a person with he-mophilia	44		346	
With transfusion recipient	342		525	
Not specified	11,519		16,137	
Recipient of blood transfu-sion	4,634	1	3,441	4
Other risk/unidentified risk	32,854	6	11,823	13
Total	511,934	100	92,242	100

Table A.4

Cumulative Adult/Adolescent Cases of AIDS by Categories of Multiple Modes of HIV Transmission Through June 1997

Multiple Modes of Exposure	AIDS Cases	
	Number	%
Men who have sex with men and inject drugs	33,600	6
Injection drug user and heterosexual contact	27,251	5
Men who have sex with men and women	8,366	1
Men who have sex with men and a transfusion	3,260	1
Men who have sex with men and women and use injection drugs	4,528	1

Table A.5

Total Number of Possible Health Care Occupationally Acquired AIDS/HIV Infection in the United States Through June 1997

Occupation	Number of Possible Transmission Cases
Dental worker	7
Embalmer/morgue technician	2
Emergency medical technician/paramedic	10
Health aide	12
Housekeeper	7
Laboratory technician	17
Nurse	29
Nonsurgical physician	10
Surgical physician	6
Respiratory therapist	2
Dialysis technician	3
Surgical technician	2
Other technicians	5
Other health care occupations	2
Total	114

Glossary

accelerated approval: Expedited FDA approval of a new treatment that is based on early surrogate marker data from clinical studies. The purpose of accelerated approval is to hasten the availability of new drugs for serious or life-threatening conditions.

acquired immune deficiency syndrome (AIDS): The final stage of HIV infection, characterized by clinical symptoms of severe immune deficiency. Although there are several diagnostic systems, the most widely used is the one provided by the CDC, which lists opportunistic infections and malignancies that, in the presence of HIV infection, constitute an AIDS diagnosis. In addition, a T-helper cell count below 200/mm^3 for people with HIV infection constitutes an AIDS diagnosis.

active immunity: Biological defense to stimulation by a disease-causing organism or other antigen.

acute: Refers to intense, short-term symptoms or illnesses that either resolve or evolve into long-lasting, chronic disease manifestations.

acute infection: Any infection that begins suddenly, with intense or severe symptoms.

adherence: The degree to which a patient follows drug schedules. A synonym for *compliance.* The act of following a prescribed therapeutic regimen.

adverse reaction (side effect): An unwanted negative reaction to an experimental drug or vaccine.

AIDS Clinical Trials Group (ACTG): A nationwide consortium of medical centers carrying out clinical trials to study therapies for HIV–AIDS, sponsored by the National Institute of Allergy and Infectious Disease (NIAID).

AIDS-defining illness: One of the serious illnesses that occurs in HIV-positive individuals and a basis for an AIDS diagnosis according to the CDC's definition of AIDS. Among these conditions are PCP, MAV, AIDS dementia complex, AIDS wasting syndrome, invasive cervical cancer, Kaposi's sarcoma, and CMV retinitis.

AIDS dementia complex: A brain disorder in people with AIDS that results in the loss of cognitive capacity, affecting the ability to function in a social or occupational setting. Its cause has not been determined exactly, but may result from HIV infection of cells in the brain or an inflammatory reaction to such infection.

AIDS-related complex (ARC): A variously defined term with little clinical value used to identify certain HIV-infected individuals prior to an AIDS diagnosis. Compared to earlier in the epidemic, the term *ARC* is used less often today. Instead, physicians chart HIV disease as starting with no apparent symptoms (asymptomatic) and progressing to symptoms (symptomatic). Fatigue, night sweats, fever, swollen glands, diarrhea, or unintentional weight loss were previously grouped under the term *ARC*.

alternative medicine: A catch-all phrase for a long list of treatments of medicinal systems, including traditional systems such as Chinese or Ayurvedic medicine as well as homeopathy, various herbal, and many other miscellaneous treatments that have not been accepted by the mainstream, or Western, medical establishment. Alternative medicine may be referred to as *complementary medicine*. The designation *alternative medicine* is not equivalent to *holistic medicine*, which is a more narrow term.

amoebiasis: A parasitic intestinal infection caused by tiny unicellular microorganisms called amoebas. Symptoms include diarrhea, bloating, and abdominal pain.

anabolic steroid: A synthetic steroid used to increase muscle mass and weight. Anabolic steroids are versions of the natural hormone testosterone but have fewer masculinizing, or androgenic, effects. Anabolic steroids have been used to reverse AIDS-related wasting syndrome on an individual basis, and positive trial data are slowly accumulating.

anemia: A decrease in number of red blood cells or amount of hemoglobin. Commonly called *low blood count*.

anergic: Relating to the immune system's inability to produce a marked reaction in response to foreign antigens. For example, HIV-infected individuals who did not react to the tuberculosis skin test even though they have contracted a tuberculosis infection are considered to be anergic.

angiogenesis: The process of new blood vessel growth. Tumors and Kaposi's sarcoma lesions stimulate angiogenesis to supply themselves with blood.

anorexia: A lack or loss of appetite that leads to significant decline in weight.

antibiotic: An agent that kills or inhibits the growth of microorganisms, especially a compound similar to those produced by certain fungi for destroying bacteria. An antibiotic is used to combat disease and infection.

antibodies: Molecules in the blood or secretory fluids that tag, destroy, or neutralize bacteria, viruses, or other harmful toxins. They belong to a class of proteins known as immunoglobulins, which are produced by B-lymphocytes in response to antigens.

antiretroviral: Drugs that treat retroviral infection. AZT, ddI, and ddC are examples of antiretrovirals used to treat HIV infection.

antisense drug: A synthetic segment of DNA or RNA that locks onto a strand of DNA or RNA with a complementary sequence of nucleotides. Antisense drugs are designed to block viral genetic instructions, marking them for destruction by cellular enzymes, to prevent the building of new virus or the infection of new cells.

apoptosis: A type of cellular suicide triggered by stimulation of particular receptors on a cell's surface. It is a metabolic process driven by cellular enzymes in which the cell's chromosomes and then the cell itself breaks down into fragments. In the immune system, apoptosis is a process that eliminates unneeded cells. Some researchers believe that accidental apoptosis may be the way that CD4 cells become depleted in HIV disease, rather than through direct killing by HIV.

aspergillus: A fungus that infects the lungs, causing a disease known as aspergillosis. The infection can spread through the blood to other organs and cause lesions in the skin, ear, and nasal sinuses in addition to the lungs, as well as occasionally in the bones, meninges, heart, kidneys, or spleen.

assay: A test used to detect the presence and concentration of a drug, virus, or other substance in bodily fluids or tissues.

asthenia: Weakness, debility.

asymptomatic: Having no symptoms; free of sensations of poor health.

attenuated virus: A weakened virus with reduced ability to infect or produce disease. Some vaccines are made of attenuated viruses.

autoimmune disease: An ailment caused by an immune response against an individual's own tissues or cells.

autoimmunization: A self-destructive process characterized by an immune response to one's own cells.

autologous: Referring to a naturally occurring substance derived from and used with the same individual. Compare endogenous.

bacterium: A microscopic organism composed of a single cell that often causes human disease.

bDNA (branched DNA): A test developed for measuring the amount of HIV (as well as other viruses) in blood plasma. The test uses a signal amplification technique, which creates a luminescent signal whose brightness depends on the viral RNA present. Test results are calibrated in numbers of virus particle equivalents per milliliter of plasma. bDNA is similar in results, but not in technique, to the PCR test. A test for measuring the amount to HIV (as well as other viruses) in blood plasma. The test uses a signal amplification technique, creating a luminescent signal whose brightness depends on the viral RNA present. Test results are calibrated in numbers of virus particles per milliliter of plasma.

bioavailability: The extent to which an oral medication is absorbed in the digestive tract and reaches the bloodstream.

blinded study: A clinical trial in which participants are unaware whether they are in the experimental or the control group.

B-lymphocytes or B-cells: One of two major classes of lymphocytes. During infections, these cells are transformed into plasma cells that produce large quantities of antibody directed at specific pathogens. Although HIV specifically infects cells displaying the CD4 receptor, especially T-helper lymphocytes, the disruption of immune function by HIV also affects B lymphocytes; also, B-cell lymphomas are common among HIV-positive people.

body fluids: Term usually referring to semen, blood, urine, and saliva.

bone marrow suppression: A side effect of many anticancer and anti-retroviral drugs, including AZT. Bone marrow suppression may lead to a decrease in red blood cells (erythrocytopenia or anemia), white blood cells (Leukopenia), or platelets (thrombocytopenia). Such reductions respectively result in fatigue and weakness, bacterial infections, and spontaneous or excess bleeding.

breakthrough infection: An infection that occurs during the course of a vaccine trial.

Burkitt's lymphoma: A cancerous tumor, frequently involving jaw bones, ovaries, and abdominal lymph nodes. The disease is common in Africa and has been associated with Epstein–Barr virus.

buyer's club: A nonprofit group that imports AIDS-related therapies available in other countries but not yet approved by the FDA for use in the United States. Many buyers' club products are sold abroad for purposes that are not related to AIDS or HIV infection.

candida: Yeast-like fungi, commonly found in the mouth, skin, intestinal tract, and vagina, but that can become clinically infectious with immune suppression.

CBO: Community-based organizations that provide multiple services to people affected by AIDS.

CD4: A membrane protein or receptor of T-helper lymphocytes, monocytes, macrophages, and some other cells; is the attachment site for HIV.

CD4/CD8 ratio: The ratio of CD4 to CD8 cells. A common measure of immune system status that is around 1.5 (to one) in healthy individuals and falls as CD4 counts fall in people with HIV infection.

CD4 count: The most commonly used surrogate marker for assessing the state of the immune system. As CD4 cell count declines, the risk of developing opportunistic infections increases. The normal range for CD4 cell counts is 500 to 1,500 per cubic millimeter of blood. CD4 count should be rechecked at least every 6 to 12 months if CD4 counts are greater than 500/mm^3. If the count is lower, testing every 3 months is advised.

CD4 percent: The percentage of total lymphocytes made up by CD4 cells. A common measure of immune status that is about 40% in healthy individuals and is below 20% in people with AIDS.

CD8 (T8): A membrane protein found on the surface of suppressor T-lymphocytes.

cell-mediated immunity (CMI): One type of immune system response, coordinated by Th1 cells, in which disease is controlled by specific defense cells (cytotoxic T-lymphocytes) that kill infected cells.

cellular immunity: Biological-defense principally mediated by lymphocytes acting directly on invading antigens.

426

cervical dysplasia: Changes in the lining cells of the cervix that may progress to cancer if not treated in time. Cervical dysplasia is detected through a Pap smear.

chancre: A sore or ulcer. Presence of a chancre on the genitals apparently increases the probability of being infected with HIV.

chemokine: Soluble chemical messengers that attract white blood cells to the site of infection. There are two structural categories of chemokines: alpha (CXC) and beta (cc). Examples of chemokines that interfere with HIV activity are the B chemokines MIP-1a, MIP-1B, and RANTES and the a chemokine SDF-1.

chronic infection: Persisting for longer than 2 weeks or recurring over time.

ciprofloxacin (Cipro): An antibiotic commonly used for lung and urinary infections and possibly MAC infections.

clade: One of the major, largely geographically isolated, HIV subtypes. Classification is based on differences in envelope protein. Clade B makes up the overwhelming majority of HIV in North America and Europe.

clinical trial: Scientifically governed investigations of medications in volunteer study participants. Their purpose is to seek information regarding the product's safety (Phase I) and efficacy (how well it works; Phases II–III).

clotting factors: Substances in the blood that cause the blood to change from a liquid to a coagulate or a solid to stop bleeding.

CMV polyradiculopathy: CMV infection of the spinal roots (the bundles of nerves coming out of the spinal cord), leading to generalized weakness and paralysis.

CMV retinitis: CMV infection of the retina. The lesions it causes lead to deterioration in vision and ultimately blindness if untreated.

cofactors: Substances, microorganisms, or characteristics of individuals that influence disease progression.

cohort: A group of individuals who share one or more characteristics for purposes of a clinical research study.

combination therapy (convergent combination therapies): Combined administration of drugs that are effective at different stages of the HIV viral cycle or that impact on different elements of the virus. Combined approaches reduce potential drug resistance.

compassionate use–access: A process for providing experimental drugs on an individual basis to very sick patients who have no treatment options. Often, case-by-case approval must be obtained from the FDA for compassionate use of a drug.

complimentary treatments: Unapproved substances or procedures used for therapeutic purposes.

contagious: Any infectious disease capable of being transmitted from person to person; contains several subunits called epitomes that are targets of specific antibodies and sytotoxic T-lymphocytes.

corticosteroid: Any steroid hormone obtained from the cortex or outer portion of the adrenal gland or any synthetic substitute for such a steroid. Corticosteroids are immunosuppressive and include prednisone, corticosterone, and aldosterone.

cross-resistance: The phenomenon in which a microbe that has acquired resistance to one drug through direct exposure also turns out to have resistance to one or more other drugs to which it has not been exposed. Cross-resistance arises because the mechanism of resistance to several drugs is the same, resulting from identical genetic mutations.

cryopreservation: A controversial treatment involving freezing cells, such as specific immune cells, for use by the same patient at a later time.

cytokines: Chemical messenger proteins released by certain white blood cells, including macrophages, monocytes, or lymphocytes.

cytomegalovirus (CMV): A herpes virus that causes opportunistic diseases in immune compromised patients. While CMV can infect most organs of the body, people with AIDS have been most susceptible to CMV retinitis and colitis.

cytotoxic T-lymphocyte (CTL): A type of CD8 or, less often, CD4 lymphocyte that kills diseased cells infected by a specific virus or other intracellular microbe. CTLs interact with antigen bearing MHC class I molecules or infected cells and have the prime role in cell-mediated immunity.

dendritic cells: Immune cells with long, tentacle-like branches called dendrites. Among the dendritic cells are the Langerhans cells of the skin and follicular dendritic cells in the lymph nodes. Most dendritic cells function as antigen presenting cells, although follicular dendritic cells do not.

disseminated: Disease scattered throughout several organ systems.

dormant: Inactive, as in a dormant infection.

dose-escalating: Describes a preliminary clinical trial in which the amount of a drug is either periodically increased or increased with each new trial arm that is added. Used to determine how well a drug is tolerated in people and what its optimum dose might be, given the observed balance between activity and side effects.

drug–drug interaction: The effects that occur when two or more drugs are used together. Such effects include changes of absorption in the digestive tract, changes in rate of the drugs' breakdown in the liver, new or enhanced side effects, and changes in the drugs' activity.

dyspnea: Shortness of breath or difficulty in breathing.

early HIV infection: The stage of HIV infection during which no major physical health symptoms are yet present, though psychological symptoms may be present.

encephalitis: Inflammation of the brain, acute or chronic, caused by viruses, bacteria, toxins, and so forth.

encephalopathy: A broad term used to describe metabolic, toxic, malignant, or degenerative diseases of the brain.

endemic: Continuous presence of a disease in a community or among a group of people.

endocrine gland: One of the organs in the body that produces hormones.

env gene: The gene that encodes spike proteins and glycoproteins of the envelope of HIV.

envelope: In virology, a protein covering of virus genetic material. The HIV envelope is composed of two glycoproteins, *gp*41 and *gp*120, that bind to the CD4 surface molecule.

enzyme: A cellular protein whose shape allows it to hold together several other molecules in close proximity to each other. Enzymes are able in this way to induce chemical reactions in other substances with little expenditure of energy and without being changed themselves. A protein that can cause chemical changes in other substances without being changed itself.

enzyme linked immunosorbent assay (ELISA): The blood test most often used to screen for HIV infection. ELISA detects HIV antibodies—not HIV itself. Because ELISA is sensitive, it has a high-false-positive rate and is therefore confirmed by a more specific test.

epidemic: A disease or condition that affects many persons within a population at the same time when ordinarily they are not subject to this condition.

epitope: A unique molecular shape or amino acid sequence carried on a microorganism that triggers a specific antibody or cellular immune response.

Epstein-Barr virus (EBV): A herpes-like virus that causes mononucleosis, infects the nose and throat and is contagious, lies dormant in the lymph glands, and is associated with Burkitt's lymphoma and hairy leuko-plakia.

erythropoietin: A substance that stimulates bone marrow to produce red blood cells.

first-line treatment: The optimal starting therapy for a treatment-naive patient. Because of the potential for the development of cross-resistance by HIV and other microbes, the choice of first-line medication(s) will affect the efficacy of succeeding (second-line) therapies.

floater: Drifting dark spots within the field of vision. Floaters can be caused by CMV retinitis, but also can appear in persons as a normal part of the aging process.

fungus: One of a group of primitive, nonvascular plants lacking chlorophyll. Among the fungi are mushrooms, yeast, rust, and molds. Some fungi are single-celled but differ from bacteria in that they have a distinct nucleus and other cellular structures. Reproduction is accomplished by spores.

gastroenteritis: Inflammation of the lining of the stomach or intestines; caused by bacterial or viral infection.

gene therapy: Any number of experimental treatments in which cell genes are altered. Some gene therapies attempt to provoke new immune activity; some try to render cells resistant to infection; some involve the development of enzymes that destroy viral or cancerous genetic material cells.

giant cells: Large multinucleated cells sometimes seen in granulomatous reactions and thought to result from the fusion of macrophages.

gingivitis: Swelling, bleeding, or soreness of the gums that can be especially severe in people with HIV infection; treated early, gingivitis can usually be controlled by regular brushing, flossing, and dental care.

gp120: A glycoprotein from HIV's envelope that binds to CD4 molecules on cell's outside membrane. Free *gp*120 in the body may be toxic to cells on its own, causing CD4 depletion in the immune system through apoptosis and neurological damage leading to AIDS dementia complex.

gp41: A glycoprotein from HIV's outside envelopes that complexes with *gp*120 to form the mechanism enabling HIV to latch onto and enter cells.

granulocytes: A type of white blood cell that helps kill bacteria and other microorganisms.

HAART (Highly Active Antiretroviral Therapy): Aggressive anti-HIV treatment usually including a combination of protease and reverse transcriptase inhibitors whose purpose is to reduce viral load to undetectable levels.

hairy leukoplakia: A whitish, slightly raised lesion that appears on the side of the tongue; related to Epstein–Barr virus infection during immune suppression.

helper-suppressor ratio: The number of helper (CD4+) T-cells to suppressor (CD8+) T-cells; suppressor cells outnumber helper cells in advanced HIV infection.

hemophilia: An inherited disease that keeps blood from clotting.

hepatitis A: A self-limiting virus-induced liver disease. Hepatitis A is acquired through ingesting fecal contaminated water or food or engaging in sexual practices involving anal contact. Injection drug users who share unclean needles also risk contracting hepatitis A.

hepatitis B: A virus-induced liver disease that usually lasts no more than 6 months, but becomes chronic and life-threatening in 10% of the cases. The highly contagious hepatitis B virus can be transmitted through sexual contact, contaminated syringes, and blood transfusions.

hepatitis C: A virus-induced liver disease. It appears to be more common among heterosexuals and injection drug users than hepatitis B. It is more likely than hepatitis B to become chronic and lead to liver degeneration (cirrhosis).

Heptavax: A vaccine for hepatitis B.

herbal treatments: Small amounts of plants, including roots, bark, leaves, or juices used for therapeutic purposes.

herpes simplex virus I (HSV I): Causes cold sores or fever blisters on the mouth or around the eyes and can be transmitted to the genital region; latent HSV I is reactivated by stress, trauma, other infections, or other causes of immune suppression.

herpes simplex virus II (HSV II): Causes painful sores on the anus or genitals; may lie dormant in nervous tissue and can be reactivated to produce symptoms; transmittable to infants during labor and delivery.

herpes varicella zoster virus (HVZ): Causes chicken pox in children; consists of very painful blisters on the skin that follow nerve pathways; may reappear in adulthood as herpes zoster causing shingles.

HHV-8 (KSHV, KS Herpes Virus): A herpes virus thought to trigger the development of Kaposi's sarcoma lesions. HHV-8's mode of transmission has not been determined.

holistic (wholistic) medicine: Various systems of health protection and restoration, both traditional and modern, that are reputedly based on the body's natural healing powers, the various ways the different tissues affect one another, and the influence of the external environment.

host: A plant or animal that supports the growth of a parasite or infectious organism.

HTLV-I: Human T-cell leukemia virus, a human retrovirus that causes a rare form of leukemia after a long period of asymptomatic infection. The virus spreads through sexual contact or the sharing of unclean needles by injection drug users.

Human Immunodeficiency Virus (HIV): The AIDS virus; a retrovirus of the lentivirus class; formerly called LAV or HTLV-III. HIV type 1 (HIV-1) is the common cause of HIV disease in North America; HIV type 2 (HIV-2) is prevalent in some parts of Africa and occasionally occurs in North America and Europe.

humoral immunity: Responses against disease rendered by lymphocytes where antibodies are produced and circulate in the blood stream to act against antigens.

hypericin: An experimental treatment for hepatitis B and CMV infection.

immune deficiency: A breakdown or inability of certain parts of the immune system to function; increases susceptibility to certain diseases.

immune reconstitution: The natural or therapy-induced revival of immune function in a body damaged by HIV infection, particularly after initiation of a highly potent antiviral therapy.

immune suppression: A state in which the immune system is damaged and does not perform its normal functions; can be induced by drugs or result from diseases.

immune system: The complex body function that recognizes foreign agents or substances, neutralizes them, and recalls the response later when confronted with the same antigen.

immune-based therapy (IBT): Anti-HIV treatment that aims to modulate, supplement, or extend the body's immune responses against HIV infection or other diseases. Also called immunotherapies. Examples of experimental immunotherapies for HIV include passive immunotherapy therapy (PIT), IL-2 and therapeutic vaccines.

immunity: Natural or acquired resistance to infection by virtue of previous exposure to a disease causing organism. Immunity may be partial or complete, long-lasting or temporary.

immunocompetent: Refers to an immune system capable of enveloping a normal protective response when confronted with invading microbes or cancer.

immunocompromised: Refers to an immune system in which the response to infections and tumors is subnormal.

immunodeficiency: A breakdown or an inability of certain parts of the immune system to function that renders a person susceptible to certain diseases that he or she ordinarily would not develop.

immunoglobulin (Ig): A general term for antibodies that bind onto invading organisms leading to the organisms' destruction. There are five classes: IgA, IgD, IgM, IgE, IgG.

immunoglobulin A (IgA): An immunoglobulin found in bodily fluids such as tears and saliva and in the respiratory, reproductive, urinary, and gastrointestinal tracts. IgA protects the body's mucosal surfaces from infection.

immunoglobulin G (IgG): The prominent type of immunoglobulin existing in the blood. Also called gamma globulin.

immunomodulator: A substance capable of modifying one or more functions of the immune system.

in vitro (in glass): An artificial environment created outside a living organism (for example, a test tube or culture plate) used in experimental research to study a disease or process.

in vivo (in life): Studies conducted within a living organism.

incidence: The number of new cases of disease in a defined population during a specified period of time.

incubation period: The time between infection exposure and the first physical response, such as the production of antibodies.

integrase: The HIV enzyme that inserts HIV's genes into a cell's normal DNA. Integrase operates after reverse transcriptase has created a DNA version of HIV genes present in virus particles.

interferons: Proteins originally defined by their activity against viral infections. Alpha, beta, and gamma interferons have been investigated as therapy for some opportunistic diseases.

interleukin: One of a large group of glycoproteins that acts as cytokines. The interleukins are secreted by and affect many different cells in the immune system.

invasive: Disease in which organisms or cancer cells are spreading throughout the body; or a medical procedure in which a device is inserted into the body.

isolate: A genetically homogeneous HIV close with distinguishing characteristics and extracted from a single source.

Kaposi's sarcoma (KS): A tumor of blood vessel walls or the lymphatic system; usually appears as pink or purple painless spots on the skin, but may also occur on internal organs.

Karnofsky score: A subjective measurement of an individual's functional ability to perform common activities.

killer cell: A generalized name for immune system cells that kill cancerous and virus-infected cells. Among the killer cells are killer T-cells (cytotoxic T-lymphocytes), NK (natural killer) cells, and K-cells.

Langerhans cells: The type of dendritic cell found in the skin. See dendritic cell.

latency: Latency and dormancy (which literally means sleeping) mean the same thing: A microbe is in the body but is not actively reproducing, not invading any tissues, and not causing symptoms. Examples of microbes that are latent or dormant in many or most healthy people are pneumocystis carinii, toxoplasma *gondii*, herpes simplex virus, the virus that causes herpes zoster, and cytomegalovirus. Once in the body, these microbes remain in the body. They remain latent or dormant until something tilts the balance in the immune system and permits them to become active.

lentivirus (slow virus): A virus that produces disease with a greatly delayed onset and protracted course such as HIV.

leukocyte: Any of the various white blood cells, which together make up the immune system. Neutrophils, lymphocytes, and monocytes are all leukocytes.

leukocytosis: An abnormally high number of leukocytes in the blood. This condition can occur during many types of infection and inflammation.

leukopenia: An abnormally low number of total leukocytes circulating in the blood, frequently the result of drug-induced bone marrow suppression.

ligand: Any molecule that binds to the surface of another molecule, such as an immune cell receptor.

limit of detection (limit of quantification): Refers to the sensitivity of a quantitative diagnostic test, such as the viral load assay. The limit of detection is the level below which the test can no longer accurately measure the amount of a substance, such as HIV RNA. If a person has an "undetectable" viral load, it does not mean that HIV is no longer present, but rather, that the test is not sensitive enough to measure the amount. For viral load assays, *limit of quantification* is becoming the preferred term.

log (logarithm): Formally, the number of times 10 must be multiplied with itself to equal a certain number. For example 100,000 is log 5 because it is equal to $10 \times 10 \times 10 \times 10 \times 10$. Logs are used to measure changes in viral load. For example, a reduction in viral load from 100,000 to 1,000 copies/ml is a two log (or 99%) reduction. Note that half/log change is not a fivefold difference but a change of 3.16-fold (the square root of ten).

long terminal repeat (LTR): The genetic material at each end of the HIV genome. When the HIV genes are integrated into a cell's own genome, the LTR interacts with cellular and viral factors to initiate the transcription of the HIV DNA into an RNA, for that is packaged in new virus particles. Activation of the LTR is a major step in triggering HIV replication.

long-term nonprogressor: An individual who has been infected with HIV for at least 7 to 12 years (different authors use different time spans) and yet retains a CD4 cell count within the normal range and has no evidence of disease progression.

long-term survivor: A looser term than long-term nonprogressor that indicates any person with any stage of HIV infection, including AIDS, who is stable over a period of years.

lymph: A transparent, slightly yellow fluid that carries lymphocytes to and from the lymph nodes and helps to collect foreign microbes.

Lymph is derived from tissue fluids. The fluid passes through the lymphatic ducts and then enters the bloodstream.

lymph nodes (glands): Small bean-sized organs of the immune system distributed widely throughout the body; lymph fluid is filtered through lymph nodes in which all types of lymphocytes take up temporary residence; antigens that enter the body find their way into lymph or blood and are filtered out by lymph nodes or the spleen.

lymphadenopathy: Swollen, firm, and possibly tender lymph nodes; the cause may be an infection or lymphoma.

lymphocytes: Several types of white blood cells, including helpers, suppressors, and B- and T-lymphocytes.

lymphoid interstitial pneumonitis (LIP): A type of pneumonia that affects 35% to 40% of children with AIDS and causes hardening of the lung membranes involved in absorbing oxygen. LIP is an AIDS-defining illness in children.

lymphoma: A cancer that starts in the lymph node. The two major types of lymphoma are Hodgkin's disease and non-Hodgkin's lymphoma (NHL). Lymphoma of the brain is considered an AIDS-defining illness unless HIV infection is ruled out.

MAC (Mycobacterium Avium Complex): A disease caused by two bacteria found in water, soil, and food. In people with AIDS, it can spread through the bloodstream to infect lymph nodes, bone marrow, liver, spleen, spinal fluid, lungs, and intestinal tract.

macrophage: A type of white blood cell that destroys degenerated cells; function to break down antigens.

malabsorption: Failure of the intestines to properly absorb food or nutrients.

malaise: A vague feeling of discomfort or uneasiness, often the result of infection or a drug's side effects.

MDR-TB (Multi-Drug-Resistant Tuberculosis): A strain of TB that does not respond to two or more standard anti-TB drugs. MDR-TB usually arises when treatment is intermittent, thus allowing a buildup of mutations in the TB bacteria that confer broader and broader drug resistance.

meningitis: An infection of the meninges, the coverings of the brain and spinal cord. Cryptococcus is the most frequent cause of meningitis in HIV infection.

monoclonal antibodies: Produced by a single cell, specific to a given antigen; useful as a tool for identifying specific protein molecules.

monocyte: A large white blood cell that acts as a scavenger, capable of destroying bacteria or other foreign material; precursor to the macrophage.

monotherapy: Medical treatment consisting of a single drug administered alone.

mucocutaneous: Pertaining to the mucous membranes and the skin, for example, mouth, vagina, and anal area.

mutation: Any alteration, loss, gain or exchange of genetic material within a cell or virus. Mutations are perpetuated in succeeding generations of that cell or virus (or of an entire multicellular organism if the mutated cell is a sperm, egg, or spore). They can occur spontaneously or in response to environmental factors.

mycosis: Any disease caused by a fungus.

myopathy: Any disease or abnormality of voluntary muscle groups.

naive T-cell: A T-cell arising from the immune system's production of fresh cells in the bone marrow. Naive T-cells respond to newly encountered pathogens containing antigens the immune system has not processed before. The naive T-cells' activation and proliferation create an acquired immune response to the newly encountered pathogenic agent. After the disease is eradicated, a portion of the T-cell population engendered by the activated naive T-cell constitutes a reservoir of memory cells, which proliferate and respond very quickly to any recurrence of the disease.

natural killer cells (NK cells): Large granular lymphocytes that attack and destroy tumor and infected cells; attack without first recognizing specific antigens.

nef: An HIV regulatory protein whose functions are not well understood. HIV without nef appears to have low capacity to infect new cells. Nef also blocks HIV-infected cells from expressing CD4 and MHC class I molecules on their surfaces, thus limiting the immune system's ability to recognize and kill these cells.

neucleoside analog: A type of antiretroviral drug, such as AZT, ddI, ddC, or D4T, whose makeup constitutes a defective version of a natural nucleoside. Nucleoside analogs may take the place of the natural nucleosides, blocking the completion of a viral DNA chain during infection of a new cell by HIV.

neuropathy: An illness involving the nerves. Nerves are responsible for (among other things) the movement of muscles and the sensation of touch, including the sensation of pain. The symptoms of a neuropathy can, therefore, be weakness of a muscle or pain and tingling. In people with HIV infection, the most frequent symptoms of neuropathy are painful feet and legs.

neutralizing antibody: Antibodies that can directly block the infective capacity of microorganisms, particularly a virus's ability to penetrate cells.

neutropenia: Abnormal drop in the number of a type of white cells called neutrophils.

neutrophil (polymorphonuclear neutrophils, PMNs): A white blood cell that plays a central role in defense against infection by engulfing microorganisms.

NNRTI (nonnucleoside reverse transcriptase inhibitor): A member of a class of compounds, including delavirdine and nevirapine, that acts to directly combine with and block the action of HIV's reverse transcriptase. In contrast, nucleoside analogs block reverse transcriptase by capping the unfinished DNA chain that the enzyme is constructing. NNRTIs have suffered from HIV's ability to rapidly mutate and become resistant to their effects.

opportunistic infection: An infection in an immune compromised individual that does not normally occur in healthy people; pathogens that cause disease only with immune opportunity.

p24: An HIV-related protein; indirect measurement of p24 provides an indication of HIV activity; a positive p24 antigen test suggests active HIV replication; p24 antibody levels are usually highest early and late in HIV infection.

palliative: Offering relief of symptoms or comfort without ameliorating the underlying disease process.

pancreatic enzymes: Proteins made by the pancreas that aid in digestion.

pancreatitis: Inflammation of the pancreas. Pancreatitis, an occasional side effect of ddI, can result in severe abdominal pain and death. Its onset can be predicted by rises in blood levels of the pancreatic enzyme amylase as well as increases in blood triglycerides.

pandemic: Denoting a disease affecting the population of an extensive region, that is, HIV disease is a pandemic disease, affecting an extensive area of the world.

pap smear: A microscopic examination of the surface cells of the cervix, usually conducted on scrapings from the cervical opening. This assay is used to detect tissue changes that could be forerunners of cervical cancer.

papillovirus (PMV): A virus that may cause oral, skin, anal, and genital warts or nipple-like growths on the skin.

parasite: An organism that feeds on or lives in a different organism; some parasites cause disease.

parenteral: Involving introduction into the bloodstream.

passive immunotherapy: A treatment in which high HIV antibodies from donors are infused into HIV-positive patients.

pathogen: An organism or material capable of causing disease.

pathogenesis: Description of the development of a particular disease, especially the events, reactions, and mechanisms involved at the cellular level.

PCR (polymerase chain reaction): A highly sensitive test that measures the presence or amount of RNA or DNA of a specific organism or virus (for example, HIV or CMV) in the blood or tissue. Unlike the standard blood test for HIV infection that detects antibodies to HIV, the PCR detects HIV itself. PCR tests are being used to gauge HIV disease progression and the effect of particular treatments on HIV infection.

peripheral neuropathy: A disorder of the nerves, usually involving the extremities. Symptoms include numbness, a tingling or burning sensation, sharp pain, weakness, and abnormal reflexes. In severe cases, paralysis may result.

phagocyte: A cell that destroys and ingests foreign matter, including bacteria.

phagocytosis: The process by which cells engulf material and enclose it within a vacuole (phagosome) in the cytoplasm.

pneumocystis carinii pneumonia (PCP): An infection of the lungs caused by a protozoan or fungus that has been the most common life-threatening opportunistic infection in AIDS patients.

polymerase: An enzyme that promotes synthesis of segments of DNA and RNA.

polymerase chain reaction (PCR): A technique for amplifying small amounts of DNA; PCR techniques are useful in identifying HIV-infection before an antibody response, such as in young infants.

postexposure prophylaxis (PEP): Administering drug treatment to prevent disease in an individual after exposure to an infectious organism. For example, guidelines have been established for postexposure prophylaxis of health care providers who have been exposed to HIV through needle sticks.

prednisone: An approved steroid used to reduce inflammation.

prevalence: The number of persons in a given population with a specified disease at a specified point in time; expressed as a percentage.

primary HIV infection: The flu-like syndrome that occurs immediately after a person contracts HIV. This initial infection precedes seroconversion and is characterized by fever, sore throat, headache, skin rash, and swollen glands. Also called acute infection.

prophylactic vaccines: Only work as preventives and must be given before infection.

prophylaxis: Prevention; a treatment intended to preserve health.

prospective study: Refers to studies designed to follow the progress of a cohort forward in time, rather than analyzing data from previous research.

protease: An enzyme that triggers the breakdown of proteins. HIV's protease enzyme breaks apart long strands of viral protein into separate proteins constituting the viral core and the enzymes it contains. HIV protease acts as new virus particles are budding off a cell membrane.

protease inhibitors: Compounds that block the ability of HIV to produce the enzyme protease, an essential enzyme for the HIV replication process.

protocol: A detailed plan for a clinical trial that states the trial's rationale, purpose, drug or vaccine dosages, length of study, route of administration, and who may participate.

provirus: The form of a virus in which its genetic material is incorporated into the host cell's genetic material.

pruritic: Itchy.

receptor: A cell's surface molecule that binds specifically to other particular extracellular molecules.

regulatory genes: HIV genes (e.g., nef, rev, tat) that regulate viral replication in infected cells.

resistance (to a drug): The ability of an organism, a microorganism, or a virus to lose its sensitivity to a drug. For example, after long term use of AZT, HIV can develop strains of virus in the body that are no longer suppressed by the drug, and therefore are said to be resistant to AZT. Resistance is thought to result from a genetic mutation. In HIV, such mutations can change the structure of viral enzymes and proteins so that an antiviral drug can no longer bind with them as well as it used to. Resistance detected by searching a pathogen's genetic makeup for mutations thought to confer lower susceptibility is called *genotypic resistance*. Resistance found by successfully growing laboratory cultures of the pathogen in the presence of a drug is called *phenotypic resistance*. High-level resistance reduces a drug's virus-suppressing activity hundreds of times. Low-level resistance represents only a few fold reduction in drug effectiveness. Depending on the toxicity of the drug, low-level resistance may be overcome by using higher doses of the drug in question.

retinitis: Inflammation of the retina; can diminish vision, contract visual fields, and increase light sensitivity. Cytomegalovirus (CMV) infection is a cause in immune suppressed persons.

retrovirus: A class of RNA viruses with a complex life cycle that includes an obligatory DNA intermediate and reverse transcription from RNA to DNA and is almost impossible for the body to eliminate. A retrovirus takes over cells in the body and makes them into factories that produce other infected cells, each with a slightly different retrovirus.

rev: A regulatory protein produced by HIV within infected cells. Rev helps transport HIV RNA sequences (messenger RNA) out from the nucleus into the cell's cytoplasm, where it directs construction of proteins for new virus particles.

reverse transcriptase (RT): A viral enzyme that transcribes viral RNA into DNA so that genetic material of the virus can be integrated into genetic material of the T-cell helper and other host cells. Many antivirals inhibit the action of this enzyme, including AZT, ddI, and ddC.

ribonucleic acid (RNA): A complex nucleic acid responsible for translating genetic information from DNA and transferring it to the cells' protein-making machinery.

rifampin: An approved antibiotic being used experimentally as a treatment for MAC.

seroconversion: When people exposed to an infectious disease develop antibodies to that disease causing agent; people seroconvert from antibody-negative to antibody-positive.

serologic test: Tests performed on the clear, liquid portion of blood (serum); often refers to tests that determine the presence of antibodies to antigens; ELISA and Western blot are two types of antibody tests.

seropositive or seronegative: Implying the presence or absence of antibodies determined by serological tests.

serostatus: The condition of having or not having detectable antibodies to a microbe in the blood as a result of infection. One may have either a positive or negative serostatus.

sign: Observable physical change indicating that a disease may be present. Examples include fever, bleeding, lesions, rash, and swelling.

SIV: Simian immunodeficiency virus.

stem cell: A cell in bone marrow that can grow into many types of immune system cells.

steroid: A member of a large family of structurally similar lipid molecules. Steroid molecules have a basic skeleton consisting of four interconnected carbon rings. Different classes of steroids have different functions. All the sex hormones are steroids. Cortisol and cortisone regulate many aspects of metabolism and, when administered medically, reduce swelling, pain, and other manifestations of inflammation.

subclinical infection: An infection, or phase of infection, without readily apparent symptoms or signs of disease.

suppressor T-cells (T8, CD8): Subset of T-cells that halt antibody production and other immune responses.

surrogate marker: A laboratory measurement or physical sign that does not directly show how patients feel, but rather predicts the likely effect of a medication on their future disease status. CD4 cell count is an example of a surrogate marker in HIV infection.

symptom: Feelings or sensations that may indicate disease that are not observable but are reported; examples include headache, nausea, pain.

symptomatic: A person who doesn't feel well and has medical problems that can be observed or measured.

syncytium (giant cell): A dysfunctional multicellular clump formed by cell-to-cell fusion.

syndrome: A group of symptoms and diseases that together are characteristic of a specific condition.

synergy (synergistic; adj.): The interaction of two or more treatments such that their combined effect is greater than the sum of the individual effects observed when each treatment is administered alone.

systemic: Affecting the whole body.

tat: An HIV protein that helps produce new complete HIV RNA genomes, and ultimately new virus, from the HIV proviral DNA template present in infected cells. Tat may also be involved in a) the reactivation of other latent viruses in people with AIDS, such as JC virus, the cause of PML; b) the development of AIDS-related KS by stimulating the formation of new blood vessels; and c) the triggering of anery and apoptosis in CD4 cells.

tat inhibitors: Experimental agents that block HIV's tat gene; for possible use in combination therapies.

T-helper cell count: The most commonly used laboratory marker for estimating level of immune dysfunction; also known as lymphocyte count or CD4 count; a measurement of number of T-helper cells per unit of blood.

therapeutic vaccines: Used to treat disease after infection occurs.

thrush: Caused by candidiasis, a yeast infection occurring in the mouth.

thymus: The central lymphoid organ that is present in the thorax and controls the ontogeny of T-lymphocytes.

titer: The concentration or activity of a given dissolved substance, such as a drug, antibody, or antigen, as measured by the solution's chemical reactivity in a *titration assay*. In particular, the extent to which an antibody-plasma extract can be diluted before losing its ability to protect against the corresponding antigen.

T-lymphocytes or T-cells: The class of lymphocytes derived from the thymus and involved in cell-mediated immune responses.

TMP/SMX (Bactrim, Septra): Used for prevention or treatment of PCP.

toxicity: The harmful side effects of a given drug.

toxoplasmosis: An opportunistic infection caused by the protozoan *Toxoplasma gondii*; frequently causes focal encephalitis (inflammation of the brain); may also involve the heart, lung, adrenal gland, pancreas, and testis.

transcription: The first step in protein synthesis, formation of messenger RNA, which conveys specific genetic information.

treatment-naive: Refers to patients with no history of previous treatment for a particular condition.

T-suppressor lymphocytes (T-8 cells): A group of T-lymphocytes that regulates the antibody production of B-lymphocytes.

vaccination: Immunization with antigens administered for the prevention of infectious diseases.

viral load: The amount of HIV RNA per unit of blood plasma. An indicator of virus concentration and reproduction rate, HIV viral load is increasingly employed as a predictor of disease progression. It is measured by PCR and bDNA tests and is expressed in numbers of copies of or equivalents to the HIV RNA genome per milliliter of plasma. (Note that there are two RNA copies per HIV virion.)

viremia: The presence of virus in the blood or blood plasma. Plasma viremia is a quantitative measurement of HIV levels similar to viral load but is accomplished by seeing how much of a patient's plasma is required to start an HIV infection in a laboratory cell culture.

virion: A virus particle existing freely outside a host cell.

virus: A group of infectious agents characterized by their inability to reproduce outside of a living host cell; may subvert the host cell's normal functions, causing the cell to behave in a manner determined by the virus.

wasting syndrome: Progressive, involuntary weight loss associated with advanced HIV infection.

Western blot: A test for detecting specific antibodies to a particular pathogen; in testing for antibodies to HIV, a Western blot test confirms a positive ELISA screening blood test.

APPENDIX C

HIV-Related Resources

AIDS Action Bulletin: Directory of clinical research in AIDS for Baltimore and Washington. Published by AIDS Action Baltimore, Inc., 2105 North Charles Street, Baltimore, MD 21218. Phone (410) 837-2437.

AIDS Drug Assistance Program (ADAP): Administered by the New York State Department of Health. ADAP provides access to specific drugs for the treatment of HIV infection and various opportunistic infections. Phone (518) 459-1641.

AIDS–HIV Treatment Directory: Published by the American Foundation for AIDS Research (AmFAR) and is updated quarterly. Directory is also available on a searchable database. Phone (800) 39-AmFAR, ext. 106.

AIDS Medicines In Development: An annual chart of medications as well as information on diagnostics and vaccines. Pharmaceutical Manufacturers Association, Communications Division, 1100 15th Street NW, Washington, DC 20005. Phone (202) 835-3400.

AIDS Treatment Data Network Inc.: The Network provides HIV treatment and research information, educational resources, and training to professionals, service providers, and the individuals and communities that they serve. It also assists individuals with lower English and Spanish literacy levels, in addition to those with little or no scientific background or expertise. 259 West 30th Street, 9th Floor, New York, NY 10001. Phone (212) 260-8868.

AIDS Treatment News: Developments in AIDS research, experimental therapies, and treatment options. John S. James, P.O. Box 411256, San Francisco, CA 94141. Phone (415) 255-0588.

AIDS Update: Newsletter includes general information on AIDS issues and treatments. Dallas Gay Alliance, P.O. Box 190712, Dallas, TX 75219. Phone (214) 528-4233.

AIDS Weekly: A weekly newsletter with short abstracts of AIDS-related news items, journal articles, conference reports. P.O. Box 830409, Birmingham, AL 35283-0409. Phone (800) 633-4931.

Association for Drug Abuse, Prevention and Treatment (ADAPT): AIDS oriented outreach, support groups, and education resource for users of injectable drugs. 552 Southern Boulevard, Bronx, NY 10455. Phone (718) 665-5421.

Being Alive. Medical updates, plus information on AIDS advocacy, a calendar of local events, listing of AIDS support groups, peer support, and counseling. Published by the LA Action Coalition, 3626 Sunset Boulevard, Los Angeles, CA 90026. Phone (213) 667-3262.

Body Positive. This newsletter provides a European perspective of treatment information not seen in similar U.S. publications. Published by Body Positive Group, 51B Philbeach Gardens, London, SW5 9EB, Great Britain. Information can be requested by mail or by fax at 011-71-373-5237; (212) 721-1346.

Bulletin of Experimental Treatments for AIDS (BETA): Mainly covers current AIDS research and developments in mainstream medicine. The newsletter devotes whole issues to specific topics. San Francisco AIDS Foundation, BETA Subscription Department, P.O. Box 2189, Berkeley, CA 94702. Phone (510) 596-9300 or (800) 327-9893.

Canadian AIDS News. A newsletter focusing on AIDS education in Canada, published by the Canadian Public Health Association, AIDS Education and Awareness Program, 400-1565 Carling Avenue, Ottawa, ON, Canada K1Z 8R1. Phone (613) 725-3769.

Canadian HIV Trials Network. Includes brief description of trials and locations of trial centers. Registry of Canadian HIV Clinical Trials, 200-1033 Davie Street, Vancouver, BC V6E 1M7. Phone (604) 631-5327 or fax (604) 631-5210.

Center for Natural and Traditional Medicines (CNTM): Promotes and disseminates information on indigenous and natural medicines. Resources include Ancient Roots: A Modern Medicine, Vol. 1: *A Cross Cultural Discussion on AIDS*. CNTM, P.O. Box 21735, Washington, DC 20009. Phone (202) 234-9632.

The Common Factor: A newsletter of the Committee of Ten Thousand, an organization by, for, and of people infected with HIV through blood and blood products. Includes treatment articles, early interventions, and resource lists. The Committee of Ten Thousand, c/o The Packard House, 583 Plain Street, Stoughton, MA 02072. Phone (617) 344-9634.

Critical Paths AIDS Project: Publishes in-depth information about treatments, research, and related political issues. Also contains an extensive listing of community events and support services in the Philadelphia area. 2062 Lombard Street, Philadelphia, PA 19146. Phone (215) 545-2212.

Directory of HIV Clinical Research in the Bay Area: The San Francisco Community Consortium, 3180 18th Street, Suite 201, San Francisco, CA 94110. Phone (415) 476-9554.

Facts on Alternate AIDS Compounds and Treatments (FAACTS): Provides summaries and reprints from the scientific and popular press concerning emerging treatments for HIV disease. 111 Gates Street, San Francisco, CA 94110. Phone (415) 648-1357.

Gay Men's Health Crisis: 129 West 20th Street, New York, NY 10011. Phone (212) 807-7517.

Healing Alternatives Foundation: A nonprofit buyers club organized to assist people with AIDS in obtaining medications. Alternative and not-yet-approved treatments are available, mail orders accepted. 1748

Market Street, Suite 204, San Francisco, CA 94102. Phone (415) 626-2316.

HIV Frontline: Published by the University of California San Francisco, Center for AIDS Prevention Studies, this newsletter specifically targets mental health and health care professionals who serve HIV infected persons. Discussions and commentary are directed at human service and clinical issues pertinent to persons with HIV. Articles emphasize practical approaches to complex clinical problems. Contact UCSF-CAPS, 74 New Montgomery, Suite 600, San Francisco, CA 94105. Phone (415) 597-9100.

Institute for Traditional Medicine and Preventive Health Care (ITM): Provides literature, catalogs, and video programs describing Chinese herbs and other aspects of traditional medicine. ITM, 2017 SE Hawthorne, Portland, OR 97214. 1-800-544-7504.

Life Link: Newsletter from the People With AIDS Coalition, includes AIDS information and local resources. PWAC also provides support groups, education, and a hotline for current AIDS–HIV information and service referrals. PWA Coalition of Long Island, 1170 Route 109, Lindenhurst, NY 11757. Phone (516) 225-5700.

National Association for People With AIDS: National advocacy and policy group that addresses issues facing people affected by AIDS. 1413 K Street, NW, Washington, DC 20005-3405. (202) 898-0414.

The News: A newsletter reporting on treatment issues and community outreach programs. Atlanta Gay Center, 63 12th Street, Atlanta, GA 30309. Phone (404) 876-5372.

Notes From the Underground. The newsletter reports on issues pertaining to AIDS treatments including background information about particular alternative therapies and their use. Also covered are experimental pharmaceutical treatments including those already approved but not indicated for HIV-associated diseases. The PWA Health Group (the New York City buyers' club), 150 West 26th Street, Suite 201, New York, NY 10001. Phone (212) 255-0520.

The Orphan Project: Dedicated to caring for children and families affected by AIDS. 121 Avenue of the Americas, 6th Floor, New York, NY 10013. Phone (212) 925-5290.

PAACNOTES: A news journal of the Physicians Association for AIDS Care. Features articles on clinical management, scientific research, and a diverse range of legal, ethical, psychosocial, and economic issues directly affecting the care of people with HIV disease. 101 West Grand Avenue, Suite 200, Chicago, IL 60610. Phone (800) 243-3059.

PI Perspective: Newsletter covers allopathic treatment information including pharmaceutical drug development and clinical trials, vaccine development, and AIDS research policy. It addresses broad-based community needs like standard of care, early intervention strategies, and prophylaxis for opportunistic infections. Project Inform, 1965 Market Street, Suite 220, San Francisco, CA 94103. Phone (800) 822-7422.

Positive Directions News: Published by Positive Directions, 140 Clarendon Street, Suite 805, Boston, MA 02115. Phone (617) 262-3456.

Positively Aware: Community-based newsletter covers many aspects of the AIDS epidemic. It focuses on research, mainstream and alternative treatment information, funding alerts, public policy issues, social concerns, and community events. Each edition also includes a Spanish language section. Test Positive Aware Network, 1340 West Irving Park, Box 259, Chicago, IL 60613. Phone (312) 404-8726.

Prisoners With AIDS Rights Advocacy Group (PWA Rag): Newsletter containing articles, treatment updates, and resources for prisoners. P.O. Box 2161, Jonesboro, GA 30327. Phone (404) 946-9346.

Psychology and AIDS Exchange: Updates the American Psychological Association's education, policy, and practice activities regarding AIDS. American Psychological Association, Office on AIDS, 750 First Street, NE, Washington, DC. Phone (202) 336-5500.

PWA Health Group: A nonprofit buyers club organized to assist people with AIDS in obtaining medications. 150 West 26th Street, Suite 201, New York, NY 10001. Phone (212) 255-0520.

PWA Newsline: Committed to including diverse opinions of the many different people affected by the AIDS epidemic. Newsline Coalition, 50 West 17th Street, 8th Fl., New York, NY 10011. Phone (212) 647-1415.

Ryan White Foundation: Ryan White Foundation is a national nonprofit organization established to increase awareness of personal, family, and community issues related to Human Immunodeficiency Virus (HIV) and Acquired Immune Deficiency Syndrome (AIDS). Target populations include youth, parents, and schools. 1-800-444-RYAN.

Seasons: A quarterly newsletter of the National Native American AIDS Prevention Center featuring articles and artwork by Native Americans affected by HIV–AIDS. American AIDS Prevention Center, 3515 Grand Avenue, Suite 100, Oakland, CA 94610.

SIDAhora: Original material published in Spanish. Each edition focuses on specific aspects of the AIDS epidemic and its effect within the Latino–Latina community. Comprehensive coverage includes treatment information, women's issues, pediatric concerns, public policy, art, and literature. Newsline Coalition, 50 West 17th Street, 8th Fl., New York, NY 10011. Phone (212) 647-1415.

Southern California Treatment Directory: A listing of clinical trials being conducted in Southern California. Southwest Community-Based AIDS Treatment Group (ComBAT), 1800 North Highland, Suite 610, Los Angeles, CA 90028. Phone (213) 469-5888.

STEP Perspective: Newsletter primarily covers treatment information including both mainstream and alternative approaches. Some articles address insurance and other practical concerns. A general information packet and a variety of fact sheets are available. Magazine style format allows topics to be examined thoroughly by an extensive scientific review committee. Seattle Treatment Education Project, 127 Broadway East, Suite 200, Seattle, WA 98102.

Treatment and Data Digest: This newsletter is essentially the report of the treatment and data committee of ACT UP–New York. Very current information about public policy, clinical trials, and research issues. Newsletter often covers first reports about issues not yet thoroughly known by the larger AIDS community, which usually leads to further investigations by others. ACT-UP–New York, 135 West 29th Street, New York, NY 10001. Phone (212) 564-AIDS.

Treatment Issues: Covers experimental treatment research for HIV disease and related opportunistic infections, including advances in prophylaxis and prevention strategies. Gay Men's Health Crisis, Medical Information, 129 West 20th Street, New York, NY 10011. Phone (212) 807-7517.

Treatment Update: Follows activities in the United States and Europe. Newsletter covers broad range of treatment issues abstracted from peer-review journals. Community AIDS Treatment Information Exchange, Suite 324, 517 College Street, Toronto, Ontario, Canada M6G. Phone (416) 944-1916.

Vancouver PWA: By the Vancouver Persons with AIDS Society, the newsletter includes short medical updates, local news, and a listing of upcoming events. 1107 Seymour Street, Vancouver, BC V6B 5S8. Phone (604) 681-2122.

WORLD: Written by and for HIV-positive women to address concerns specific to HIV disease and women including treatment information and psychosocial issues. Newsletters also include forums for personal testimonies, activist alerts, and events calendar. P.O. Box 11535, Oakland, CA 94611. Phone (510) 658-6930.

NATIONAL CENTERS AND HOTLINES

AIDS Clinical Trials, Information Service P.O. Box 6421, Rockville, MD 20850. 800-TRIALS-A, (800) 874-2572.

American Foundation for AIDS Research (AmFAR), 1515 Broadway, 36th Floor, New York, NY 10036. (212) 719-0033.

Burroughs Welcome Drug Information, 3030 Cornwallis Road Research Triangle Park, NC 27709. (800) 443-6763.

Center for AIDS Intervention Research (CAIR), Medical College of Wisconsin, 1201 N. Prospect Avenue, Milwaukee, WI 53202. (414) 456-7700.

Center for AIDS Prevention Studies (CAPS), University of California at San Francisco, 74 New Montgomery, Suite 600, San Francisco, CA 94105. (415) 597-9100.

Gay Men's Health Crisis (GMHC), 129 West 20th Street, New York, NY 10011. (212) 807-6655.

Hemophilia/HIV Peer Association, PO Box 931, Nevada City, CA 95959. (800) 800-5154.

HIV Center for Clinical and Behavioral Studies, Columbia University, New York, 722 West 68th Street, New York, NY 10032.

Names Project—The AIDS Quilt, Box 14573, San Francisco, CA 94114. (415) 863-1966.

National AIDS Hotline (24 hours/day), (800) 342-AIDS (1-800-342-2437), 800-344-SIDA (800 344-7432, Spanish).

National AIDS Information Clearinghouse, (800) 458-5231.

National Hotline for Experimental Drug and Treatment Center, (800) 874-2572.

Native American Indian AIDS Hotline, (800) 283-2437.

People with AIDS Hotline, (800) 828-3280.

Project Inform Hotline (Treatment), 347 Delores Street, Suite 301, San Francisco, CA 94110. (800) 334-7422 (within California), (800) 822-7422 (outside California).

Sexually Transmitted Disease Hotline, Test Positive Aware Network, 1340 West Irving Park, Box #259, Chicago, IL 60613. (312) 404-8726; (800) 227-8922.

KEY INTERNET WEBSITES

Comprehensive websites with multiple links to other sites

American Medical Association HIV/AIDS
http:/www.ama-assn.org/insight/spec_con/hiv_aids/hiv_aids.htm

Centers for Disease Control and Prevention
www.dc.gov

HIV Insite
University of California at San Francisco
http://hivinsite.ucsf.edu

National Insitutes of Health
www.nih.gov

AIDS Advocacy

AIDS Action
1875 Connecticut Avenue, NW, Suite 700,
Washington, DC 20009
Phone: (202) 986-1300
www.aidsaction.org

AIDS Coalition to Unleash Power (ACT-UP)
New York www.actupny.org
San Francisco www.actupgg.org

American Psychological Association Office on AIDS
http://www.apa.org/pi/aids.html

Mothers' Voices
165 West 46th Street, Suite 701
New York, NY 10036
Phone: (212) 730-2777
Executive Director: Ann Kirth
www.mvoices.org

National AIDS Treatment Advocacy Project
580 Broadway, Suite 403
New York, NY 10012
Phone: (212) 219-0106 or 1-888-26-NATAP
www.natap.org

People With AIDS Coalition
286 NE 39th Street
Miami, FL 33137
(305) 573-8777
users.aol.com/hapizo/pwac

Stop AIDS Worldwide
2261 Old Middlefield Way
Mountain View, CA 94043 USA
Phone: (415) 988-0878
www.stopaidsworldwide.org

Author Index

Numbers in italics indicate names that appear in the reference list.

Avron, J., *340*
Ayehunie, S., 31, *327*
Ayotte, D., *368*
Azen, S., *345*

Baba, T. W., 28, 35, *327*
Bacchetti, P., 59, 65, 68, 69, 73, 83,
    327, 363, 367, 383
Bacellar, H., 88, *327*
Bagellar, H., *361*
Baggett, L., *326*
Bahr, G. R., 32, 156, 160, 163, 244,
    245, 249, 250, 254, 263, 305,
    306, 310, *368*
Baily, M. C., *390*
Baird, B. F., *380*
Bakal, D. A., 172, *328*
Bakeman, R., 144, *389–390*
Baker, C., 149, *362*
Balan, M., 247, *365–366*
Balfour, H. H., *357*
Ballard, K., 282, 300, *352*
Balsley, C. M., *353*
Balson, P., *410–411*
Balson, P. M., *383*
Bandura, A., 253, 255, 256, *328, 387*
Bangsberg, D., 131, *328*
Barbarini, G., *330–331*
Barbour, R. S., *328*
Barcherini, S., *407*
Barditch-Crovo, P., *340*
Barnhart, J. L., 57, *396*
Baron, D., 298, *374*
Barrett, D. C., *333*
Barrett, R. L., *328*
Barrows, L., *383*
Barsky, A. J., 173, 174, *328*
Bartelli, D., *382*
Barter, G., 303, *377*
Bartholow, B. N., 237, *328, 345*
Bartlett, J., *408*
Bartlett, J. A., 13–14, 69, 103, *384*
Bartlett, J. G., 41, 60, 62, 66, 73, 77,
    84, 85, 104, 105, 106, 125, *328*
Barton, S., *335*

Barton, S. E., 110, *398*
Bartrop, R. W., 177, *328*
Batchelor, W. F., 141, *383*
Batki, S. L., 317, *345*
Battjes, R. J., *358*
Baum, A., 176, 177, *329, 397, 411*
Baum, B., 29, *350*
Baum, M. K., *354*
Baumberger, C., *370*
Bayer, R., 240, 246, *328*
Beatty, D. C., 159, *395*
Beck, A. T., 307, *328–329*
Beck, C. K., 175, *358*
Beck, E. J., 30, 290, 292, *328–329*
Beck, K., 246, *410*
Becker, J., *327*
Becker, J. T., *382, 394*
Becker, K., *348*
Beckett, A., 310, 320, *325, 329*
Bednarik, D. P., 17, *329*
Beecham, M., *329*
Beevor, A., *335*
Beevor, A. S., 150, *329*
Belcher, L., 52, 242, 244, 245,
    364–365
Belkin, G. S., 156, 158, 161, 167, 169,
    190, 285, *329*
Belman, A., 88–89, 200, *372*
Benator, D., *354*
Bendiksen, R., *342*
Benight, C. C., 180, 256, *329*
Benjamin, A. E., 302, 303, *329*
Bennett, C., 52, *385*
Bennett, L., 300, *329*
Beral, V., 71, 83, *329*
Berenson, A. B., 237, *329*
Bergam, K., *347*
Berger, T. G., 15, 94, *329–330*
Bergey, E., 29, *330*
Berkelman, R. L., 53, 70, 97, *339, 349*
Berns, D. S., *385*
Bernstein, B. M., *368*
Bertini, M., *402*
Besch, C. L., 131, 133, 136, *330, 354*
Beschorner, W., *361*

Subject Index

About the Author

Seth C. Kalichman is an associate professor in the Department of Psychiatry and Behavioral Medicine at the Medical College of Wisconsin and a senior scientist at the Center for AIDS Intervention Research (CAIR). Dr. Kalichman has published extensively on the psychological aspects of the HIV–AIDS epidemic. His research focuses on identifying factors that determine HIV risk behavior, testing theoretically derived intervention models, and examining the psychological adjustment of people with HIV infection. His work has been published in the *Journal of Consulting and Clinical Psychology*, the *American Journal of Public Health*, the *American Journal of Psychiatry*, and *Health Psychology*. Dr. Kalichman is the author of *Mandated Reporting of Suspected Child Abuse; Ethics, Law, and Policy* and *Answering Your Questions About AIDS*, published by the American Psychological Association, and *Preventing AIDS: A Sourcebook for Behavioral Interventions*, published by Erlbaum. He was the 1997 recipient of the Distinguished Scientist Award for Early Career Contribution to Psychology in Health from the American Psychological Association.

Dr. Kalichman received his PhD in Clinical Community Psychology from the University of South Carolina and did his undergraduate work at the University of South Florida. His research and clinical interests include the psychosocial aspects of AIDS, human sexuality, sexual violence, child maltreatment, and public policy. Dr. Kalichman currently dedicates all of his effort to developing behavioral strategies to impede the spread of HIV infection in urban settings and to addressing the psychological needs of people affected by HIV and AIDS.